The Complete Guide for the Development and Implementation of Health Promotion Programs

Werner W. K. Hoeger
Boise State University

Morton Publishing Company
925 W. Kenyon Ave., Unit 12
Englewood, Colorado 80110

ISBN: 0-89582-165-6

Preface

The cost of health care in the United States dramatically increased from about $12 billion in 1950 to $243.4 billion in 1980. By the middle 1980s, these costs were expected to reach $500 billion, which is in excess of 10 percent of the Gross National Product. Experts believe that if this trend continues, the cost of health care expenditures will double every five years.

These spiraling increments in health care costs over the last few decades have motivated many corporations to implement health promotion programs with the intent of containing or decreasing health expenditures. Preventive medicine is becoming the main objective of most corporate health programs. In this regard, the biggest challenge faced by corporations is to teach their employees how to take control of personal health habits by practicing positive lifestyle activities that will decrease the risk of illness and help achieve total well-being.

Realizing that investments in health and fitness make good business sense, over 400 major corporations in the United States are now offering on-site health promotion programs to their employees. These organizations devote resources to these programs because they know that they can expect less absenteeism, on-the-job injury, hospitalization, disability, job turnover rates, premature death, and health care costs, as well as an increase in employee morale and job productivity. Furthermore, several organizations are using health promotion programs as an incentive to attract, hire, and retain their employees. In addition, young executives are looking for such organizations, not only for the added health benefits, but because it shows an attitude of concern and care by corporate officers.

The main focus of this textbook is to teach individuals how to set up and implement a comprehensive health promotion program. Information is presented on the importance, justification, and development of worksite health and fitness programs, including clinical and field testing, data analysis, disease risk reduction counseling, and implementation of programs aimed at achieving the highest level of wellness.

The textbook presents the recommended guidelines and testing protocols for the establishment of coronary heart disease risk profiles, physical fitness profiles, and cancer risk screening. Also included are the educational materials necessary to effectively counsel and help individuals achieve total well-being. Information on such topics as exercise prescription, diet and nutrition, cardiovascular disease and cancer risk reduction, smoking cessation, and stress management is given.

This book is dedicated to my lovely wife, beautiful children, and loving parents.

ACKNOWLEDGMENTS

The author wishes to acknowledge the valuable help of Richard K. Riley in the preparation of the final manuscript. Special gratitude is expressed to Dr. LaVon Johnson for his professional leadership; to Linda Blanksma, Jeff Anderson, Dr. Glenn R. Potter, Dr. David R. Hopkins, Kenneth A. Hyde, Charles B. Scheer, and Lisa Olson for their valuable contributions and support; and to everyone else who helped to make this work possible.

The textbook plan is also a reflection of the author's experiences at the Fitness Monitoring Preventive Medicine Clinic in Lake Geneva, Wisconsin; The University of Texas of The Permian Basin Wellness Center in Odessa, Texas; and the Boise State University Employee Fitness and Wellness Program in Boise, Idaho. Additionally, parts of this textbook include materials that are reproduced with permission from the author's previous textbook, *Lifetime Physical Fitness & Wellness: A Personalized Program,* also published by Morton Publishing Company (1986).

Table of Contents

Introduction to Health Promotion

During the last two decades there has been a tremendous increase in the number of people participating in fitness and wellness programs. From an initial fitness fad in the early 1970s, physical fitness and wellness programs have become a trend that is now very much a part of the American way of life. The increase in the number of participants is primarily attributed to scientific evidence linking vigorous exercise and positive lifestyle habits to better health, improved quality of life, and total well-being.

Research findings in the last few years have shown that physical inactivity and negative lifestyle habits are a serious threat to the health of the nation. Advances in modern technology have almost completely eliminated the need for physical exertion in most everyone's daily life. The automated society that we live in no longer provides the human body with sufficient physical activity to insure adequate health. Additionally, as the American people started to enjoy the so-called "good life" (sedentary living, alcohol, fatty foods, excessive sweets, tobacco, drugs, etc.), a parallel increase was seen in the incidence of chronic diseases such as hypertension, coronary heart disease, atherosclerosis, strokes, diabetes, cancer, emphysema, and cirrhosis of the liver. As the incidence of chronic diseases increased, it became clear that prevention was the best medicine. Consequently, a new health/fitness/wellness trend has gradually developed over the last two decades. People have begun to realize that good health is largely self-controlled and that the leading causes of premature death and illness in the United States could be prevented through adherence to positive lifestyle habits.

PHYSICAL FITNESS, HEALTH PROMOTION, AND WELLNESS

Over the years, physical fitness has been defined in several ways. The President's Council on Physical Fitness and Sports has indicated that physical fitness is the measure of the body's strength, stamina, and flexibility. According to the American Medical Association, physical fitness is the general capacity to adapt and respond favorably to physical effort; implying that individuals are physically fit when they can meet the ordinary as well as the unusual demands of daily life safely and effectively without being overly fatigued, and still have energy left for leisure and recreational activities.

From a health point of view, there are four basic components to total physical fitness: cardiovascular endurance, muscular strength and endurance, muscular flexibility, and body composition. To develop overall fitness, an individual has to engage in separate programs aimed at improving each one of the four basic components of fitness.

During the late 1960s and in the 1970s, we began to realize that good physical fitness was an important factor in the fight against chronic diseases, particularly those of the cardiovascular system. Because of increased participation in physical fitness programs in the last few years, we have begun to see a reduction in cardiovascular mortality rates. It was estimated that in the year 1983 alone there were 165,000 fewer cardiovascular deaths than expected. This decrease in mortality is attributed to increased fitness and better health care in the country. Furthermore, several studies have shown an inverse relationship between exercise and premature cardiovascular mortality rates. In one study conducted among 16,936 Harvard alumni linking exercise habits and mortality rates, results indicated that as the amount of weekly physical activity increased, the risk of cardiovascular deaths decreased. The greatest decrease in cardiovascular deaths was observed among alumni who used in excess of 2,000 calories per week through physical activity (Table 1.1). Another study conducted in the late 1960s also seemed to indicate a lower mortality rate from coronary heart disease for men and women who participated in moderate and heavy exercise (Table 1.2).

Although there is a definite improvement in the quality of life and most likely an increase in

longevity for those who participate in physical fitness programs, in the early 1980s it became obvious that just improving the four basic components of physical fitness was not always sufficient to decrease the risk for disease and insure better health. For example, an individual who is running three miles per day, lifting weights regularly, participating in stretching exercises, and watching his/her body weight can easily be classified in the good or excellent category for each one of the fitness components. However, if this same individual suffers from high blood pressure, smokes, is under constant stress, consumes excessive alcohol, and/or eats too many fatty foods, he/she is probably developing several

Table 1.1.

Cause-Specific Death Rates[a] per 10,000 Man-Years of Observation Among 16,936 Harvard Alumni, 1962-1978, by Physical Activity Index

Cause of Death (n = 1,413)	% of Total Deaths	Physical Activity Index, Kcal/week		
		<500	500-1,999	2,000+
Cardiovascular Diseases	45.3	39.5	30.8	21.4
Cancer	31.6	25.7	19.2	19.0
Accidents	5.5	3.6	3.9	3.0
Suicides	4.8	5.1	3.2	2.9
Respiratory Diseases	4.3	6.0	3.2	1.5

From Paffenbarger, R. S., R. T. Hyde, A. L. Wing, and C. H. Steinmetz. "A Natural History of Athleticism and Cardiovascular Health." *JAMA* 252(4): 491-495, 1984. Copyright 1985, American Medical Association.

[a]Adjusted for differences in age, cigarette smoking, and hypertension.

Table 1.2.

Deaths from Coronary Heart Disease per 100 Men and Women by Amount of Physical Exertion

Sex	Age	Degree of Exercise			
		None	Slight	Moderate	Heavy
Men	40-49	1.46	1.17	1.12	1.00
	50-59	1.43	1.17	1.06	1.00
	60-69	1.91	1.64	1.19	1.00
	70-79	2.91	2.03	1.45	1.00
Women	40-49	—	1.29	1.07	1.00
	50-59	—	1.21	1.06	1.00
	60-69	2.01	1.86	1.11	1.00
	70-79	3.15	2.30	1.33	1.00

From Hammond, E. C., and L. Garfinkel. "Coronary Heart Disease, Stroke, and Aortic Aneurysm." *Archives of Environmental Health* 19(8):174, 1969. A publication of the Helen Dwight Reid Educational Foundation. (Table based on data of more than 1 million men and women studied over a period of six years).

risk factors for cardiovascular disease and may not be aware of it. A risk factor is defined as an asymptomatic state that may lead to disease.

One of the best examples that good physical fitness is not always a risk-free guarantee for a healthy and productive life was the tragic death in 1984 of Jim Fixx, author of *The Complete Book of Running*. At the time of his death by heart attack, Fixx was fifty-two years old. He had been running between sixty and eighty miles per week and had felt that anyone in his type of condition could not die from heart disease. At age thirty-six, Jim Fixx had been smoking two packs of cigarettes per day, weighed about 215 pounds, did not engage in regular cardiovascular exercise, and had a family history of heart disease. His father had experienced a first heart attack at age thirty-five and later died at age forty-three. Perhaps in an effort to decrease his risk of heart disease, Fixx began to increase his fitness level. He started to jog, lost fifty pounds, and quit cigarette smoking. Nevertheless, Fixx declined on several occasions to have an exercise electrocardiogram (ECG) test done, which would have most likely revealed his cardiovascular problem. This unfortunate death is a good example that exercise programs by themselves will not make high-risk people immune to heart disease, other than probably delaying the onset of a serious or fatal problem.

Once it became clear that good fitness by itself would not always decrease the risk for disease and insure better health, a new "wellness" concept developed in the 1980s. Wellness has been defined as the constant and deliberate effort to stay healthy and achieve the highest potential for well-being. The wellness concept goes well beyond absence of disease and optimal physical fitness. It incorporates other aspects such as proper nutrition, smoking cessation, stress management, alcohol and drug abuse control, regular physical examinations, health education counseling, and environmental support. Not only must the individual be physically fit and manifest no signs of disease, but there must also be an absence of risk factors for disease (hypertension, hyperlipedimea, cigarette smoking, negative stress, faulty nutrition, etc.). The relationship between physical fitness, health, and wellness is illustrated in the wellness continuum in Figure 1.3.

Figure 1.1. *Health-Related Components of Physical Fitness.*

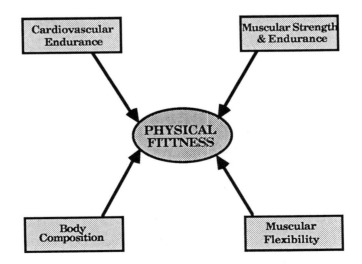

Figure 1.2. *Wellness Components.*

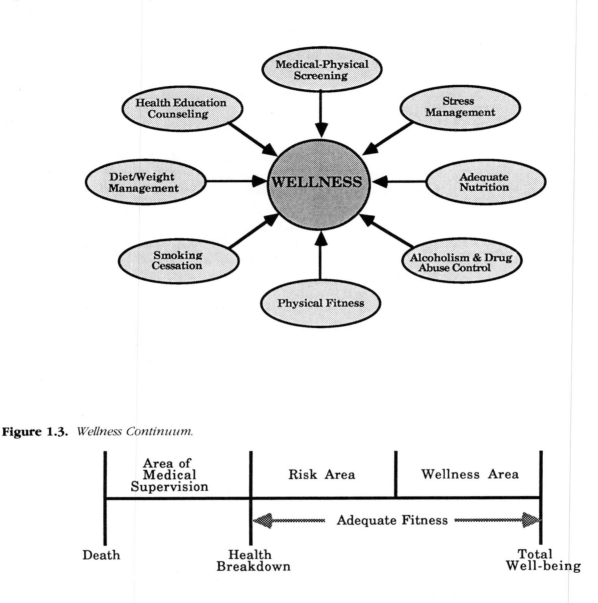

Figure 1.3. *Wellness Continuum.*

Along with the wellness concept, the term "health promotion" has also gained significant popularity in recent years. Health promotion is defined by experts as any combination of activities either educational, organizational, economic, and/or environmental that are conducive to good health. Both terms — health promotion and wellness — are often used interchangeably. They imply an all-inclusive umbrella composed of a variety of activities aimed at helping individuals recognize components of lifestyle that are detrimental to their health, and then implement principles and programs to change their behavior so as to improve the quality of life and achieve total well-being. Perhaps the difference between the two terms is that health promotion refers to the actual program, while wellness may refer to the program or to the outcome of the program that is enjoyed by the participant (total well-being or wellness).

MAJOR HEALTH PROBLEMS IN THE UNITED STATES

The most prominent health problems in the United States today are basically lifestyle related (*see* Table 1.3). According to some research, 53

Table 1.3.
Leading Causes of Death in the United States: 1984 Estimates*

Cause	Total Number of Deaths	Percent of Total Deaths
1. Major cardiovascular diseases	973,418	47.7
2. Cancer	453,492	22.2
3. Accidents	92,941	4.6
4. Chronic and obstructive pulmonary disease	69,100	3.4
5. All other causes	450,448	22.1

*Source: National Center for Health Statistics. U.S. Public Health Service, DHHS.

percent of all disease is self-controlled, 64 percent of factors contributing to mortality are caused by lifestyle (48 percent) and environmental (16 percent) factors, and 83 percent of deaths prior to the age of sixty-five are preventable. Most Americans are threatened by the very lives they lead today.

Current statistics indicate that 70 percent of all deaths in the United States are caused by cardiovascular disease and cancer. Close to 80 percent of these deaths could be prevented through a positive lifestyle program. Accidents are the third leading cause of death. While not all accidents are preventable, many are. A significant amount of fatal accidents are related to drug abuse and lack of use of seat belts. The fourth cause of death, chronic and obstructive pulmonary disease, is largely related to tobacco use.

Cardiovascular Disease

The most prevalent degenerative diseases in the United States are those of the cardiovascular system. Approximately half of all deaths in this country are attributed to heart and blood vessel disease. According to the 1983 estimates by the American Heart Association, 63.2 million Americans were afflicted by cardiovascular disease, including almost 58 million suffering from hypertension and almost 5 million affected by coronary heart disease. The 1986 estimated cost of heart and blood vessel disease exceeded $78.6 billion. Heart attacks alone cost American industry 132 million workdays annually, including $13.6 billion in lost productivity because of physical and emotional disability.

It must also be noted that more than 1.5 million people suffer heart attacks each year, with over half a million of them dying as a consequence of the attack. About 50 percent of the time, the first symptom of coronary heart disease is a heart attack itself, and 40 percent of the people who suffer a first heart attack die within the first twenty-four hours. In one out of every five cardiovascular deaths, sudden death is the initial symptom. Over half of those who die are men in their most productive years — between the ages of forty and sixty-five. Additionally, the American Heart Association estimates that over $700 million a year is spent in replacing employees suffering heart attacks. Oddly enough, most coronary heart disease risk factors are reversible and can be controlled by the individual through appropriate lifestyle modifications.

Cancer

Even though cancer is not the number-one killer, it is the number-one health fear of the American people. Cancer is defined as an uncontrolled growth and spread of abnormal cells in the body. Some cells grow into a mass of tissue called a tumor which can be either benign or malignant. A malignant tumor would be considered a "cancer." If the spread of cells is not controlled, death ensues. Approximately 22 percent of all deaths in the United States are due to cancer. Over 450,000 people died of this disease in 1986, and an estimated 930,000 new cases were expected the same year. The overall medical costs for cancer were estimated to be in excess of $20 billion for 1986. Figure 1.5 shows the 1986 estimated new

Figure 1.4. *Cardiovascular Disease Incidence: From* **Heart Facts,** *American Heart Association, 1986.*

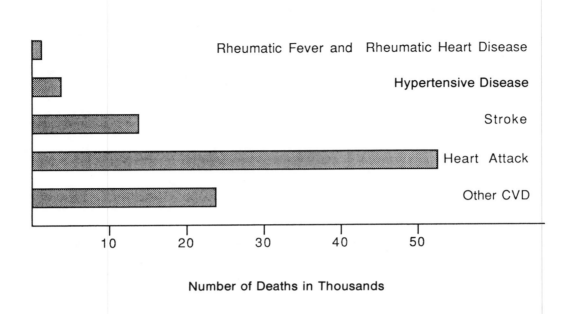

Number of Deaths in Thousands

Figure 1.5. *Estimated Deaths and New Cases for Major Sites of Cancer: 1986. From 1986* **Cancer Facts and Figures** *by the American Cancer Society.*

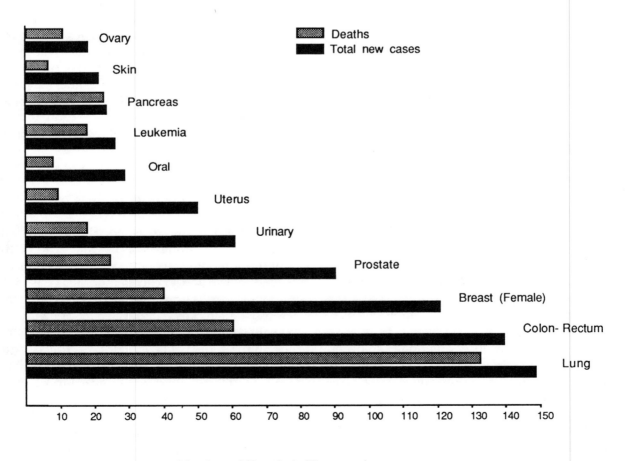

Number of People in Thousands

cases and deaths for major sites of cancer, excluding non-melanoma skin cancer and carcinoma in situ.

Scientific evidence and testing procedures for the early detection of cancer are continuously changing and improving. Cancer is now viewed as the most curable of all chronic diseases. Over 5 million Americans with a history of cancer are now alive, and close to 3 million of them are considered cured. In fact, the American Cancer Society maintains that the biggest factor in fighting cancer today is prevention through health education programs. Evidence indicates that as much as 80 percent of all human cancer can be prevented through positive lifestyle modifications. The basic recommendations include a diet high in cabbage-family vegetables, in fiber, in vitamins A and C, and low in fat. Alcohol and salt-cured, smoked, and nitrite-cured foods should be used in moderation. Cigarette smoking and tobacco use in general should be eliminated, and obesity should be avoided.

BENEFITS OF HEALTH PROMOTION PROGRAMS

As the need for physical exertion steadily decreased in the last century, the nation's health care expenditures dramatically increased. Health care expenditures in the United States totaled $12 billion in 1950. In 1960 this figure reached $26.9 billion, by 1970 it increased to $75 billion, and by 1980 health care costs accounted for $243.4 billion. At that trend, this cost was estimated to reach $500 billion in 1986, which would be in excess of 10 percent of the Gross National Product. At the current rate of escalation, experts have indicated that health care expenditures will double every five years.

Current estimates indicate that over half of the health care expenditures in the United States are presently being absorbed by American business and industry. The cost of insurance premiums to industry also continues to increase each year. For example, the cost of insurance premiums for 15,000 employees of the Kimberly-Clark Corporation in 1977 was $14.3 million. This figure had increased by 75 percent in only four years. At the Ford Motor Company, health benefits are the most expensive fringe benefit to the employee. From 1977 to 1979 alone, these costs increased from $450 million to $600 million. Since 1975, General Motors has been spending more for health benefits than for steel used in building automobiles.

Many organizations that carefully assess every expenditure often ignore health care costs and lost production due to the poor lifestyle and health practices of their employees. Medical data from the Massachusetts Mutual Insurance Company showed in 1983 that an average cardiovascular event (heart attack, myocardial infarction, cardiovascular aneurysm, or stroke) would cost $35,000. A study by the Blue Cross and Blue Shield Association indicated that the average medical bill for patients who died of cancer in 1983 exceeded $22,000 during the final year of life. Since medical costs have been inflating at an approximate 20 percent annual rate, these figures could easily double in a matter of four to five years. Such staggering medical costs are bringing companies to the realization that it costs less to keep an employee healthy than treating him/her once sick. Consequently, health care cost containment through the implementation of health promotion programs has become a major issue for many organizations around the country.

There is now strong scientific evidence linking fitness and wellness program participation to decreased medical costs, better health, and improved job productivity. Most of this research is being conducted and reported by organizations that have already implemented fitness or wellness programs. Let's examine the evidence:

The backache syndrome, usually the result of physical degeneration (inelastic and weak muscles), cost American industry over $1 billion annually in lost productivity and services alone. An additional $250 million is spent in workmen's compensation. The Adolph Coors Company in Golden, Colorado, which initiated a wellness program in 1981 for employees and their families, reported savings of more than $319,000 in 1983 alone through a preventive and rehabilitative back injury program.

A 1981 survey of the 1,500 largest employers in the United States showed that organizations that offered prevention/health promotion programs to their employees had an average annual health care cost per employee of $806. This compared with an average per employee cost of $1,015 for all companies, representing a $209 savings per employee per year (an approximate 20 percent difference).

Figure 1.6. *Health Care Cost Increments in the Last Four Decades.*

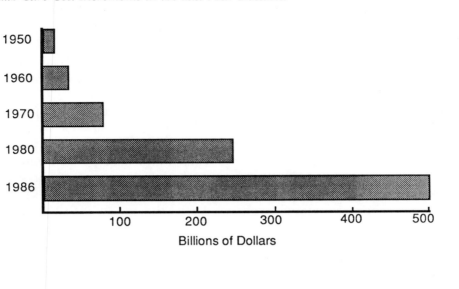

Figure 1.7. *Average Annual Health Care Cost Per Employee for the 1,500 Largest Employers in the United States: 1981.*

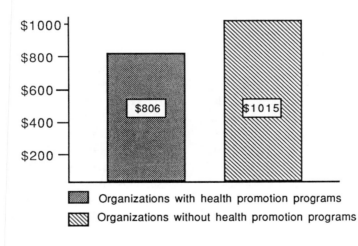

☒ Organizations with health promotion programs
☒ Organizations without health promotion programs

From July 2, 1979 until June 27, 1980, Prudential Insurance Company of Houston, Texas, conducted a study of its 1,386 employees. Those who participated for at least one year in the company's fitness program averaged 3.5 days of disability, as compared to 8.6 days for nonparticipants. A further breakdown by level of physical fitness (determined by treadmill times) showed no disability days for those in the high fitness group, 1.6 days for the good fitness group, and 4.1 disability days for the fair fitness group. If the entire Home Office staff's disability days were to decrease to 3.5 days per year, the study estimated that the direct savings from salary paid out during sickness would average $204 per employee, or $282,744 a year. Additionally, the company would save three to four times that amount in indirect costs due to replacements, productivity loss, overtime, etc. Decreased absenteeism is perhaps the most significant short-term cost/benefit of fitness/wellness programs, since absent employees are nonproductive and represent dollars paid out without return to the organization.

The Mesa Petroleum Company in Amarillo, Texas, has been offering an on-site fitness program since 1979 to its 350 employees and their family members (approximately 64 percent of the employees were using the fitness center on a regular basis). A 1982 survey showed an average of $434 per person in medical costs for the nonpartic-ipating group in the company, while the participating group averaged only $173 per person per year. This represents a yearly reduction of $200,000 in medical expenses. Sick leave time was also significantly less for the physically active group — twenty-seven hours per year as compared to forty-four for the inactive group.

Figure 1.8. *Relationships Between Medical Claims, Absenteeism, and Exercise Participation at the Mesa Petroleum Company in Amarillo, Texas: 1982. From "Reduced Costs, Increased Worker Production Are Rationale For Tax-Favored Corporate Fitness Plans."* **Employee Benefit Plan Review,** *November 1983:20.*

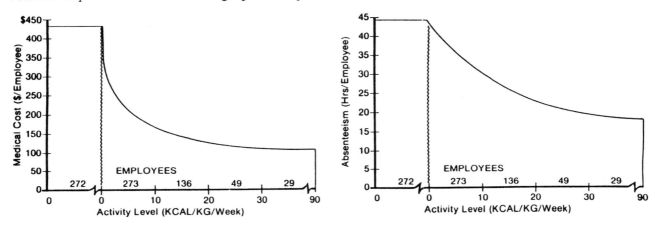

Figure 1.9. *Annual Medical Care Costs for Tenneco Incorporated, Houston, Texas: 1982-83. From "New Fitness Data Verifies: Employees Who Exercise Are Also More Productive."* **Athletic Business** *8(12):24-30, 1984.*

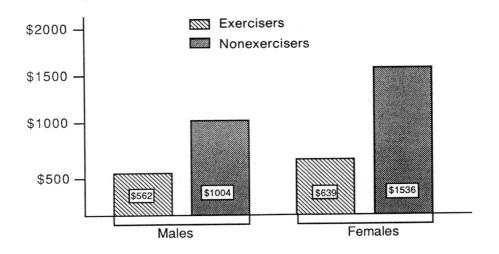

Data analysis conducted by Tenneco Incorporated in Houston, Texas, in 1982 and 1983 showed a significant reduction in medical care costs for men and women who participated in an exercise program. Annual medical care costs for male and female exercisers were $562 and $639, respectively. For the nonexercising group, the costs were reported at $1,004 for the men and $1,536 for the women. Sick leave was also reduced in both the men and women participants. The greatest difference was seen between female exercisers and nonexercisers — 22.5 fewer hours for the exercisers. The difference between men exercisers and nonexercisers was 5.5 fewer hours for the exercising group. Furthermore, a survey of the more than 3,000 employees found that job productivity is related to fitness. The company reported that individuals with high ratings of job performance also rated high in exercise participation.

In 1980, the New York Telephone Company spent $2.84 million on wellness and prevention programs for 80,000 of its employees. As a direct result of the program, the company saved $5.54 million in employee absence and treatment costs. This represented a health care cost reduction of $69.25 per employee.

An independent research project of the Canadian government in 1981 documented an $84 per employee savings in health care costs for Canada Life Assurance Company in the first year of its wellness program. An additional $210 per employee savings in absenteeism and turnover was also calculated. The results were obtained by comparing figures with the North American Life Company, which offered no fitness or lifestyle programs.

Similar evidence was found in another study conducted at two large Toronto insurance corporate offices. One served as the experimental site, while the second (demographically similar) served as the control site. Approximately 50 percent of the employees at the experimental site participated in a fitness and lifestyle education program. The exercise group used the health care system half as often as compared to the nonexercisers within the experimental site or the control site. Absenteeism was decreased by 42 percent for the exercise group, while only a 22 to 23 percent decrease was seen in the nonexercisers or the control group. At the experimental site, employee turnover rate among the exercise group was only 1.5 percent against 15 percent for the nonexer-

cisers. Company estimates indicated that the total cost of the program was $192,000. Savings resulting from absenteeism costs and decreased job turnover rate were reported at $660,000, which resulted in an annual net cost/benefit of $468,000.

Strong data is also coming in from Europe. Research in West Germany reported a 68.6 percent reduction in absenteeism by workers with cardiovascular symptoms who participated in a physical fitness program. The Goodyear Company in Norrkoping, Sweden, indicated a 50 percent reduction in absenteeism following the implementation of a fitness program. Studies in the Soviet Union report increased physical work capacity and motor coordination, lower incidence of disease, shorter illness duration, and fewer relapses among individuals participating in industrial fitness programs. In the Federal Republic of Germany, the law mandates that corporations employing workers with jobs sedentary in nature must provide an in-house facility for physical exercise.

Another reason why some organizations are offering health promotion programs to their employees, and one that is overlooked by many because it does not seem to directly affect the bottom line, is simple concern by top management for the physical well-being of the employees. Whether the program helps decrease medical costs is not the primary issue for its implementation. The only reason that really matters to top management is the fact that health promotion programs help individuals feel better about themselves and help improve quality of life. Such is the case of Mannington Mills Corporation, which recently invested $1.8 million in an on-site fitness center. The return on investment is secondary to the company's interest in happier and healthier employees. The center is also open to dependents and retirees. As a result of this program, Mannington Mills feels that the participants, about 50 percent of the 1,600 people eligible, can enjoy life to its fullest potential, and the employees will most likely be more productive simply because of the company's caring attitude.

Although the evidence on cost/benefits of health promotion programs is already substantial, the greatest impact will not be felt for another ten to fifteen years. Most middle-age and older people already have chronic health problems related to poor lifestyle patterns. It takes years to reverse many of these problems, and a large number of them may be irreversible because of advanced stages of disease. Nevertheless, even during late stages of disease, health and quality of life can be improved. Those who are already using the health care system will continue to do so until negative lifestyle behaviors are reversed and health is restored. The real reduction in costs will come when our younger people reach middle and older age with considerably fewer health problems. If we can keep this younger generation healthy and well through active participation in health promotion programs, the long-term savings in health care costs will be many, many times greater than what has already been reported.

In addition to the financial and physical benefits described, many corporations are using health promotion programs as an incentive to attract, hire, and retain employees. Many companies are now taking a hard look at the fitness and health level of potential employees and are seriously using this information in their screening process. As a matter of fact, some organizations refuse to hire smokers and/or overweight individuals. On the other hand, many executives feel that an on-site health promotion program is the best fringe benefit they can enjoy at their corporation. Young executives are also looking for such organizations, not only for the added health benefits, but because an attitude of concern and care is being shown by the head corporate officers.

THE WELLNESS CHALLENGE FOR THE 1980s AND 1990s

Since a better and healthier life is something that every person needs to strive to attain individually, the biggest challenge that we face in the next few years is to teach people how to take control of their personal health habits by practicing positive lifestyle activities that will decrease the risk of illness and help achieve total well-being. With such impressive data available on the benefits of health promotion programs, no longer can organizations, the health profession, or individuals themselves ignore the value of these programs in the development and maintenance of good health. Investments in wellness make good sense, and organizations that devote resources to these programs do so because they know they can expect less absenteeism, on-the-job injury, hospitalization, disability, job turnover rates, premature death, and health costs, as well as an increase in employee morale, job productivity, and physical well-being.

REFERENCES

1. Allsen, P.E., J. M. Harrison, and B. Vance. *Fitness for Life: An Individualized Approach.* Dubuque, IA: Wm. C. Brown, 1984.

2. American Cancer Society. *1986 Cancer Facts and Figures.* New York: The Society, 1986.

3. American Heart Association. *Heart Facts.* Dallas, TX: The Association, 1986.

4. Bowne, D. W., M. L. Russell, J. L. Morgan, S. A. Optenberg, and A. E. Clarke. "Reduced Disability and Health Care Costs in an Industrial Fitness Program." *Journal of Occupational Medicine* 26(11):809-816, 1984.

5. Colacino, D. "A Fitness Program that was Designed to Fit." *Business and Health* 23-25, December 1983.

6. Duncan, D. F., and R. S. Gold. "Reflections: Health Promotion — What is it?" *Health Values* 10(3): 47-48, 1986.

7. Fielding, J. E. "Preventive Medicine and the Bottom Line." *Journal of Occupational Medicine* 21(2):79-82, 1979.

8. Gatty, B. "How Fitness Works Out." *Nation's Business* 18-24, July 1985.

9. Gettman, L. R. "Cost/Benefit Analysis of a Corporate Fitness Program." *Fitness in Business* 1(1):11-17, 1986.

10. Hammond, E. C., and L. Garfinkel. "Coronary Heart Disease, Stroke, and Aortic Aneurysm." *Archives of Environmental Health* 19(8):174, 1979.

11. Herbert, H. R., L. Montgomery, and H. P. Wetzler. "Planning a Fitness Program for Industry." Washington, D.C.: President's Council on Physical Fitness and Sports, 1983. Contained in Federal Fit Kit.

12. Hoeger, W. W. K. *Lifetime Physical Fitness & Wellness: A Personalized Program.* Englewood, CO: Morton Publishing Company, 1986.

13. Kaufman, J. E. "State of the Art: Physical Fitness in Corporations." *Employee Services Management* 26(1):8-9, 26-27, 1983.

14. Leepson, M. "Staying Healthy." *Congressional Quarterly Inc.* 635-651, 1983.

15. Marcotte, B., and J. H. Price. "The Status of Health Promotion Programs at the Worksite, A Review." *Health Education* 4-8, July/August 1983.

16. Paffenbarger, R. S., R. T. Hyde, A. L. Wing, and C. H. Steinmetz. "A Natural History of Athleticism and Cardiovascular Health." *JAMA* 252(4):491-495, 1984.

17. Parkinson, R., and Associates. *Managing Health Promotion in the Workplace.* Palo Alto, CA: Mayfield Publishing Company, 1982.

18. Perham, J. "Check-Up Centers for Physical Exams." *Dun's Business Month* 110-112, October 1984.

19. *Physical Fitness in Business and Industry.* Washington, D.C.: President's Council on Physical Fitness and Sports, 1972.

20. Shephard, R. J. "Practical Issues in Employee Fitness Programming." *Physician and Sports Medicine* 12(6):161-166, 1984.

21. Shilstone, S. "The Fitness Renaissance: Will It Stand The Test of Time." *Sunbelt Executive* 54-56, third quarter 1984.

22. Smith, L. K. "Cost-Effectiveness of Health Promotion Programs." *Fitness Management* 2(3):12-15, 1986.

23. Sorochan, W. D. *Promoting Your Health.* New York: John Wiley & Sons, Inc., 1981.

24. Staff. "America's Fitness Binge." *U.S. News & World Report* 58-61, May 3, 1982.

25. Staff. "Fitness, Corporate Style." *Newsweek* 96-97, November 5, 1984.

26. Staff. "Health Benefits Come Under the Knife." *Fortune* 100-110, May 2, 1983.

27. Staff. "New Fitness Data Verifies: Employees Who Exercise Are Also More Productive." *Athletic Business* 8(12):24-30, 1984.

28. Staff. "Reduced Costs, Increased Production are Rationale for Tax-Favored Corporate Fitness Plans." *Employee Benefit Plan Review* 20-22, November 1983.

29. Van Camp, S. P. "The Fixx Tragedy: A Cardiologist's Perspective." *Physician and Sports Medicine* 12(9): 153-155, 1984.

30. Wright, C. C. "Cost Containment Through Health Promotion Programs." *Journal of Occupational Medicine* 22:36-39, 1980.

Designing A Health Promotion Program

Spiraling increments in medical costs over the last few decades have motivated many organizations to implement health promotion programs with the intent of containing or decreasing health expenditures. Over 400 major corporations in the country are now offering health/fitness programs. Organizations have begun to realize that there is a substantial financial return in this type of investment. A similar trend is seen in hospitals across the country, with more than 2,250 offering some kind of health promotion program. Close to 500 have constructed in-house fitness facilities, with services available not only to their staff but to the community in general.

Organizations considering the implementation of health promotion programs should observe several steps in the development phase:

1. Secure management support (also medical, where necessary)

2. Establish a wellness committee

3. Assess needs and priorities

4. Define goals and objectives

5. Identify and/or hire adequate personnel

6. Secure adequate fitness facilities

7. Determine incentives for program participation

MANAGEMENT SUPPORT

The first step in designing a worksite health promotion program is to have the full support by the top levels of management. It is practically impossible to launch a successful program without their total commitment and enthusiastic support. Management must perceive the need for such a program, and it should be a part of the overall philosophy and mission of the organization. Management participation in the developing stages and later in the program itself is critical and will significantly enhance employee interest and participation. An employee is more likely to participate when the leadership of the organization sets high standards and leads the way through their own example.

Along with management support, the commitment of the company's physician (if such exists) and any other medical staff is also crucial to launch a successful program. Some medical personnel may be somewhat skeptical at first because of their lack of experience in this area. The wellness movement, however, is difficult to disassociate from the medical profession. Working in close association with companies' physicians and bringing out the value of professionally conceived health programs will help in gaining their support.

WELLNESS COMMITTEE

Once total support from management has been given, a wellness committee needs to be established. This committee should have a representative from each key division in the organization and should be chaired by a program coordinator assigned by management. The coordinator is usually a fitness enthusiast within the company who has skills to coordinate all available resources in the developing stages of the program. The committee will be responsible for assessing the needs and priorities of the program. This is a crucial step because the program must be designed to meet the specific needs of the organization. The committee will also have the responsibility of searching for a health/fitness director (for qualifications, *see* Personnel). In small organizations with a relatively small number of participants, the coordinator may continue to lead the program. Once the needs and priorities have been established, the committee, in cooperation with the health/fitness director, must define the intended goals and objectives of the program.

ASSESSING NEEDS AND PRIORITIES

One of the primary responsibilities of the wellness committee is to identify the company's and the employees' needs and priorities for the program. This information will help in defining the magnitude of the program and its goals and objectives and can be used to measure program success after the implementation. Examples of needs assessment questionnaires are given in Figures 2.1 and 2.2. These questionnaires can be adapted to obtain specific information, which may vary from one organization to the other. However, when assessing needs and priorities, three aspects should be taken into consideration:

1. Medical care. Includes patterns of medical problems and services provided to employees and dependents. Trends in health risk such as cardiovascular disease, obesity, smoking, cancer, etc. should be considered.

2. Health care costs. All expenditures resulting from medical care, disability benefits, lost productivity, replacement costs, and insurance premiums need to be considered.

3. Perceived needs by employees and dependents. This information can be collected through a simple questionnaire in which employees and dependents are surveyed as to whether they perceive a need for the program, whether or not they would participate, how and when they would like the program offered, and what type of health education and fitness activities they would like to see implemented. If the perceived needs are not met, program interest will significantly decrease.

Another important factor is to plan for and allow employee dependents into the program. Since health care benefits are usually extended to all dependents, they should be included in order to increase family health and have a greater impact on health care cost containment. Family participation will contribute to the success of the program. Total well-being involves more than just the individual. It incorporates many aspects, including physical training, nutrition, weight control, stress management, substance abuse, smoking cessation, recreation, and other environmental factors that extend well beyond the company's doors — many of which are best implemented in the home. Consequently, needs assessment questionnaires should be made available to all potential participants.

In some instances, it is advisable to have a guest speaker (or program director if already hired) discuss the benefits of health promotion programs prior to surveying employees and dependents. This will increase health awareness, which may be the most immediate need of a wellness program. Increasing awareness of positive health habits will increase interest and motivate individuals to participate. This initial contact is most significant, as often times it may be the only opportunity to sell the program to potential participants. Therefore, the information must be presented in a clear, concise, well-documented, and easily understood manner to the intended audience.

GOALS AND OBJECTIVES

The justification, success, and evaluation of the program will largely depend on how well needs and priorities of employees, dependents, and the organization are met. In this respect, program goals and objectives must be realistic and clearly

Figure 2.1. *Company Needs Assessment Questionnaire.*

I. General Information

1. Company name: _____

2. Company address: _____

    City: _____ State: _____

3. Chief executive officer: _____

4. Medical director: _____

5. Does management perceive a need for the program? _____

6. Are funds available for a wellness program? _____

7. Does (or would) management allow time off for program participation? _____

II. Employee Information

1. Total number of employees: _____

2. Number of locations: _____

3. Number of shifts: _____

4. Number of employees by age and sex:

Age	Men	Women
29 and younger:	_____	_____
30 to 39:	_____	_____
40 to 49:	_____	_____
50 to 59:	_____	_____
60 and over:	_____	_____

5. Total number of dependents 18 and over: _____

6. Number of dependents by age and sex:

Age	Men	Women
29 and younger:	_____	_____
30 to 39:	_____	_____
40 to 49:	_____	_____
50 to 59:	_____	_____
60 and over:	_____	_____

7. Total number of retirees: _____

III. Health/Fitness Program Information

1. Worksite program director or coordinator available: _____

2. Other health promotion/fitness personnel available: _____

3. Fitness testing available? _____
    Number tested: employees _____ dependents _____ retirees _____
    Total cost: $_____

4. Medical screening available? _____
    Number tested: employees _____ dependents _____ retirees _____
    Total cost: $_____

Figure 2.1. *Company Needs Assessment Questionnaire (continued).*

5. Activity program (fitness training) available? _____
   If so, is it in-house: _____ or corporate membership: _____
   In-house, indicate type of facilities and equipment available:

   _____
   _____
   _____

6. Smoking policy available? _____

7. Health education programs available? _____
   If so, indicate: _____ Blood pressure screening and management
   _____ Smoking cessation
   _____ Stress management
   _____ Nutrition
   _____ Weight control
   _____ Coronary heart disease risk management
   _____ CPR training
   _____ Cancer prevention
   _____ First aid training
   _____ Substance abuse control
   _____ Healthy food selection at cafeteria
   _____ Wellness education newsletter
   Others, indicate: _____
   _____

IV. Identifying Health Care Cost

1. Total annual health care cost: $_____
   Cost by gender: Men $_____ Women $_____

2. Health care cost by category and gender:

Category	Total Cost	Men	Women
Cardiovascular	$_____	$_____	$_____
Cancer	$_____	$_____	$_____
Low-back	$_____	$_____	$_____
Respiratory	$_____	$_____	$_____
Accidents	$_____	$_____	$_____
Gastrointestinal	$_____	$_____	$_____
All-others	$_____	$_____	$_____

3. Total sick days per year: _____
   Sick days by gender: Men_____ Women_____

4. Sick days by category and gender:

Category	Total Days	Men	Women
Cardiovascular	_____	_____	_____
Cancer	_____	_____	_____
Low-back	_____	_____	_____
Respiratory	_____	_____	_____
Accidents	_____	_____	_____
Gastrointestinal	_____	_____	_____
All-others	_____	_____	_____

5. Total replacement cost: $_____
   Replacement cost by gender: Men $_____ Women $_____

Figure 2.2. *Participant Needs Assessment Questionnaire.* *

A. Check the items you would like to improve.
   _____ Your health
   _____ Your fitness level
   _____ Your weight/appearance
   _____ Your energy level

B. Are you currently involved in any regular activity or program designed to improve or maintain your health?   _____ Yes   _____ No

C. If yes, check the activities in which you participate and the times of day they occur.
   _____ Walking   _____ Jogging
   _____ Cycling   _____ Exercise classes
   _____ Aerobic dance   _____ Weight training
   _____ Racquetball   _____ Tennis
   _____ Health education seminars _____ Other activities (list)
                                      _____
                                      _____

   Times: _____ Before work   _____ Mid-morning
          _____ Lunch time   _____ Mid-afternoon
          _____ After work

D. If offered, would you participate in a company-sponsored health/fitness program on a regular basis?   _____ Very likely   _____ Likely   _____ Not likely

E. If activities could be offered by the company, which would interest you the most and what times during the day would you participate?
   _____ Walking   _____ Jogging
   _____ Cycling   _____ Exercise classes
   _____ Aerobic dance   _____ Weight training
   _____ Racquetball   _____ Tennis
   _____ Health education seminars _____ Other activities (list)
                                      _____
                                      _____

   Times: _____ Before work   _____ Mid-morning
          _____ Lunch time   _____ Mid-afternoon
          _____ After work

F. If other aspects of the program could be offered, which would interest you the most and what times of the day would you participate?
   _____ Blood pressure screening
   _____ Smoking cessation
   _____ Nutrition education
   _____ Weight control classes
   _____ Other activities (list)
   _____
   _____

   Times: _____ Before work   _____ Mid-morning
          _____ Lunch time   _____ Mid-afternoon
          _____ After work

*Reproduced with permission. *Heart at Work*. American Heart Association.

Figure 2.2. *Participant Needs Assessment Questionnaire. (continued)*

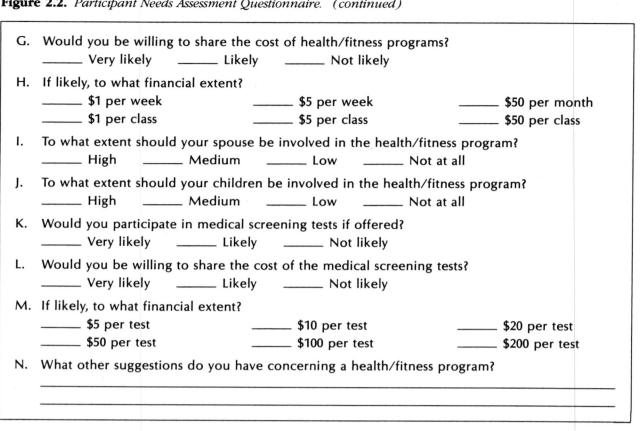

G. Would you be willing to share the cost of health/fitness programs?
_____ Very likely _____ Likely _____ Not likely

H. If likely, to what financial extent?
_____ $1 per week _____ $5 per week _____ $50 per month
_____ $1 per class _____ $5 per class _____ $50 per class

I. To what extent should your spouse be involved in the health/fitness program?
_____ High _____ Medium _____ Low _____ Not at all

J. To what extent should your children be involved in the health/fitness program?
_____ High _____ Medium _____ Low _____ Not at all

K. Would you participate in medical screening tests if offered?
_____ Very likely _____ Likely _____ Not likely

L. Would you be willing to share the cost of the medical screening tests?
_____ Very likely _____ Likely _____ Not likely

M. If likely, to what financial extent?
_____ $5 per test _____ $10 per test _____ $20 per test
_____ $50 per test _____ $100 per test _____ $200 per test

N. What other suggestions do you have concerning a health/fitness program?
_____
_____

defined. All too often programs are launched with total management support, but if goals and objectives have not been established, evaluation of the respective programs becomes difficult. For example, in 1980 Johnson & Johnson implemented a "Live for Life" program with the general goals of encouraging employees to exercise, practice good nutrition, achieve ideal body weight, stop smoking, and reduce alcohol intake. The specific objectives to be accomplished in five years were:

1. To increase to 70 percent the number of people who exercised a minimum of two times per week.

2. To increase from 25 percent to 50 percent the number of employees who practiced sound nutritional habits.

3. To have 60 percent of the employees within 10 percent of ideal body weight.

4. To decrease the smoking rate and the number of individuals with alcohol problems by 50 percent.

When writing worksite wellness objectives, the leadership must keep in mind that in some cases, objectives may be difficult to evaluate. For instance, job productivity is difficult to measure in executives whose main responsibility is that of decision making. However, in assembly line work, productivity can easily be determined. Similarly, if the corporate goal is to increase morale or feelings of well-being, the specific objectives may not be measurable. Whenever possible, objectives should be quantifiable, allowing for easier and more accurate program evaluation.

Objectives can also be classified into short-, intermediate-, or long-range objectives. If the general goals are to decrease the incidence of heart disease and health care costs, some examples of short-range objectives could be:

• Cardiovascular endurance: 30 percent of employees and 10 percent of dependents will participate in aerobic exercise during the first three months of the program.

- Nutrition: 40 percent of all employees and their spouses will be given a dietary analysis during the initial month of the program and will receive follow-up counseling on optimal nutrition.

- Blood chemistry analysis: 50 percent of employees and adult dependents (eighteen years and older) will receive a blood test for blood lipid analysis (total cholesterol, HDL-cholesterol, and triglycerides) during the first sixty days of the program. All (100 percent) employees and dependents showing abnormal results will be followed up by the company's physician and will receive nutrition counseling and an aerobic exercise prescription.

- Smoking cessation: 50 percent of all smokers (employees and dependents) will participate in a smoking cessation seminar during the third month of the program.

Intermediate-range objectives could be defined as follows:

- Cardiovascular endurance: 20 percent improvement in cardiovascular fitness by all exercise participants six months into the program, and an increase in exercise participation rate to 40 and 20 percent, respectively, for employees and dependents by the end of the first year.

- Nutrition: 20 percent of all program participants will have decreased their total fat intake to less than 30 percent of total calories six months into the program.

- Blood chemistry analysis: 10 percent reduction in total cholesterol and 20 percent reduction in serum triglycerides for all hyperlipedimic participants by the end of the first year of exercise and nutrition programs.

- Smoking cessation: 30 percent smoking cessation among program participants in the initial year of the program.

Finally, the long-range objectives could be:

- Health benefits: 10 percent reduction in cardiovascular events five years into the program.

- Health care cost reduction: 20 percent reduction in health care costs at the end of five years.

- Smoking cessation: A smoke-free organization at the end of the fifth year of the program.

Based on some of the previous examples, it is clear that in order to set goals and objectives, certain preliminary data must be collected. Information on health care costs and heart disease risk must be obtained. Costs can be obtained through the benefits or personnel department. Risk for heart disease can be obtained through heart disease risk profiles or appraisals. This initial information is also valuable in justifying the implementation of a wellness program.

PERSONNEL

It is essential that good leadership be provided to ensure adequate participation. With few exceptions, employee fitness programs in the United States report a participation rate of approximately 20 percent of all eligible employees. Unfortunately, in many cases individuals who have the greatest risk for illness are the least likely to participate. To have a significant impact on risk reduction, health improvement, and cost containment, employees who need intervention most must be reached. In this regard, the leadership will have its greatest challenge — that of motivating the high-risk group to participate.

The health/fitness director has the responsibility of administering and supervising the entire program. This includes leadership, budget, personnel, equipment, health/fitness assessments, health education, implementing and supervising the exercise programs, and providing personal attention and encouragement to all participants. This person becomes the central figure of the program, and much of the success is based on the quality of this leadership.

While initially most health/fitness directors were professionals with an exercise physiology background, the scope of wellness programs now indicates that this type of training by itself is not sufficient to provide adequate leadership. An ideal program director, in addition to having a solid foundation in exercise physiology, fitness testing, data processing, and statistical analysis, needs to have knowledge in areas related to nutrition and weight control, stress management, smoking cessation, business management, and human relations. He/she needs to be a role model and a real motivator and have excellent communication skills. The latter is vital, as often times out-of-condition employees do not want to be laughed at or be intimidated when participating in the program. The director has to work with such individuals and emphasize that it will take some time to get into condition and reap the benefits of wellness, but he/she also needs to reassure them that it can be accomplished. In many instances, the director may only have one opportunity — the initial contact — to reach these individuals.

Although no single curriculum will insure adequate professional preparation, health promotion directors and other health/fitness staff are usually prepared through a combination of academic and practical experience. Practical experience is a key factor, because although potential health promotion leaders may have extensive academic preparation, they may not feel at ease when working directly with people, such as in health/fitness testing and counseling. Previous job experience is often a good indicator of how well a given individual will perform in this type of setting. Student internships are also a valuable tool in determining how well a person enjoys and carries out job responsibilities in corporate wellness programs. Furthermore, several organizations offer professional certification for fitness and health promotion staff, and it is highly recommended that all individuals working in this field hold such certifications.

Perhaps the most comprehensive and difficult certification program is offered by the American College of Sports Medicine, which requires both a sound academic background and practical experience for certification application. Two types of certification programs are offered. The preventive tract, first implemented in 1987, is primarily designed for individuals working in corporate

wellness settings. Three certification levels are given in this tract: (1) exercise leader/aerobics (leads exercise/aerobics classes), (2) health fitness instructor (leads exercise and health-enhancement programs for individuals with no history of disease or those who have controlled disease), and (3) health/fitness director (holds leadership position in a wellness program). The second certification program, the rehabilitative tract, is intended for those involved in graded-exercise testing (stress ECG) and cardiac rehabilitation. Three certification levels are also given in this tract: (1) exercise test technologist (administers graded-exercise testing), (2) exercise specialist (conducts exercise testing, prescribes exercise, and provides exercise leadership), and (3) program director (holds a leadership position in a cardiac rehabilitation program). A list of several organizations providing one or more levels of certification is given in Figure 2.3. In addition, all health promotion personnel should be active in the Association for Fitness in Business, the national organization that provides educational support to work site fitness and health promotion programs.

Since health promotion programs need to be medically sound, the support of medical personnel is required in many programs. This is especially necessary for high-risk participants, particularly for heart disease. Based on the scope of the assessment phase, medical personnel are often required to perform and interpret certain tests. For example, all maximal graded-exercise testing performed on symptomatic individuals, that is, those with known disease, or coronary disease risk factors, requires the physical presence of a physician (the actual test is usually carried out by an

Figure 2.3. *Exercise Certification and Training Organizations.*

Organization	Location	
• Aerobics and Fitness Association of America	Sherman Oaks, California	
• American Aerobics Association	Durango, Colorado	
• American College of Sports Medicine	Indianapolis, Indiana	
• Institute for Aerobics Research	Dallas, Texas	
• International Dance — Exercise Association	San Diego, California	
• National Dance — Exercise Instructors Training Association	Minneapolis, Minnesota	
• The Aerobic Way National Certification Agency, Inc.	Lake Quivira, Kansas	
• The International Exersafety Association	Cleveland, Ohio	
• Universal Gym Equipment, Inc.	Cedar Rapids, Iowa	

exercise test technologist). Blood samples for blood chemistry analysis should be drawn by a nurse or medical technician. The interpretation of test results in both cases can only be done by a physician.

Other supportive personnel that may be used in addition to those previously described are dieticians and behavioral psychologists. The use of their services will depend on the needs and priorities perceived by the participants, the size of the program, and the wellness goals and objectives established by the organization. Supportive personnel (including physicians and nurses) could be volunteers, consultants, or part-time staff, unless the program is of such magnitude that full-time employment is justified. Recommended guidelines for required personnel to implement an in-house health promotion program are given in Table 2.1.

FACILITIES

Current costs of facilities for employee fitness programs in the United States have been estimated between $150 and $1,000 per participant per year. The cost varies depending on the size and luxury of the facility. However, an impressive facility is not required to run an effective exercise program. An in-house facility can be established without an inordinate amount of space, equipment, or cost.

As a minimum, a facility should include locker rooms, showers, a meeting room for educational seminars, and an open area of about 1,500 to 2,000 square feet. The size of the facility and the amount of equipment is often determined by needs, participants, and funds available. If the company decides to build a fitness center or develop one using existing available space, professional guidance (a fitness expert and an architect) should be employed.

All facilities should include some equipment for cardiovascular fitness development. Such equipment can range from jump ropes and rebounders to bicycle ergometers, rowing machines, cross-country skiing simulators, or treadmills. The bicycle ergometer is probably the most basic piece of equipment, since it is relatively inexpensive (as compared to treadmills), uses little space, and can be used for training as well as for simple cardiovascular endurance assessment (oxygen uptake estimation).

A small amount of strength training equipment and some mats are necessary for muscular strength and flexibility development. In choosing strength training equipment, "fixed" weights are recommended over free weights for safety reasons and lower risk for injury. Strength training equipment, however, can be expensive, and if funds are limited, it may not be necessary in the initial stages of a program. With some creativity, a large

Table 2.1.
Recommended In-House Staff Needs for Health Promotion Programs.

Personnel	Program Size (based on total number of participants)*		
	<50	50-250	250>**
● Wellness Coordinator	x	x	x
● Health/Fitness Instructor	x	x	x
● Wellness Director (Health/Fitness Director)		x	x
● Exercise Leader/Aerobics		x	x
● Exercise Test Technologist			x
● Physician			x
● Support Personnel			x

*Actual number of participants, not total number of employees.
**When the number of participants exceeds 250, most of the medical testing (e.g. stress-ECGs, blood analysis, medical/physical exams) can be done in-house. For smaller programs these services should be contracted with other agencies.

variety of strength training exercises can be performed using the individual's own body weight as resistance to increase muscular tone and stamina. Additional information on companies that offer different types of fitness equipment is given in Figure 2.4.

One piece of equipment crucial for data processing and analysis is a computer system to produce individual/group risk and fitness profiles, exercise prescriptions, nutritional evaluations, health/fitness records, and exercise logs. The type of system to be used should be determined according to the software requirements, which are, in turn, determined by the magnitude of the assessment phase, the total number of participants, and the various health education programs to be offered.

Some organizations committed to the wellness movement have exercise and sport complexes which far exceed those offered at many private clubs and colleges. An example is the Xerox Corporation, which runs seven exercise centers across the country, including a $3.5 million facility at their International Center for Training and Management in Leesburg, Virginia. This center includes two gymnasiums, a weight training room, a swimming pool, four tennis courts, two racquetball courts, a soccer field, a putting green, and 2,300 wooded acres for jogging and recreation. Most companies with established fitness programs are constantly expanding to greater and better training facilities — an indication of the firm belief that fit participants are healthier and more productive workers. Some organizations have reported that employees are often more impressed by fitness facilities than by other fringe benefits offered by the company. Some simple guidelines for in-house fitness facilities have been developed by the American Heart Association and are presented in Table 2.2.

Nevertheless, from a cost standpoint, it is practically impossible for many organizations to establish elaborate health/fitness centers. As a result, some companies that do have fitness centers share their facility with other corporations housed in the same building complex. Furthermore, there is a growing trend among many companies to use facilities and personnel already available in downtown areas like YMCAs, Boys Clubs, Jewish Centers, health clubs, schools, colleges and universities, and local hospitals with fitness facilities. Membership fees are either paid in full by the company or shared with the employees and de-

pendents. When implementing this type of arrangement, the exercise facility should be conveniently located. Most employees will not drive across town for a fitness workout. Studies indicate that compliance is enhanced when the fitness facility is close to the workplace.

The one drawback at this point with many outside facilities is that very few of them conduct comprehensive health/fitness assessments and subsequent health education programs aimed at behavior modification and health enhancement. If these programs are unavailable, an organization could purchase these services from other external providers such as hospitals, private consultants, health/fitness clinics, and even colleges and universities. Another alternative is for a company to hire its own health/fitness director or health/fitness instructor to develop a screening and health education program based on existing equipment at local clubs. In some instances, minor additional equipment such as skinfold calipers, metronomes, blood pressure sphygmomanometers, stopwatches, etc. may be required to do a thorough assessment. More information on specific equipment needed for different assessment options is discussed in Chapter 3.

INCENTIVES

It is well accepted that regular participation is the key to bring about lifestyle modifications that will result in healthier individuals. Motivating people to initiate a positive lifestyle program and then maintaining a high level of interest is the biggest challenge faced in any wellness program. Even when initial interest in the program is high, regular participation in most organizations only runs around 20 percent of all eligible employees. One of the highest rates of participation in the country has been reported by The Mesa Petroleum Company in Amarillo, Texas, with a 64 percent participation rate.

The most important factor affecting program adherence is adequate leadership. The health/fitness director must be able to present the benefits of a fit and healty lifestyle to all potential participants in a convincing manner. In this regard, the intial contact with the employees is most crucial in terms of motivating them to participate. Once an individual decides to enroll, the quality of the program, individual attention, and the creativity of the leadership play a significant role

Figure 2.4. *Fitness-Equipment Manufacturers.* *

Company	Equipment
Allegheny International Exercise Company P.O. Box 778 Lincolnton, NC 28092	Vitamaster bikes Rowers Treadmills
AMF 200 American Avenue Jefferson, IA 50129	Recumbent bike Rower
Amerec Corporation 1776 136th Pl. NE Bellevue, WA 98005	Tunturi bikes Rowers Treadmills
Bally Fitness Products Corporation 10 Thomas Rd. Irvine, CA 92718	Lifecycle bike Liferower
Bollinger Industries, Inc. 222 W. Airport Freeway Irving, TX 75062	Bikes Rowers Treadmills
Concept II R. R. 1, Box 1100 Morrisville, VT 05661	Concept II rower
Diversified Products P.O. Box 100 Opelika, AL 36803	Bikes Rowers Weight systems
Excelsior Fitness Equipment Co. 615 Landwehr Rd. Northbrook, IL 60062	Schwinn Air-Dyne bike
Fitness Master, Inc. 1387 Park Rd. Chanhassen, MN 55317	Fitness Master ski simulator
Genesis Inc. 7920 Silverton Ave. San Diego, CA 92126	Treadmills
Heart Rate, Inc. 3186-G Airway Ave. Costa Mesa, CA 92626	Versa-Climber
J. Oglaend, Inc. 40 Radio Circle Mt. Kisco, NY 10549	Bodyguard bikes Rowers
Landice Treadmills 269 E. Blackwell St. Dover, NJ 07801	Treadmills
M & R Industries 7140 180th Ave. Redmond, WA 98052	Avita bikes Rowers Treadmills

*Reprinted by permission of Rodale's *Runner's World Magazine.* Copyright 1986.

Figure 2.4. *Fitness-Equipment Manufacturers.*

Company	Equipment
MAI 17635 Northeast 67th Ct. Redmond, WA 98052	Monark bikes Rowers Treadmills
Marcy Gymnasium 2801 W. Mission Rd. Alhambra, CA 90031	Bikes Free weights Gym systems
Nautilus Equipment P.O. Box 1783 Deland, FL 32720	Weight systems
PSI 141 Jonathon Blvd. North Chaska, MN 55318	Nordic-Track ski simulator
Pacer Industries 1121 Crowley Rd. Carrolton, TX 75006	Treadmills
Paramount Fitness 6636 E. 26th St. Los Angeles, CA 90040	The Chair recumbent bike
ProForm 8170 SW. Nimbus Ave. Beaverton, OR 97005-6423	The Aerobot
Sportech 401 Euclid Ave. Cleveland, OH 44114	Treadmills
Triangle Health & Fitness P.O. Box 2000 Morrisville, NC 27560	CVex recumbent bike/rower
Trotter Treadmills, Inc. P.O. Box 103 Hopedale, MA 01747	Treadmills
Universal Fitness Products Universal Gym Equipment P.O. Box 1270 Cedar Rapids, IA 52406	Aerobicycle Tredex Treadmills Weight training equipment
West Bend Co. 400 Washington St. West Bend, WI 53095	Bikes Rowers Treadmills

Table 2.2.
Guidelines for In-House Facilities.*

Facility	Program Size (based on total number of employees)		
	Small <50	Medium 50-1000	Large 1000>
● Existing space used as exercise class area (e.g. cafeteria)	x	x	x
● Showers and dressing areas	x	x	x
● Outdoor track		x	x
● Exercise room with equipment		x	x
● Indoor track			x
● Multi-purpose gymnasium			x
● Courts			x
● Swimming pool			x

*Reproduced with permission. Heart at Work. American Heart Association.

in maintaining program participation. Since different things motivate different people, a good director must try to find out what motivates a given person and then implement principles that will help program adherence.

To encourage and increase employee participation, companies are continuously designing new and creative incentive programs. Medical-physical assessments, individualized exercise prescriptions, and behavior modification counseling are initially used to get employees involved in the program. Physiological measurements (cardiovascular fitness, percent body fat, blood lipid profile, blood pressure, stress ECGs, etc.) help determine potential risk for disease and serve as a motivator to start lifestyle changes aimed at health enhancement. A trained and enthusiastic counselor, in conjunction with the participant, will use this information to prescribe personalized programs to achieve the desired objectives. The results also serve as a starting point to monitor changes and evaluate progress realized through intervention programs. Such assessments are commonly offered to employees and often to their relatives at little or no cost. Some companies charge a certain fee with the incentive that if the individual continues in the program and shows progress, part or all of the paid fees are reimbursed at the end of the year.

Participants also enjoy regular follow-up assessments, as they provide a means to ascertain fitness changes, and risk reduction, and maintain motivation for program participation.

Other types of incentives that have been successfully used by different organizations are:

· Individuals are paid by the number of miles that they walk, run, cycle, or swim. Hospital Corporation of America in Nashville, Tennessee, paid the participants sixteen cents per mile walked or run, four cents per mile cycled, and sixty-four cents per mile swum.

· The Schwartz Meat Company in Norman, Oklahoma, encouraged participation by allowing employees to earn as much as a month's extra pay per year if husband and wife both participated in the fitness program.

· Annual health insurance premiums are often reimbursed to employees adhering to the exercise program.

· Davidson Louisiana, Inc. offered a free trip to Rome or Mexico to regular fitness participants. Eighty percent of the company's employees joined the program, with 80 percent of them qualifying for the free vacation in the initial year.

- Some companies have developed a point system whereby an individual accumulates points based on predetermined goals such as participation time, percent improvement in cardiovascular fitness, decrease in percent body fat, calories burned through exercise, decrease in total cholesterol or improvement in total cholesterol HDL-cholesterol ratio, quitting cigarette smoking, etc. Monetary bonuses or gifts including exercise clothing, shoes, books, cookbooks, and vegetable steamers are given according to the total number of points earned.

- Most organizations do charge a minimal annual fee for equipment repair and maintenance. The fee is then either fully or partially reimbursed to regular program participants. This benefit is also made available to dependents as well. The Phillips Petroleum Company in Bartlesville, Oklahoma, has one of the finest employee fitness facilities in the country. The center is popular because the entire family can join for only a small fee of twelve dollars per year. This fee is quite insignificant when compared to health club memberships which can run anywhere from $300 to over $1,000 per year, not including initial registration fees.

Other incentives that have also been used to increase exercise participation and adherence are awards such as trophies, plaques, logo-emblazoned shirts and jackets, and t-shirt patches. Several organizations have elite groups (e.g., 500 Mile Club) and provide social activities or a company picnic-day after certain objectives are met. Equally motivating are individual computerized exercise logs. Participants can enter basic information on heart rate, weight, and type and duration of the physical activity done. The computer will produce a weekly/monthly/yearly report on total number of miles (run, walked, swum, cycled), hours exercised, calories burned, weight lost, aerobic points, average training intensity, average oxygen uptake during training, etc. Many individuals feel such an incentive, along with regular fitness follow-ups, to be the best motivators to exercise adherence.

A final way of maintaining a high level of interest is by providing a health-oriented environment. Newsletters, health/fitness magazines, behavior modification seminars, regular presentations on current wellness topics, offering healthy foods with nutritional information at the organization's cafeteria, etc. all increase wellness awareness and help maintain and/or improve program adherence.

While most incentive programs add a small cost to the employer, it has been shown that these costs are rather insignificant when compared to the benefits derived from a healthier, more productive, and less absent employee.

PROGRAM IMPLEMENTATION

Upon completion of the planning phase, the program director, in conjunction with the wellness committee, will need to decide the scope of the program. This decision should be based on the results of the needs assessment questionnaires and the personnel, facilities, and funds available. The scope of the program may include any or all of the following:

1. Health/fitness assessments. This may include medical/physical examinations, fitness profiles, heart disease risk profiles, cancer risk profiles, nutritional evaluations, and tension and stress evaluations. The frequency of such assessments will depend on funds available and needs based on initial test results and nature of the intervention program.

2. Behavioral modification seminars. May include smoking cessation, stress management, blood pressure control, nutrition, weight control, etc.

3. Physical activities and daily workout schedule. A decision should be made as to which activities (jogging, cycling, swimming, aerobic dance, weight training, etc.) will be offered and whether the activities will be conducted prior to or after work, during lunch hours, or if employees will be given release time during work hours to participate.

When motivating, registering, or selecting participants for the wellness program, they need to be reassured of the confidentiality of all test results. If this is not done, some individuals may perceive poor test results or abnormal findings as a threat to their job security.

Following the assessment phase, group and/or individual consultations must take place to interpret test results, counsel on risk reduction, give exercise prescriptions, and set individual goals and objectives. Furthermore, participants are assigned to respective behavioral modification seminars according to their respective test results. The information obtained from the various assessments is also used to better determine the goals and objectives of the program.

PROGRAM EVALUATION

The purpose of evaluation in health promotion programs is to measure behavioral change, health and fitness improvement, and cost effectiveness. Traditionally, organizations measured success based on the number of individuals participating. While this will determine whether the specific objective on program participation is being met, it fails to detect positive lifestyle changes, health improvement, increased fitness, and cost savings as a result of participation. Program evaluation is best accomplished when initial goals and objectives are clearly defined.

Health and fitness changes can be assessed through the administration of pre- and post-tests (knowledge tests, health/fitness assessments, nutrition evaluations, number of employees who quit smoking, etc.). Cost/benefit is frequently measured through the number of health insurance claims, job-related injuries, absenteeism, and productivity, and then statistically compared to previous years and/or nonparticipating employees.

Detailed program evaluation as previously described is important because it will show management a return on the investment. It also reinforces the need for wellness programs to increase the health of our national working force. Perhaps a greater number of companies have not implemented wellness programs because of the relatively few scientific studies showing the direct relationship between active participation and cost savings. Unfortunately, many organizations see these programs as requiring expensive facilities, equipment, supervisory personnel, and valuable time spent away from work. These companies feel justified in sparing their bottom lines until even greater evidence conclusively proves that the programs are cost effective. As more research becomes available, an even greater trend in organizations implementing health promotion programs across the country can be expected.

REFERENCES

1. American College of Sports Medicine. "1987 ACSM Certification Programs." *Sports Medicine Bulletin* 21(4):7-8, 1986.
2. American Heart Association. *Heart at Work*. Dallas, TX: The Association, 1984.
3. Barnes, L. "AAFDBI: Bringing Fitness to Corporate America." *Physicians and Sports Medicine* 11(1):127-133, 1983.
4. Blue Cross Association, Blue Shield Association, President's Council on Physical Fitness and Sports, and American Association of Fitness Directors in Business and Industry. *Building a Healthier Company*. Chicago, April 1978.
5. Bowne, D. W., M. L. Russell, J. L. Morgan, S. A. Optenberg, and A. E. Clarke. "Reduced Disability and Health Care Costs in an Industrial Fitness Program." *Journal of Occupational Medicine* 26(11):809-816, 1984.
6. Brennan, A. J. "How to Set Up a Corporate Wellness Program." *Management Review* 41-47, May 1983.
7. Colacino, D. "A Fitness Program that was Designed to Fit." *Business and Health* 23-25, December 1983.
8. Ebel, H. "Let's Put The Personal touch Back Into Fitness." *Athletic Purchasing and Facilities* 7(12):12-18, 1983.
9. Fleischman, B., and L. Wade. "A Small Company Takes Time Out for Life." *Fitness in Business* 1(1):25-27, 1986.
10. Gatty, B. "How Fitness Works Out." *Nation's Business* 18-24, July 1985.
11. Herbert, H. R., L. Montgomery, and H. P. Wetzler. "Planning a Fitness Program for Industry." Washington D.C.: President's Council on Physical Fitness and Sports, 1983. Contained in Federal Fit Kit.
12. Howell, P. "Inside Corporate Fitness." *Athletic Business* 9(7):22-25, 1985.
13. Leepson, M. "Staying Healthy." *Congressional Quarterly Inc.* 635-651, 1983.
14. Moore, M. "Are Employee Fitness Programs for Everyone." *Physician and Sports Medicine* 11(1):143-148, 1983.
15. Parkinson, R., and Associates. *Managing Health Promotion in the Workplace*. Palo Alto, CA: Mayfield Publishing Company, 1982.
16. Perham, J. "Fitness Programs Down the Line." *Dun's Business Month* 106-110, October 1984.
17. Redding, B. "Opportunity in Corporate Fitness." *Fitness Management* 2(3):8-10, 22, 1986.
18. Shephard, R. J. "Practical Issues in Employee Fitness Programming." *Physician and Sports Medicine* 12(6):161-166, 1984.
19. Shephard, R. J., P. Morgan, R. Finucane, and L. Schimmelfing. "Factors Influencing Recruitment to an Occupational Fitness Program." *Journal of Occupational Medicine* 22(6):389-398, 1980.
20. Staff. "As Companies Jump on Fitness Bandwagon." *U.S. News and World Report* 36-39, January 28, 1980.
21. Staff. "New Fitness Data Verifies: Employees Who Exercise Are Also More Productive." *Athletic Business* 8(12):24-30, 1984.
22. Sylvester, N. "Marketing Fitness: Sell the Imagery Not the Agony." *Athletic Business* 8(7):8-16, 1984.
23. Tiersten, S. "First Steps to Corporate Fitness." *Fitness Management* 2(3): 17-19, 1986.
24. Wood, D. "Idea Foundation Certification." *Fitness Management* 2(4):44-46, 1986.

CHAPTER THREE

Coronary Heart Disease and Fitness Profiles

Most people may initiate an exercise program without any risks to their health. Nevertheless, for some people there is a slight increased risk of exercise-related injury or even sudden death if not properly screened. Therefore, it is recommended that individuals who wish to start an exercise program undergo a pre-participation evaluation. This evaluation in some cases may be conducted by nonmedical personnel. The extent of the evaluation and the type of personnel required to conduct the evaluation depends on the age, health status, and level of physical activity of the person.[1] Pre-exercise evaluations are especially important for sedentary adults, for those with one or more cardiovascular risk factors, and for all symptomatic or diseased individuals. The results of the evaluation are used to identify areas of risk so that appropriate action can be taken to decrease the incidence of illness and/or premature death. The data are also used for exercise prescription purposes and serve as a starting point from which future changes in health and fitness can be determined.

Basic screening for adults prior to initiating an exercise program should include a comprehensive review of their health history (*see* example wellness questionnaire, Appendix B) and a limited medical evaluation to determine current risk for cardiovascular disease and other possible contraindications to exercise. As a part of the medical evaluation, the assessment of the following parameters is recommended:

body composition, blood lipids, blood glucose, resting blood pressure, and, whenever possible or required, a resting and stress ECG. The results can then be easily compiled and presented in the form of a profile. A health profile is an inventory of genetic factors and lifestyle-related behaviors used in predicting a person's future risk of having a major or fatal health breakdown.

In this chapter, the different components involved in the establishment of coronary heart disease risk and fitness profiles are introduced. The discussion will focus on personnel, equipment, test protocols, measurement techniques, and data analysis used in determining the components of each profile. A detailed definition and interpretation of test results for each risk factor and the various physical fitness components are given in Chapter 4. Since more than one test protocol may be used to establish some of the components of the profiles (e.g., cardiovascular fitness, body composition, flexibility, stress ECG, etc.), only a brief introduction may be given in this chapter to each test. A detailed description is presented in various appendices at the back of the book. The purpose for discussing more than one protocol is to offer a choice of tests, since not every facility has the availability of the same equipment and/or personnel to conduct a given test. A selection of different tests will also allow for greater flexibility in designing the assessment phase of the program.

WELLNESS QUESTIONNAIRE AND INFORMED CONSENT FOR EXERCISE TESTING AND/OR PARTICIPATION

In most instances, a health/fitness director has little information concerning the medical history and health-related behaviors of first-time program participants. In this regard, a standard procedure in health evaluation programs is to have all participants fill out a health history or wellness questionnaire and sign an informed consent form for exercise testing and/or participation.

The wellness questionnaire becomes a valuable tool in the total evaluation process since it can be used to identify potential areas of risk for disease as well as contraindications to exercise testing and participation. The questionnaire should provide information on personal and family history of cardiovascular disease, general health history, nutrition, smoking history, tension and stress evaluation, and physical activity habits. A sample wellness questionnaire is provided in Appendix B.

The information collected through the wellness questionnaire will also aid in determining the extent of the pre-exercise evaluation, and consequently should be carefully reviewed by the program director or a physician. If the information is reviewed by the program director, any medical concerns must be brought to the attention of qualified medical personnel before any testing or exercise participation is initiated. Furthermore, some of the data provided are used to determine several of the risk factors for the coronary profile (personal and family history, smoking, tension and stress, diabetes, estrogen use, and age). This information will be discussed later on in the chapter under the respective coronary risk factors. Much of the remaining data gathered in the questionnaire will help in counseling individuals toward risk reduction and health enhancement. For example, the physical activity section can provide guidelines for writing the exercise prescription. The nutrition section will give a general idea of the individual's diet. While it will not provide a comprehensive dietary analysis, it can identify potential problem areas for initial counseling. If needed or desired, a more complete nutritional analysis can be conducted at a later date (see Appendix J). Similarly, the tension and stress section can reveal problem areas that may require counseling.

In addition, all program participants should sign an informed consent form prior to initiating exercise testing and/or exercise participation. The intent of this form is to make sure that participants realize the small, but real risk of exercise-related injuries, and in rare instances, sudden death. When individuals are given this form to sign, the possible risks, the testing protocols, the objectives of testing, the reasons for exercise participation, and any other concerns or questions that they may have should be clarified. A sample informed consent for exercise testing, developed by the American College of Sports Medicine, is shown in Figure 3.1. A form for exercise participation, developed by the American Heart Association, is given in Figure 3.2.

CORONARY HEART DISEASE RISK PROFILE

In establishing a coronary heart disease (CHD) risk profile, data must be obtained for each CHD risk factor. A risk factor has been defined as an asymptomatic state that may cause disease. A thorough CHD profile should include all of the following risk factors: cardiovascular fitness, resting and exercise electrocardiograms, total cholesterol/high density lipoprotein (HDL) cholesterol ratio, triglycerides, diabetes mellitus, blood pressure, body composition, cigarette smoking, tension and stress, personal and family history of heart disease, estrogen use, and age. The corresponding value for each test can be obtained through a battery of medical-, fitness-, and lifestyle-related tests.

The CHD risk profile is normed according to age, sex, and potential contribution of each risk factor toward the development of the disease. The norm tables for the different risk factors and respective risk categories are found in Appendix A. Since the contribution of each factor in the development of the disease differs, a weighing system assigns the highest number of risk points to the most significant risk factors (see Table 4.1, Chapter 4). This weighing system is based on current research and according to work done at leading preventive medicine facilities in the United States.

The maximum number of risk points ranges from two points for estrogen use and elevated

Figure 3.1. *Informed Consent for an Exercise Test (Sample).*

1. Explanation of the Exercise Test

   You will perform an exercise test on a cycle ergometer or a motor-driven treadmill. The exercise intensity will begin at a level you can easily accomplish and will be advanced in stages, depending on your fitness level. We may stop the test at any time because of signs of fatigue or you may stop when you wish because of personal feelings of fatigue or discomfort.

2. Risks and Discomforts

   There exists the possibility of certain changes occurring during the test. They include abnormal blood pressure, fainting, disorder of heart beat. Every effort will be made to minimize these through the preliminary examination and by observations during testing. Emergency equipment and trained personnel are available to deal with unusual situations which may arise.

3. Benefits to be Expected

   The results obtained from the exercise test may assist in the diagnosis of your illness or in evaluating what type of physical activities you might engage with no or low hazards.

4. Inquiries

   Any questions about the procedures used in the exercise test or in the estimation of functional capacity are encouraged. If you have any doubts or questions, please ask us for further explanations.

5. Freedom of Consent

   Your permission to perform this exercise test is voluntary. You are free to deny consent if you so desire.

I have read this form and I understand the test procedures that I will perform. I consent to participate in this test.

_____
Signature of Patient

_____   _____
Date   Witness

Questions: _____

_____

_____

Response: _____

_____

_____

Physician signature (optional):

Reproduced with permission from *Guidelines for Exercise Testing and Prescription.* American College of Sports Medicine. Philadelphia: Lea & Febiger, 1986.

Figure 3.2. *Informed Consent for Exercise (Sample).*

I desire to engage voluntarily in the _____
exercise program in order to attempt to improve my physical fitness.

I understand that these activities are designed to place a gradually increasing workload on my circulation and thereby attempt to improve its function. The reaction of the cardiovascular system to such activities cannot be predicted with complete accuracy. There is the risk of certain changes occurring during or following the exercise. These changes include abnormalities of blood pressure or heart rate, ineffective "heart function", and possibly, in some instances, a "heart attack" or "cardiac arrest."

I realize that it is necessary for me to promptly report to the exercise supervisor any signs or symptoms indicating any abnormality or distress. I consent to the administration of any immediate resuscitation measures deemed advisable by the exercise supervisor.

I have read the foregoing and I understand it. My questions have been answered to my satisfaction.

Participant signature _____

Date _____

Reproduced with permission. *Heart at Work: Exercise Program Coordinator's Guide.* American Heart Association.

serum triglycerides, to ten points for an elevated total cholesterol/HDL-cholesterol ratio. Each factor has also been given a zero risk level, where any particular factor will not increase the risk for disease. After the values for each factor are established, individual risk points are assigned by referring to Appendix A. The risk points for each factor are then totaled, and the final score will give an indication of overall cardiovascular risk within the next few years (*see* Table A.15 in Appendix A).

A simple version of the comprehensive risk profile is shown in Figure 3.3. This self-assessment cardiovascular risk factor analysis can be used as an initial screening tool and to educate people regarding the risk factors that lead to the development of the disease. When interpreting the results of this self-assessment form, people need to be reminded that it is only an estimated analysis. More precise testing is required for an accurate prediction. Also, note that this simple analysis should never take the place of a comprehensive evaluation. Nevertheless, the final score is a good indicator of whether a person is taking good care of his/her cardiovascular health and practicing appropriate preventive medicine techniques. Furthermore, since the guidelines for zero

risk are outlined, it provides a guide to identify potential risk, help raise awareness, and initiate steps for risk reduction.

CARDIOVASCULAR ENDURANCE

Cardiovascular endurance, cardiovascular fitness, or aerobic capacity is determined by the maximal amount of oxygen that the human body is able to utilize per minute of physical activity. This value can be expressed in liters per minute (L/min) or milliliters per kilogram per minute (ml/kg/min). The latter is most frequently used because it takes into consideration total body mass (weight). When comparing two individuals with the same absolute value, the one with the lesser body mass will have a higher relative value, indicating that a greater amount of oxygen is available to each kilogram (2.2 pounds) of body weight. Since all tissues and organs of the body utilize oxygen to function, a higher amount of oxygen consumption indicates a more efficient cardiovascular system.

The most precise way to determine maximal oxygen uptake is through direct gas analysis. This

Figure 3.3. *Cardiovascular Risk Factor Analysis: Self-Evaluation Form.*

		Score
1. CARDIOVASCULAR FITNESS	Do you participate in a regular aerobic exercise program (brisk walking, jogging, swimming, bicycling, jazzercise etc.) for more than 20 minutes:	
	Once a week or less......................................	6
	Two times per week.....................................	3
	Three or more times per week	0 _____
2. BLOOD PRESSURE	Blood pressure reading is (score applies to each reading, e.g. 150/86 score = 5):	
	Systolic Diastolic	
	161 or higher.... (4) 101 or higher.... (4)	4-8
	141 - 160........ (3) 91 - 100........ (3)	3-6
	121 - 140........ (2) 81 - 90......... (2)	2-4
	Unknown ...... (1) Unknown ..... (1)	1-2
	120 or less ...... (0) 80 or less ...... (0)	0 _____
3. BODY COMPOSITION	Body Fat Percentage	
	Men Women	
	28% or higher 33% or higher	4
	23% - 27% 28% - 32%	3
	18% - 22% 23% - 27%	2
	13% - 17% 18% - 22%	1
	12% or less 17% or less.............................	0 _____
4. TOTAL CHOLESTEROL-HDL RATIO	Ratio is 10.0 or higher	10
	Ratio is between 6.6 - 9.9	7
	Ratio is between 5.6 - 6.5	4
	Ratio is between 4.6 - 5.5	2
	Ratio is less than 4.5	0
	If unknown answer question 6	_____
5. TRIGLYCERIDES	Level is above 250	2
	Level between 101 and 249.............................	1
	Level less than 100	0
	If unknown answer question 6	_____
6. DIET	Do not answer if 4 and 5 have been answered.	
	Does your normal diet include (high score if all apply):	
	One or more daily servings of red meat, 7 or more eggs/week, daily butter-cheese-whole milk, daily sweets and alcohol...	8-12
	Four to six servings of red meat/week, 4-6 eggs/week, margarine, 1 or 2% milk, some cheese, sweets and alcohol	3-7
	Fish (no hard-shell), poultry, red meat less than three times/week, less than 3 eggs/week, skim milk and skim milk products, moderate sweets and alcohol	0 _____
7. DIABETES	Are You:	
	Diabetic and blood sugar is out of control	6
	Diabetic and blood sugar controlled with medication	3
	Diabetic and blood sugar controlled with diet alone	2
	Non-diabetic	0 _____
	Sub Total Risk Score _____	

Adapted from Hoeger, W. W. K. "Self Evaluation of Cardiovascular Risk." *Corporate Fitness & Recreation* 5(6):13-16, Oct/Nov 1986.

Figure 3.3. *Cardiovascular Risk Factor Analysis: Self-Evaluation Form. (continued).*

	Subtotal Risk Score (from previous page) _____
8. ECG	Add scores for both ECG's Resting ECG Stress ECG Abnormal...... (3) Abnormal...... (8) .... 3-11 Equivocal ...... (1) Equivocal ...... (4) .... 1-5 Normal........ (0) Normal........ (0) .... 0 Unknown and age 35 or older and never had resting ECG.. 2 _____
9. SMOKING	Smoke 40 or more cigarettes per day .... 8 Smoke 30-39 cigarettes per day......................... 6 Smoke 20-29 cigarettes per day......................... 5 Smoke 10-19 cigarettes per day......................... 4 Smoke 1-9 cigarettes per day........................... 3 Smoke less than 1 cigarette per day.................... 1 Pipe, cigar smoker or chew tobacco .... 2 Ex-smoker less than one year .... 1 Non-smoker, but live or work in smoking environment .... 2 Ex-smoker over one year .... 0 Lifetime non-smoker .... 0 _____
10. TENSION AND STRESS	Are you: Always tense, uptight, on the run, easily angered .... 4 Nearly always tense, quite impatient, often hurried .... 3 Often tense, impatient when waiting, moody .... 2 Sometimes tense, slight impatience, seldom rushed .... 1 Hardly ever tense, easygoing, not rushed .... 0 _____
11. PERSONAL HISTORY	Have you ever had a heart attack, stroke, coronary bypass surgery or any type of KNOWN heart problem: During the last year .... 8 1-2 years ago .... 6 2-5 years ago .... 3 More than 5 years ago................................. 2 Never had heart problems .... 0 _____
12. FAMILY HISTORY	Have any of your blood relatives (parents, uncles, brothers, sisters, grandparents) suffered from cardiovascular disease (heart attack, strokes, bypass surgery): One or more before age 50 .... 4 One or more between ages 51 and 60 .... 2 One or more after age 61............................. 1 None have suffered from cardiovascular disease .... 0 _____
13. AGE	55 or older .... 4 45-54 .... 3 35-44 .... 2 25-34 .... 1 24 or younger .... 0 _____
14. ESTROGEN USE (Birth control pills and certain hormone drugs)	Are you: 35 or older and using estrogen .... 2 Any age and used estrogen for over 5 years .... 2 35 or younger and used estrogen for less than 5 years ...... 1 Do not use estrogen .... 0 _____
	Total Risk Score _____

CARDIOVASCULAR RISK CATEGORIES

Very low ....5 or less points
Low .... Between 6 and 15 points
Moderate .... Between 16 and 25 points
High........................ Between 26 and 35 points
Very High .... 36 or more points

is done with the use of a metabolic cart through which the amount of oxygen consumption can be directly measured. However, this technique is very sophisticated, and the test requires costly equipment that is not readily available in most health/fitness centers. As a result, several alternate methods of estimating maximal oxygen uptake using limited equipment have been developed.

Even though most cardiovascular endurance tests are probably safe to administer to apparently healthy individuals, that is, those with no major coronary risk factors, the general guidelines issued by the American College of Sports Medicine should always be followed to assure the safety of the participants. These guidelines are shown in Table 3.1.

Several tests used to estimate maximal oxygen uptake will now be introduced. The actual protocols to conduct each one of these tests are given in Appendix C. However, keep in mind that these are different testing protocols and that each test will not necessarily yield the same results. Therefore, to make valid comparisons, the same protocol should be used in pre- and post-assessments.

1. The 1.5-mile run test. This test is most frequently used to predict cardiovascular fitness according to the time it takes to run/walk a 1.5-mile course. Maximal oxygen uptake is estimated based on the time it takes to cover the distance (*see* Table C.1 in Appendix C).

The only equipment necessary to conduct this test is a stopwatch and a track or premeasured 1.5-mile course. It is perhaps the easiest test to administer, but caution should be taken when conducting the test. Since the objective is to cover the distance in the shortest period of time, it is considered to be a maximal exercise test. The use of this test should be limited to conditioned individuals who have been cleared for exercise. At least six weeks of aerobic training are recommended before a person should be allowed to take the test. It is contraindicated for unconditioned beginners, symptomatic individuals, and those with known disease and/or CHD risk factors.

2. Astrand-Ryhming test. Because of its simplicity and practicality, the Astrand-Ryhming test has become one of the most common techniques used when estimating maximal oxygen uptake in the laboratory setting. The test requires little time and equipment and can be administered to most everyone, since submaximal workloads are used to estimate maximal oxygen uptake. All that is required for the test is a technician who knows how to take exercise heart rate, a bicycle ergometer that allows for the regulation

Table 3.1.
Guidelines for Exercise Testing.

	APPARENTLY HEALTHY		HIGHER RISK			WITH DISEASE
	Below 45	45 and Above	Below 35 No Symptoms	35 and Above No Symptoms	Symptoms	Any Age
Maximal Exercise Test Recommended Prior to an Exercise Program	No	Yes	No	Yes	Yes	Yes
Physician Attendance Recommended for Maximal Testing	No (under 35)	Yes	Yes	Yes	Yes	Yes
Physician Attendance Recommended for Sub-maximal Testing	No	No	No	Yes	Yes	Yes

Reproduced with permission from *Guidelines for Exercise Testing and Prescription.* American College of Sports Medicine. Philadelphia: Lea & Febiger, 1986.

of workloads, a stopwatch, and six minutes in which to conduct the test.

Good judgment is essential when administering the test. Heart rates are taken each minute. To predict maximal oxygen uptake, the average of the fifth- and sixth-minute heart rates should fall in the range of 120 to 170 beats per minute (bpm). The test is most accurate when an individual reaches the higher heart rates (around 150 to 170 bpm). However, in older people, such rates could be near or at maximal heart rate, which could make it an unsafe test to perform without additional equipment (ECG unit) and/or the presence of a physician. When choosing workloads for older people, final exercise heart rates should not exceed 130 to 140 bpm.

A limitation of this test is that it cannot be given to individuals on medications that lower heart rate (such as Beta blockers) and/or those with a chronotropic heart rate response (a heart rate that increases slowly during exercise and never reaches maximum). The test has also been found to overestimate maximal oxygen uptake on highly conditioned individuals and those with very low resting heart rates (especially genetically determined), as well as underestimate maximal oxygen uptake on highly unfit people. In spite of these limitations, it still remains one of the most popular and practical tests.

3. The step test. Similar to the Astrand-Ryhming test, step tests require submaximal workloads, are quite simple, and require little time to administer. Over the years, several step test protocols have been developed, and most of them are used to directly classify people into cardiovascular fitness categories according to recovery heart rates. Some tests, however, do allow estimation of maximal oxygen uptake through the use of predicting equations.

The three-minute step test included in Appendix C gives as good an estimate of maximal oxygen uptake as the Astrand-Ryhming test. The equipment required is a bench or gymnasium bleacher 16¼ inches high, a stopwatch, and a metronome. One of the advantages of this test is that if individuals are taught to take their own heart rate, a large group of people can be tested at once when using gymnasium bleachers.

4. Maximal treadmill graded exercise tests. Most maximal exercise protocols require the presence of a physician during administration of the test. It is usually conducted with the individual hooked up to an electrocardiographic monitor. Maximal oxygen uptake can be estimated through the use of predicting equations based on the duration of the test.

The two most common protocols used in treadmill exercise testing are the Bruce and the Balke protocols. The workload increments on the Bruce protocol are quite demanding; consequently, few nonathletic individuals go beyond the fourth stage. The Balke protocol is not as strenuous; thus, it takes longer to complete. Several leading physicians in the field of preventive medicine feel that the Balke protocol is a safer test because lower increments in workloads are used. This, in turn, reduces the amount of strain on the cardiovascular system, perhaps decreasing the risk for abnormal heart function. A third testing protocol, used primarily with highly trained individuals, is the Ellestad protocol. This test is perhaps even more demanding than the Bruce protocol. A graphic illustration of all three protocols is given in Figure 3.4, and a complete description and the predicting equations for maximal oxygen uptake for each test are contained in Appendix C.

Figure 3.4. *Treadmill Protocols for Exercise Testing.*

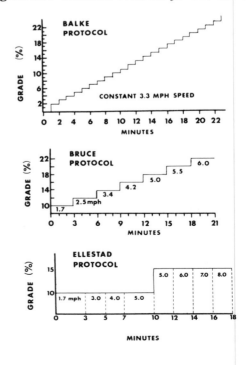

5. Submaximal treadmill exercise tests. These tests are conducted using the same maximal treadmill protocols, except that the tests are terminated at 85 percent of maximum heart rate range (85 percent of the difference between maximum and resting heart rates, plus the resting heart rate). Either the Bruce, Balke, or Ellestad protocols may be used, and maximal oxygen uptake is estimated through the use of similar predicting equations (also found in Appendix C).

Once maximal oxygen uptake has been determined, the CHD risk points and respective risk category for cardiovascular endurance can be looked up in Table A.1, found in Appendix A. For example, the number of risk points assigned to a thirty-four-year-old male with a maximal oxygen uptake of 37 ml/kg/min is 3.6 points, and this person would be classified in a "high risk" category for this particular factor. A maximum of six risk points can be given for a very high risk (or poor fitness) category for cardiovascular endurance.

RESTING ELECTROCARDIOGRAM

The electrocardiogram (ECG) is a recording of the electrical activity as it passes through the heart muscle. It is a useful tool in diagnosing cardiac abnormalities. The resting ECG can be administered by a trained technician or nurse, but the interpretation of the results can only be done by a physician.

The ECG is obtained by placing electrodes against the skin surface on standard body landmarks. The electrical current going through the heart muscle is picked up by these electrodes, and different leads or "pictures" of this activity are recorded on an electrocardiograph. As the number of leads used is increased, the sensitivity to detect abnormalities is also increased. Most facilities use a standard twelve-lead ECG to study heart function.

Based on the findings, a physician can interpret the ECG as either normal, equivocal, or abnormal. An abnormal ECG is assigned three risk points. One point is assigned to an equivocal resting ECG, and no points are given to a normal tracing (*see* Appendix A, Table A.2).

EXERCISE STRESS ELECTROCARDIOGRAM

An exercise stress ECG, also referred to as a maximal exercise tolerance test, is used to predict or evaluate abnormal heart function in either apparently healthy, symptomatic, or diseased individuals. The stress ECG is a much better test for the discovery of coronary heart disease as compared to the resting ECG. It can be used to evaluate changes in heart function due to disease, exercise, medications, and/or surgery. This test is also used to ascertain the safety of exercise prior to initiating an exercise program, as well as to determine cardiovascular functional capacity (expressed as maximal oxygen uptake or in MET* units).

During an exercise stress ECG, an individual is exercised using progressive workload increments until maximum capacity is reached or contraindications are found that require termination of the test. Depending on the purpose for conducting the test, stress ECGs are classified as either functional or diagnostic. A functional test is basically used to determine an individual's maximal functional or aerobic capacity, while a diagnostic test is administered to establish abnormal responses to exercise. A diagnostic stress ECG is valuable in evaluating exercise-induced myocardial ischemia (lack of blood flow to the heart muscle), left ventricular dysfunction, dysrrhythmias of the heart, and abnormal heart rate and blood pressure responses.

While not every adult who wishes to start an exercise program needs a stress ECG, the following guidelines can be used to determine when this type of test should be administered:

1. Adults forty-five years or older.

2. A total cholesterol level above 200 mg/dl, or a total cholesterol/HDL-cholesterol ratio above 4.0 for women and 4.5 for men.

3. Hypertensive and diabetic patients.

4. Cigarette smokers.

---

*One MET equals the resting oxygen uptake, which is approximately 3.5 ml/kg/min. METs are multiples of the resting oxygen consumption rate (e.g., 2 METs= 7.0 ml/kg/min).

Figure 3.5. *Exercise Tolerance Test with Twelve-lead Electrocardiographic Monitoring (courtesy of the University of Texas of the Permian Basin Wellness Center, Odessa, Texas).*

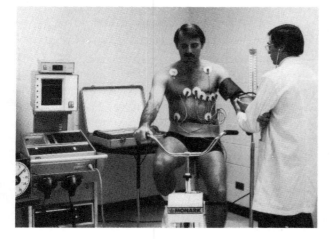

5. Individuals with a family history of coronary heart disease, syncope, or sudden death before age sixty.

6. All individuals with symptoms of chest discomfort, dysrrhythmias, syncope, or chronotropic incompetence (a heart rate that increases slowly during exercise and never reaches maximum).

Although the predictive value of a stress ECG has been at times questioned, it must be remembered that at present it is the most practical, inexpensive, noninvasive procedure available in diagnosing latent coronary heart disease. The sensitivity of the test is increased as the severity of the disease increases. Test protocols, number of leads, electrocardiographic criteria, and the quality of the technicians administering the test further increase its sensitivity. It therefore still remains a very useful tool in identifying those at high risk for exercise-related sudden death.

Graded exercise stress ECG tests are commonly administered on a treadmill or on a bicycle ergometer but can also be given using an arm ergometer or a step test. They can be continuous or discontinuous in nature. The choice of modality is dependent upon time, expense, physical handicaps, and/or physical condition of the participant. A discontinuous test protocol is one in which workloads are alternated with intervals of rest. Discontinuous tests are recommended for individuals with claudication (severe leg pain), angina, and poor muscular fitness. This type of protocol

will allow a greater amount of work to be accomplished prior to the onset of symptoms or fatigue that may require test termination. The arm-crank ergometer is an example of such a test. In continuous tests, workloads are gradually increased without intervals of rest, until complete exhaustion or contraindications make it necessary to stop.

While most testing centers in the United States prefer the use of treadmills for graded exercise tests, there are some advantages for using a bicycle ergometer. During a bicycle test there is less upper body movement, which allows for easier blood pressure assessment and better ECG tracings (less interference related to skeletal muscle activity). Another advantage of bicycle ergometry is that people do not have to support their own body weight, which makes it useful for testing overweight individuals and those with joint problems in the lower extremities. Bicycles are also less expensive and can be easily transported for testing at different locations. The disadvantage is that most subjects do not achieve their true maximal oxygen uptake values (about 10 percent lower as compared to treadmill tests), nor their maximal heart rates. The main reason for these lower values is attributed to the fact that many people do not ride bicycles. In cycling, most of the work is performed by the quadriceps muscle group, and localized muscle fatigue probably sets in before the individual is able to achieve maximal functional capacity.

In addition to a treadmill, bicycle ergometer, or arm ergometer, other equipment necessary to administer a stress test includes an ECG recorder, an oscillosope (allows visual observation of the ECG at all times), a cardiotachometer (provides a constant heart rate readout), blood pressure equipment (sphygmomanometer and stethoscope), and emergency equipment and drugs (*see* Table 3.2).

With regard to emergency equipment and personnel required for exercise stress testing, the American Heart Association's committee on exercise has issued the following guidelines:[2]

Emergency equipment and qualified personnel should be available for exercise testing of all persons. Patients with known or suspected heart disease or dysfunction should not be tested without a qualified physician at the site or in the immediate area (within thirty seconds) in order to provide life-saving emergency care. In the case of

Table 3.2.
Emergency Equipment and Drugs.

1. Defibrillator with electrode paste	1. Aromatic ammonia
2. Airway	2. Metaraminol (aramine)
3. Oxygen	3. Furosemide (lasix)
4. Intravenous sets including fluids	4. Epinephrine
5. Intravenous canulas	5. Atropine
6. Intravenous stand	6. Isoproterenol (isuprel)
7. Syringes and needles in multiple sizes	7. Calcium chloride
8. Adhesive tape	8. Sodium bicarbonate
9. AMBU bag with pressure release valve	9. Lidocaine
10. Suction equipment	10. Amyl nitrate ampule
	11. Digoxin-I.V. and tablets
	12. Nitroglycerin tablets
	13. Verapamil (isoptin)
	14. I.V. Propranolol (inderal)
	15. I.V. Diazepam (valium)
	16. Dopamine
	17. I.V. Nitroglycerin

Reproduced with permission from *Guidelines for Exercise Testing and Prescription*. American College of Sports Medicine. Philadelphia: Lea & Febiger, 1986.

younger individuals (under age thirty-five), free of clinical abnormalities or increased risk factors, the untoward responses to exercise are extremely uncommon. Direct physician presence is not considered necessary provided the health care personnel directing the sessions are trained to the satisfaction of the responsible physician in cardiopulmonary resuscitation (CPR) and emergency cardiac care (ECC) according to standards set by the American Heart Association and the Committee on Emergency Medical Services of the National Academy of Sciences — National Research Council, Division of Medical Sciences.

Unless exercise stress testing is conducted by a physician, it is recommended that all stress tests be administered by qualified personnel such as a preventive and rehabilitative exercise test technologist, an exercise specialist, or a program director. This type of personnel, certified by the American College of Sports Medicine, is required to have adequate knowledge and practical experience in exercise physiology, electrocardiography, pathophysiology, selection and administration of proper test protocols, and emergency procedures related to stress testing. They are also aware of the recommended guidelines set out by the American College of Sports Medicine to screen individuals for stress testing and to determine whether the test can be done with or without the physical presence of a physician. They are capable of identifying contraindications to testing, abnormal responses during the test, and termination points based on physiological and clinical data. Regardless of whether a stress test is conducted with or without the supervision of a physician, the final ECG and blood pressure interpretation can only be done by a physician.

The risk points for the stress ECG are assigned based on the interpretation of the results. A normal test is given no risk points, an equivocal test is given four points, and an abnormal test is awarded eight risk points (*see* Table A.2 in Appendix A).

BLOOD CHEMISTRY ASSESSMENT

A blood chemistry analysis is a minimum requirement for all individuals wishing to initiate an exercise program. It should also be a yearly test for all individuals who have a personal and/or family history of heart disease. A basic blood lipid analysis should include total cholesterol, HDL-cholesterol, triglycerides, and glucose levels.

Blood can be drawn by a medical technician or a registered nurse. The analysis can usually be done at a local hospital or community blood lab that specializes in such work. These labs usually provide all of the equipment necessary for drawing the blood. The cost for this analysis ranges from about twelve to twenty-five dollars per analysis. Depending on the capabilities of the lab, turn-around rates are anywhere from one to three days.

Risk points for blood chemistry are assigned as follows (these are contained in Appendix A, Tables A.3, A.4, and A.5):

• Total cholesterol/HDL-cholesterol ratio: up to ten points

• Triglycerides: up to two points

• Glucose: up to three points (an additional three points are assigned to known diabetics, regardless of current blood sugar level).

BLOOD PRESSURE

Blood pressure is assessed with a sphygmomanometer and a stethoscope. The sphygmomanometer consists of an inflatable bladder contained within a cuff and a mercury gravity manometer or an aneroid manometer from which the pressure is read. The appropriate size cuff must be selected in order to get accurate readings. The size is determined by the width of the inflatable bladder, which should be about 40 percent of the circumference of the midpoint of the arm.

The blood pressure is usually measured in the sitting position with the forearm and the manometer at the same level as the heart. Initially, the pressure should be recorded from each arm, with subsequent pressures recorded from the arm with the highest reading. The cuff should be applied approximately one inch above the antecubital space (natural crease of the elbow), with the center of the bladder applied directly over the medial (inner) surface of the arm. The stethoscope head should be applied firmly but with little pressure over the brachial artery in the antecubital space. The arm should be slightly flexed and placed on a flat surface. The bladder can be inflated while feeling the radial pulse to about 30 to 40 mmHg above the disappearance of the pulse. Avoid overinflating the cuff, as it may cause blood vessel spasm, resulting in higher blood

pressure readings. The pressure should be released at a rate of 2 mmHg per second. As the pressure is released, systolic blood pressure is determined at the point where the initial pulse sound is heard. The diastolic pressure is determined at the point where the sound disappears. The recordings should be made to the nearest 2 mmHg (even numbers) and expressed as systolic over diastolic pressure, i.e., 124/80. The person measuring the pressure should also note whether the pressure was recorded from the left or the right arm.

Figure 3.6. *Blood Pressure Assessment Using a Mercury Gravity Manometer.*

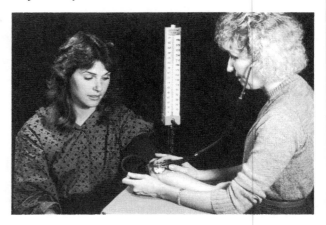

In some cases, the loudness of the pulse sounds decreases in intensity (point of muffling of sounds) and can still be heard at a lower pressure (50 or 40 mmHg) or even all the way down to zero. In this situation, the diastolic pressure is recorded at the point where there is a clear/definite change in the loudness of the sound (also referred to as fourth phase), and at complete disappearance of the sound (fifth phase), e.g. 120/78/60 or 120/82/0.

A final consideration when measuring blood pressure is that several readings by different people or at different times of the day should be taken to establish the real values. One single reading may not be an accurate value, since many factors can affect blood pressure. Excitement, nervousness, food, smoking, pain, temperature, exertion, etc. can all significantly alter the pressure. Whenever possible, readings should be taken in a quiet, comfortable room following a few minutes of rest in the recording position. When more than one reading is taken, the bladder should be completely deflated and at least one minute should be allowed before the next recording is made.

The respective risk points and risk categories for the measured blood pressure are contained in Table A.6, also in Appendix A. A maximum of eight risk points (four points for systolic and four points for diastolic) can be assigned for elevated blood pressure.

BODY COMPOSITION ASSESSMENT

The term "body composition" is used in reference to the fat and nonfat components of the human body. The nonfat component is usually referred to as lean body mass. The fat component is referred to as fat mass or percent body fat. Body composition can be determined by several different procedures. The most common are: (a) hydrostatic or underwater weighing, (b) skinfold thickness, and (c) circumference measurements.

While hydrostatic weighing is the most accurate technique, it also requires a significant amount of time, skill, equipment, and complex procedures. This technique is based on the Archemedian principle of water displacement to determine the density of the human body. Percent fat is then calculated from the obtained body density through the use of predicting equations.

During underwater weighing, the air left in the lungs has an effect on the buoyancy of the human body. Therefore, residual lung volume (the volume of air left in the lungs following complete expiration) has to be determined while the person is in the water to account for the exact amount of air left in the lungs during immersion. This volume must be taken into consideration to accurately compute the density of the body. However, many health/fitness centers and laboratories estimate residual volume because they lack the necessary equipment and/or personnel for actual measurement. This practice will affect the accuracy of this technique. The psychological factor of being weighed underwater also affects the precision of the assessment. The procedure can be uncomfortable, difficult, and often impossible to perform. Many individuals are unable to completely force all of the air out from the lungs and then immerse for

a period of five to ten seconds to obtain the underwater weight. Other procedures using different lung volumes have been developed and published, but their validity is questionable. Hence, the residual volume method still remains the most precise protocol to determine body density. In view of the previous discussion, fitness experts agree that unless the correct hydrostatic weighing procedures are followed, the use of the skinfold thickness technique is a more practical choice to determine body composition in adult fitness programs.

Figure 3.7. *Hydrostatic Weighing Technique for Body Composition Assessment (courtesy of Fitness Monitoring Preventive Medicine Clinic, Lake Geneva, Wisconsin).*

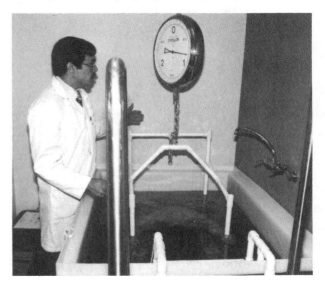

The assessment of body composition using skinfold thickness is based on the principle that 50 percent of the fatty tissue in the body is deposited directly beneath the skin. If this tissue is measured validly and reliably, a good indication of percent body fat can be obtained. This procedure is performed with the aid of pressure calipers, and several sites are measured to reflect the total percentage of fat. This technique correlates well with hydrostatic weighing (when done correctly) and provides a quick, easy, and inexpensive technique to estimate body composition.

Exercise technicians need to keep in mind that even with the skinfold technique, a minimum amount of training is necessary to achieve accurate measurements. Experts recommend that technicians administering skinfold thickness tests need to measure about fifty subjects under qualified supervision to achieve proficiency. Also, variations in measurements on a same subject are often found when these are taken by different observers. Therefore, it is advisable that pre- and post-measurements be conducted by the same technician. Additionally, measurements should be taken at the same time of day, preferably in the morning, since water hydration changes due to activity or exercise can increase skinfold girth up to 15 percent.

Figure 3.8. *Skinfold Thickness Technique for Body Composition Assessment.*

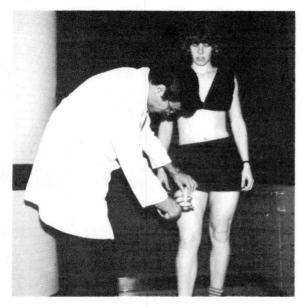

Circumference measurement techniques are also used in assessing percent body fat. With the aid of a cloth measuring tape, percent body fat is estimated according to selected body site measurements. However, the current circumference measurement techniques available, although easy to administer, have questionable validity.

As with maximal oxygen uptake, technicians collecting data on body composition should be aware that all pre- and post-assessments should be done using the same technique. Results obtained through one method will not necessarily compare favorably with a different technique. The various risk categories and risk points for body composition are given in Tables A.7 (men) and A.8 (women) in Appendix A. Procedures for body composition assessment are included in Appendix D.

SMOKING

Information on tobacco use (cigartte smoking, chewing and dipping tobacco, and pipe or cigar smoking) is supplied by the participant, usually through a questionnaire. A sample question to gather this information is found in the wellness questionnaire contained in Appendix B (*see* general health history section, question F). Up to eight risk points are assigned for this factor, and the number of points and specific risk category depend on the type and amount of tobacco used (*see* Table A.9 in Appendix A).

TENSION AND STRESS

The precise assessment of this risk factor is perhaps among the most difficult to establish, since all of the information is based on a subjective evaluation of how much stress is encountered in daily life, and how well a person copes with that stress. A series of surveys on recent life experiences, behavior patterns, stress vulnerability, and symptoms experienced during stress are frequently used to help individuals make a better prediction of their current level of stress. Several of these surveys are found in the wellness questionnaire (*see* Appendix B) under the tension and stress section. Based on the person's reply to the different surveys, a final stress rating is established by the participant in conjunction with the person conducting the pre-test interview. The final rating will classify the individual in one of five tension and stress categories: "hardly ever tense," "sometimes tense," "often tense," "nearly always tense," and "always tense" (*see* wellness questionnaire, tension and stress section, question D). Risk points are progressively assigned from zero points for "hardly ever tense" to four points for the "always tense" category (*see* Table A.10, Appendix A).

PERSONAL AND FAMILY HISTORY OF HEART DISEASE

Risk points for personal and family history of cardiovascular disease are determined according to previous cardiovascular problems encountered by the individual or by blood relatives who suffer or have suffered from this disease. Personal history points range from zero points for no previous history to a maximum of eight for a significant problem within the last year. A maximum of four points is assigned for family history, depending on the age at which blood relatives first suffered from cardiovascular disease. The earlier the incidence, the higher the number of points. The data on personal and family history are obtained through questions A, B, C, and D in the cardiovascular disease history section of the sample wellness questionnaire in Appendix B. The respective risk points and risk categories are found in Tables A.11 and A.12 in Appendix A.

ESTROGEN USE

The use of birth control pills and certain other estrogen-containing drugs have been linked to increased risk for heart disease. Risk has been found to increase with age and number of years of estrogen use. Since the increase in risk is not as significant as other factors, such as an elevated total cholesterol/HDL-cholesterol ratio, hypertension, or cigarette smoking, only a maximum of two risk points is assigned to women over thirty-five who use estrogen, or to those who have used such for over five years. As with the last four risk factors, this information can be gathered with the use of the questionnaire (*see* question K in the general health history section). Risk points and risk categories are given in Table A.13. in Appendix A.

AGE

Age has been identified as a risk factor for heart and blood vessel disease because of the higher incidence of this disease among older people. In terms of risk points, one tenth of a point is given for each year after the age of twenty, up to four points at age sixty (*see* Table A.14, Appendix A).

OVERALL CHD RISK CATEGORY

Upon completion of data collection and establishment of risk points for each factor, the overall CHD risk category is determined by adding together the risk points from all factors. After all points have been totaled, an individual is placed in one of five risk categories for potential development of coronary heart disease. These overall risk categories are given in Appendix A, Table A.15.

The interpretation of the meaning of the overall risk category and the test results on each CHD risk factor, as well as the guidelines for risk reduction and cardiovascular health enhancement, are discussed in Chapter 4. The contents of Chapter 4 are presented in such a way that they can be used not only to interpret the results of the profile, but also to prescribe personalized risk reduction programs.

FITNESS PROFILE

From a health point of view, the basic components of physical fitness are cardiovascular endurance, muscular strength and endurance, muscular flexibility, and body composition. In the following fitness profile, assessment of the strength and flexibility components will be explained. The cardiovascular fitness and body composition components are determined in the same manner as explained under the heart disease profile. In addition to the fitness components, a posture test and a pulmonary function test will be discussed. While these are not considered components of physical fitness, they are frequently used as screening and motivational tools for fitness and health enhancement.

The test results for the fitness components are interpreted according to normative and criterion standards. The percentile ranks for each component of physical fitness are contained in Appendix A, Tables A.16 to A.23. The fitness categories for muscular strength and endurance and muscular flexibility are based on normative data and are also given in Appendix A (Tables A.18 to A.21). However, the fitness categories for cardiovascular endurance and body composition are determined according to criterion standards and are given in Tables 4.3 and 4.9 in Chapter 4. Normative data are used for strength and flexibility because most experts still do not know what constitutes an ideal fitness level for these two components, while minimum standards (in terms of health benefits) have been clearly defined for cardiovascular endurance and body composition.

MUSCULAR STRENGTH AND ENDURANCE

Muscular strength and endurance are important components of physical fitness. Although muscular strength and endurance are interrelated, a basic difference exists between the two. Strength is defined as the capacity of a muscle to exert maximal force against resistance. Endurance is the capacity of a muscle to exert submaximal force repeatedly over a period of time. Keeping these two principles in mind, strength tests and training programs have been designed to measure and develop absolute muscular strength, muscular endurance, or a combination of both.

Muscular strength is usually determined by the maximal amount of resistance (one repetition maximum or 1 RM) that an individual is able to lift in a single effort. This assessment gives a good measure of absolute strength, but it does require a considerable amount of time since the 1 RM is determined through trial and error. There is also a slight increased risk for injury among adults who do not regularly engage in strength training exercises because the 1 RM determination requires a maximal effort.

Another choice of test, one that requires submaximal resistance, is a better alternative when testing nonathletic adults. An example of such a test is contained in Appendix E. With this test, a person is required to lift a submaximal resistance based on selected percentages of body weight. This test is quite simple and less time consuming to administer. The objective of the test is to perform as many repetitions as possible on three different exercises (leg extension, bench press, and sit-up). For individuals who perform a low number of repetitions, the test will primarily measure absolute strength. For those who are able to perform a large number of repetitions, the test will be an indicator of muscular endurance. A percentile rank for each exercise is given based on the number of repetitions performed (*see* Table A.18), and the overall strength/endurance rating is obtained by calculating the average percentile rank from all three exercises. The final strength/endurance fitness category is based on the average percentile rank obtained. A score over 80 percentile is excellent, between 60 and 79 percentile is good, from 40 to 69 percentile is average, from 20 to 39 percentile is fair, and a score of 19 percentile or less is poor.

Another problem encountered when testing adult populations is that almost all strength tests are normed for younger people only, usually less than thirty years old. However, the selected percentages of body weight used in the strength and endurance test in Appendix E vary according to the age of the person, and the norms in Appendix A are based on the different age categories. This strength test should be conducted on a Universal Gym machine (using fixed resistance), since this type of equipment was used to develop the norms.

FLEXIBILITY

Flexibility is defined as the ability of a joint to move freely through its full range of motion. The contribution of good muscular flexibility to overall fitness and preventive health care has been generally underestimated and overlooked by health care professionals and practitioners. Sports medicine specialists have indicated that many muscular-skeletal problems and injuries, especially among adults, are related to a lack of flexibility. Improving and maintaining adequate levels of flexibility are important to enhance the quality of life.

Most of the flexibility tests developed over the years have little application in health and fitness programs. For example, the back hypertension test, the front-to-rear splits test, and the bridge-up test all may have applications in sports like gymnastics and several track and field events, but they are not indicative of actions encountered by most people in daily life. Because of the lack of practical flexibility tests, most health/fitness centers have relied strictly on the sit-and-reach test as an indicator of overall flexibility. However, flexibility is joint specific, and a high degree in one joint does not necessarily indicate a high degree in other joints. As a result, two additional tests were recently developed to obtain a better indication of overall body flexibility.* These tests are the trunk rotation (right and left) test and the shoulder rotation test. The procedures and norms for the battery of flexibility tests (including the sit-and-reach test) are described in Appendix F.

Similar to the strength component, a percentile rank for each flexibility test is given based on each test score (*see* Tables A.19 through A.21), and the overall flexibility rating is obtained by calculating the average percentile rank from all four tests. The final flexibility fitness category is based on the average percentile rank obtained (over 80 percentile is excellent, 60 to 79 percentile is good, 40 to 69 percentile is average, 20 to 39 percentile is fair, and 19 percentile or less is poor).

---

*From Hoeger, W. W. K. Lifetime Physical Fitness & Wellness: A Personalized Program. Morton Publishing Co., 1986.

Figure 3.9. *Battery of Flexibility Tests (from top to bottom: Sit-and-Reach Test, Trunk Rotation Test, and Shoulder Rotation Test).*

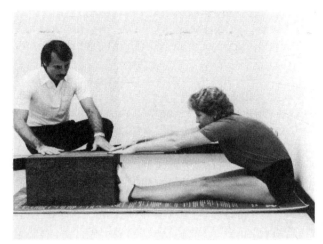

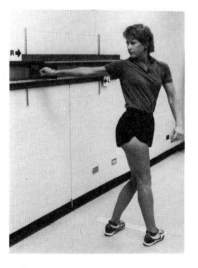

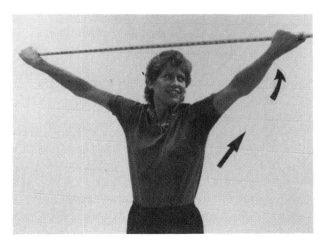

POSTURE ANALYSIS

Posture tests are used to detect deviations from normal body alignment and prescribe corrective exercises or procedures to improve alignment. Determining proper body alignment has been difficult to evaluate because most experts still don't exactly know what constitutes good posture. To objectively analyze a person's posture, an observer must be adequately trained to identify abnormalities and give ratings according to the amount of deviation from "normal" posture.

The use of a posture rating chart as shown in Appendix H provides simple and easy guidelines for better evaluation. Assuming the drawings in the left column as proper alignment, and the drawings in the right column as extreme deviations from normal, an observer is able to rate each body segment on a scale from one to five. A rating of one constitutes poor alignment, while a rating of five indicates good alignment. The precision of the analysis can be increased with the aid of a plumb line, two mirrors, and a camera. The mirrors are placed at an eighty- to eighty-five-degree angle, and the plumb line is centered in front of the mirrors. Another line is drawn down the center of the mirror on the right. The person should stand with the left side to the plumb line (*see* Figure 3.10). The plumb line is used as a reference to divide the body into front and back halves, and the line on the back mirror to divide the body into right and left sides. A picture is then taken that can be compared to the rating chart given in Appendix H. This procedure allows for a better comparison of the different body segment alignments. This technique will not only allow for a more objective analysis, but the picture by itself really seems to motivate people to engage in physical activity as a means to improve posture. Fitness Monitoring, a preventive medicine clinic in Wisconsin, reported that its clients rated posture analysis as one of the most interesting tests conducted at the clinic. Most clients rated it second only to the graded exercise stress test. The ratings for posture analysis are given in Table A.24, Appendix A.

PULMONARY FUNCTION

Even though lung volumes and capacities are not directly related to physical fitness or heart disease, the assessment of pulmonary function as

Figure 3.10. *Photographic Technique for Posture Analysis (courtesy of Fitness Monitoring Preventive Medicine Clinic, Lake Geneva, Wisconsin).*

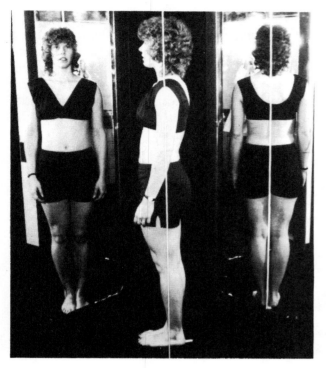

part of a wellness program is valuable in screening individuals for lung disease. One of the most common tests used to detect lung disease is known as spirometry. With this test, the amount of air that a person can inhale and exhale, including how fast the air is moved from the lungs (flow rate), is measured. The values measured through spirometry are subsequently compared to predicted norms based on age, height, and sex.

Based on guidelines by the American Thoracic Society, when spirometry tests are conducted for screening purposes only, a graphic recording of the forced expiratory curve is not required (although highly recommended), unless the test results are abnormal. Graphic recordings are required for all diagnostic spirometry. In addition, a point of critical concern in spirometry testing is adequate training of all pulmonary technicians. A large number of physicians supervising spirometry tests in community hospitals lack proper training themselves, and spirometry equipment manufacturers may not be providing adequate training in the use of this equipment either. Consequently, the need for proper training under qualified

supervision and "hands-on live patient capabilities" is most significant to obtain reliable spirometric results.[7] At least three acceptable tests should be performed, and the values of the two best tests should not vary by greater than 5 percent or approximately 100 ml (whichever is greater).

Among the most common parameters assessed through spirometry are forced vital capacity (FVC), forced expiratory volume at one second (FEV1) and/or three seconds (FEV3), forced mid-expiratory flow (FEF25-75%), and forced expiratory flow at 75 to 85 percent of FVC (FEF75-85%). FVC represents the maximal amount of air that a person can forcefully exhale after a maximal inspiration. FEV1 is the volume of air moved from the lungs during the first second of FVC. These two volumes are used to determine the FEV1/FVC ratio, which is used as an indicator of airway obstruction. FEF25-75% represents the average flow across the middle half of the forced expiration (FVC). In the past, this test was referred to as maximal mid-expiratory flow rate (MMEF). FEF75-85% measures the average flow between 75 and 85 percent of FVC. Significant reductions in these flow rates are also used as indicators of airway obstruction. FEF75-85% seems to be especially valuable in detecting early airway obstruction. The benefit of detecting airway obstruction in the early stages lies in the increased probability of reversing the obstructive process.

The procedures for determining the different spirometric parameters and the predicting equations for normal values are given in Appendix I. Since the computation of actual volumes requires technical expertise, it is perhaps much easier to obtain a computerized spirometer which automatically analyzes all parameters and is capable of producing a printout with actual, predicted, and percent of predicted values (*see* sample printout in Figure 3.11). The spirometer should also be capable of producing a graphic recording of the forced expiratory curve. Nevertheless, the test should still be administered by properly trained personnel to make sure that reproducible data have been generated.

Sample coronary heart disease and fitness profiles are shown in Figure 3.12. To obtain practical expertise, it is recommended that at first the computations to obtain the respective profiles be carried out by hand (a sample case study is contained in Appendix K). However, the process is significantly simplified with the use of the

Figure 3.11. *Computerized Lung Function Spirometry Test Results Using an Eagle II Spirometer (courtesy of Warren E. Collins, Inc. 220 Wood Road, Braintree, MA 02184).*

```
SPIROMETRY
12/30/86 BP:688 RC:N
PT:290463142 TEMP:19
HT: 70 AGE:38 SEX:M

PRE      ACT   PRED   %

FVC      5.22  4.99  105      INTERPRETATION
FEV1     4.27  4.01  106
RATIO      82    83   99      PRELIMINARY REPORT
FEV3     5.19  4.77  109      SUGGESTS
RATIO      99    96  103      MILD OBSTRUCTIVE
PEFR     10.7  9.48  113      AIRWAYS
MMEF     4.21  4.94   85      BASED ON THESE
FEF25    10.3  8.73  118      DECISIONS:
FEF50    4.77  6.28   76      FVC %PRED > 80
FEF75    1.83  3.24   56      FEV1/FVC %PRED < 100
```

computer software available with this textbook. As mentioned previously in this chapter, the interpretation of the test results for both profiles and guidelines for cardiovascular risk reduction and fitness development are given in Chapter 4.

ASSESSMENT OPTIONS

The implementation of the testing phase for the previous profiles can be done entirely as described in this chapter or offered in parts only. Different assessment options can be administered depending on the type of population that is being screened, the goals and objectives of an organization, and the funds, personnel, and facilities available. A total of five different options could be implemented using a combination of the CHD risk factors and fitness components discussed.

Type I assessment:
Comprehensive CHD risk profile and fitness profile (all test elements, including posture analysis and lung function).

Type II assessment:
Comprehensive CHD risk profile (no fitness profile, posture analysis, or lung function).

Type III assessment:
Basic CHD risk profile (all test elements under the comprehensive profile with the exception of the resting and stress ECGs) and complete fitness profile.

Type IV assessment:
Basic CHD risk profile (no fitness profile, posture analysis, or lung function).

Type V assessment:
Fitness profile, posture analysis, and lung function.

The most effective way to administer any of the assessment options is by organizing the test elements into different stations. For example, assessment options I and III could be organized into eight or nine stations with an approximate team of eleven to fourteen people. Some of the technicians (such as for flexibility and strength testing) could be upper-level college students who could be hired on a part-time basis. By organizing the testing phase into stations, individuals could be scheduled every five minutes (twelve per hour), and they would just move along from one station to the other. The following is an example of how this would work:

Station 1.
Pre-test interview by the program director (for wellness questionnaire review).

Station 2.
Blood drawing: one technician (two technicians if a relatively large number of people are to be tested). Since a twelve-hour fast is required prior to blood drawing, all of the bloods could be drawn early in the morning so that the last

Figure 3.12. *Sample Coronary Heart Disease Risk Profile and Physical Fitness Profile (also includes posture analysis and spirometry results).*

```
                    CORONARY HEART DISEASE RISK PROFILE

  Jane Doe                              Soc. Sec.: 999-99-9999
  1111 Golden Street                        Date: 03-12-1987
  Boise, ID  83725

                                    Test       Risk       Risk
  CHD Risk Factors                 Results    Points     Category
  --------------------------------------------------------------------
   1. Cardiovascular Endurance       31.6       2.4       Moderate
   2. Resting ECG                     1.0       0.0       Very Low
   3. Stress ECG                      2.0       4.0       Moderate
   4. Total Cholesterol             224.0
      HDL-Cholesterol                24.0
      Total Cholesterol-HDL Ratio     9.3       9.8       Very High
   5. Triglycerides                 134.0       0.4       Low
   6. Glucose                        97.0       0.0       Very Low
   7. Systolic Blood Pressure       144.0       2.4       High
   8. Diastolic Blood Pressure       86.0       0.7       Low
   9. Body Fat Percentage            27.1       1.4       Moderate
  10. Smoking                         9.0       5.0       High
  11. Tension and Stress             3.0        2.0       Moderate
  12. Personal History of Heart Disease  1.0    0.0       Very Low
  13. Family History of Heart Disease    4.0    4.0       Very High
  14. Age Factor                     42.0       2.2       High
  15. Estrogen                        4.0       2.0       Very High
      Current Body Weight           144.5
      Ideal Body Weight             131.6
  --------------------------------------------------------------------
      Total Risk                                36.3      Very High


                    PHYSICAL FITNESS PROFILE

  --------------------------------------------------------------------
   1. Cardiovascular Endurance       31.6              Average
   2. Muscular Strength              37%               Fair
      Upper Body Strength            10.0              Average
      Abdominal Strength              6.0              Fair
      Lower Body Strength             7.0              Average
   3. Muscular Flexibility           35%               Fair
      Sit-and-Reach                  14.0              Average
      Right Trunk Rotation           12.0              Fair
      Left Trunk Rotation            14.0              Fair
      Shoulder Rotation              25.0              Fair
   4. Body Composition               27.1              Average
  --------------------------------------------------------------------
   5. Posture                        35.0              Average
   6. Pulmonary Function
      Forced Vital Capacity           4.1              98% Predicted
      Forced Exp. Vol. 1 Sec.         2.6              79% Predicted
      FEV1/FVC Ratio                 63%
      Forced Exp. Flow 25-75%         2.1              60% Predicted
      Forced Exp. Flow 75-85%         0.8              67% Predicted
  --------------------------------------------------------------------
```

*Computer software available through Morton Publishing Company. Englewood, Colorado.

group of people will not have to wait until later in the day to have their first meal.

Station 3.

Resting heart rate and blood pressure: one technician.

Station 4.

Body composition: one technician if skinfolds are used (for hydrostatic weighing, a separate appointment should be made).

Station 5.

Posture analysis: one technician.

Station 6.

Flexibility tests: two technicians to conduct the three flexibility tests.

Station 7.

Pulmonary function screening: one technician.

Section 8.

Cardiovascular endurance: two or three technicians. For an Astrand-Ryhming test, three bicycles and three technicians are needed. For a step test, two are sufficient. (For assessment option I, which includes resting and stress ECGs, a separate appointment must be made unless several treadmills and ECG recording equipment are available. A physician is also required to supervise most stress ECGs.)

Station 9.

Muscular strength: one or two technicians to administer all three tests.

As you may have noticed, if hydrostatic weighing and graded exercise tests are included, separate appointments must be made because each test requires between twenty and sixty minutes to administer. Otherwise, the order of stations can be followed quite easily at five-minute intervals. In the case of assessment option IV (basic CHD profile — no ECGs and no fitness profile), using the Astrand-Ryhming test or the step test to assess cardiovascular endurance, the stations are reduced to five and the number of technicians to seven. One technician is used for the pre-test interview, one for blood drawing, one for resting heart rate and blood pressure, one for body composition (skinfolds), and three for cardiovascular endurance assessment. Using this type of arrangement, an experienced team could evaluate three people every ten minutes (eighteen per hour) or approximately one hundred people in six hours of actual testing.

Another point of interest is that since not every person is required to have a stress ECG prior to exercise participation, the basic CHD profile (type IV) can be used as a screening tool to determine who should be given a stress ECG. The basic CHD profile is still comprehensive because it includes all of the CHD risk factors with the exception of resting and stress ECGs. This type of assessment can be administered at a rather small cost to an organization. If the equipment is available (three bicycle ergometers or benches for cardiovascular endurance, a blood pressure sphygmomanometer and stethoscope, four stopwatches, a set of skinfold calipers, and computer capabilities to analyze the data), the actual cost per participant would run about thirty to fifty dollars (including technicians' compensation). Of course, the cost would increase if strength, flexibility, lung function, and posture analysis are included, as an additional number of technicians would be required.

A sample case study of an individual given a complete type I assessment is presented in Appendix K. In this appendix, the reader will be guided through the necessary steps and computations needed to establish the profiles. An additional data collection form is also included in this appendix.

REFERENCES

1. American College of Sports Medicine. *Guidelines for Graded Exercise Testing and Exercise Prescription.* Philadelphia: Lea & Febiger, 1986.
2. American Heart Association Committee on Exercise. *Exercise Testing and Training of Apparently Healthy Individuals: A Handbook for Physicians.* New York: The Association, 1972.
3. American Heart Association. *Coronary Risk Handbook: Estimating Risk of Coronary Heart Disease in Daily Practice.* Dallas, TX: The Association, 1973.
4. American Heart Association. *Heart at Work.* Dallas, TX: The Association, 1984.
5. American Heart Association. *Recommendations for Human Blood Pressure Determination by Sphygmomanometers.* Dallas, TX: The Association, 1980.
6. American Heart Association. *Risko: A Heart Hazard Appraisal.* Dallas, TX: The Association, 1981.
7. American Thoracic Society. "ATS Statement — Snowbird Workshop on Standardization of Spirometry." *American Review of Respiratory Disease,* Volume 119:831-838, 1979.

8. Astrand, P.O., and K. Rodahl. *Textbook of Work Physiology.* New York: McGraw-Hill, 1977.
9. Cooper, K. H. "A Critical Look at Exercise Research." *Aerobics* 6(2):3, 1985.
10. Cooper, K. H. *The Aerobics Program for Total Well-Being.* New York: Mount Evans and Co., 1982.
11. Hoeger, W. W. K. "Self-Evaluation of Cardiovascular Risk." *Corporate Fitness & Recreation* 5(6):13-16, 1986.
12. Hoeger, W. W. K. *University of Texas of The Permian Basin Wellness Center: Unpublished Test Protocols.* Odessa, TX: U.T. Permian Basin, 1984.
13. Johnson, L. C. "Fitness Testing: The Basic Ingredients." *Athletic Purchasing and Facilities* 7(3):36-42, 1983.
14. Johnson, L. C. *Interpreting Your Test Results.* Lake Geneva, WI: Fitness Monitoring Preventive Medicine Clinic, 1983.
15. Kannel, W. B., D. McGee, and T. Gordon. "A General Cardiovascular Risk Profile: The Framingham Study." *American Journal of Cardiology* 38(7):46-51, 1976.
16. McArdle, W. D., F. I. Katch, and V. L. Katch. *Exercise Physiology: Energy, Nutrition and Human Performance.* Philadelphia: Lea & Febiger, 1986.

17. Morris, J. F., A. Koski, and J. Breese. "Normal Values and Evaluation of Forced End-Expiratory Flow." *American Review of Respiratory Disease.* Volume 111:755-762, 1975.
18. New York State Education Department, Division of HPER. *The New York State Physical Fitness Test: A Manual for Physical Education Teachers.* New York: The Department, 1958.
19. Pollock, M. L., R. L. Bohannon, K. H. Cooper, J. J. Ayres, A. Ward, and S. R. Linnerud. "A Comparative Analysis of Four Protocols for Maximal Treadmill Stress Testing." *American Heart Journal* 92(1):39-46, 1976.
20. Pollock, M. L., J. H. Wilmore, and S. M. Fox III. *Health and Fitness Through Physical Activity.* New York: John Wiley & Sons, 1978.
21. Ruppel, G. *Manual of Pulmonary Function Testing.* St. Louis: The C. V. Mosby Company, 1975.
22. Van Camp, S. P. "The Fixx Tragedy: A Cardiologist's Perspective." *Physician and Sports Medicine* 12(9):153-155, 1984.

Interpretation of Coronary Heart Disease and Fitness Profiles

Cardiovascular disease is the leading cause of death in the United States, accounting for nearly one-half of the total mortality rate in 1984. The disease refers to any pathological condition that affects the heart and the circulatory system (blood vessels). Some examples of cardiovascular diseases are coronary heart disease, peripheral vascular disease, congenital heart disease, rheumatic heart disease, atherosclerosis, strokes, high blood pressure, and congestive heart failure. Although heart and blood vessel disease is still the number one health problem in the country, the incidence has declined by 36 percent in the last twenty years. The primary cause for this dramatic decrease has been health education. More people are now aware of the risk factors for cardiovascular disease and are making significant changes in their lifestyles to lower their own potential risk of suffering from this disease.

The major form of cardiovascular disease is coronary heart disease (CHD), a condition where the arteries that supply the heart muscle with oxygen and nutrients are narrowed by fatty deposits such as cholesterol and triglycerides. The narrowing of the coronary arteries diminishes the blood supply to the heart muscle, which can eventually lead to a heart attack. CHD is the single leading cause of death in the United States, accounting for approximately one-third of all deaths, and more than half of all cardiovascular deaths. Oddly enough, almost all of the risk factors for CHD are preventable and reversible, and risk reduction can be accomplished by the individual himself.

CORONARY HEART DISEASE PROFILE INTERPRETATION

Although genetic inheritance plays a role in the development of CHD, the most important determinant in whether an individual will suffer from this disease is his/her own personal lifestyle. In this regard, CHD risk factor analyses are administered to evaluate the impact of a person's lifestyle and the genetic endowment as potential factors contributing to the development of coronary disease. The specific objectives of a CHD risk factor analysis are: (a) to screen individuals who may be at high risk for the disease, (b) to educate regarding the leading risk factors that lead to its development, (c) to implement programs aimed at risk reduction, and (d) to use as a starting point to ascertain changes induced by the intervention program.

The leading risk factors that contribute to the development of CHD have been identified and are listed in Table 4.1. To provide a meaningful CHD risk score, a weighing system was developed according to the impact that each risk factor has on the development of the disease.* As was mentioned in Chapter 3, this weighing system was developed based on current research available in this area, and according to the work done at leading preventive medicine facilities in the

---

*The weighing system for the coronary heart disease risk factor analysis has been adapted with permission from Fitness Monitoring Preventive Medicine Clinic, Lake Geneva, Wisconsin.

Figure 4.1. *The Heart and its Blood Vessels. Top: a normal/healthy heart. Bottom: myocardial infarction (heart attack) as a result of acute reduction in the blood flow through the anterior descending coronary artery.*

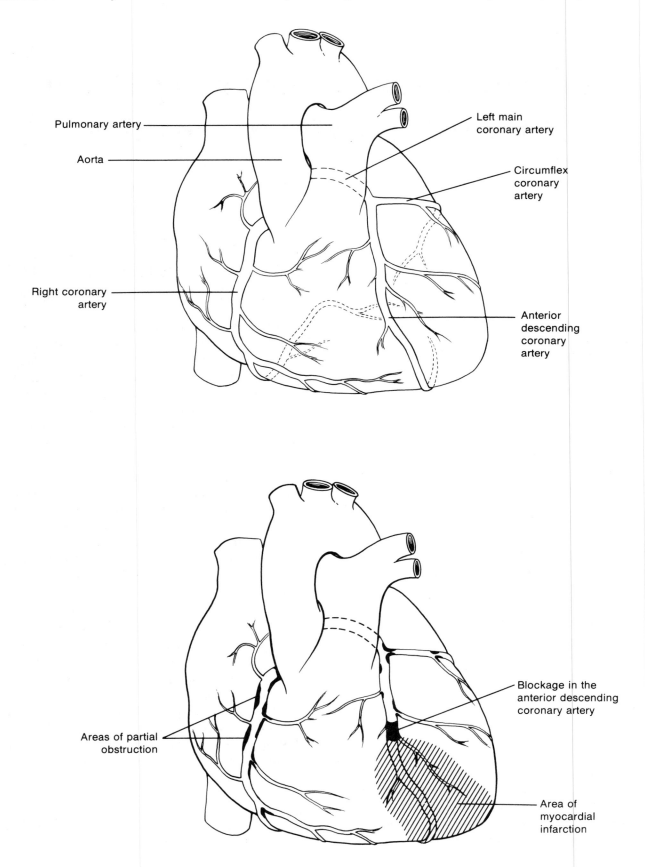

United States. The most significant risk factors are given the heaviest numeric weight. For example, the total cholesterol/HDL-cholesterol ratio seems to be the best predictor for CHD development. Consequently, up to ten risk points are assigned to a "very high" ratio. On the other hand, the least heavily weighted risk factors are estrogen use and triglycerides. Only a maximum of two risk points is assigned to these two factors. Each risk factor is also given a zero risk level, or the level at which a particular factor does not increase the risk for disease. Based on the actual test results, a person receives a score anywhere from zero to the maximum number of points for each factor. When the risk points obtained from all of the risk factors are totaled, the final number is used to rate an individual in one of five overall risk categories for potential development of coronary heart disease.

The overall CHD risk categories are given in Table 4.2. Additionally, a condensed table of the risk categories for each factor given in Appendix A is included in this chapter for quick reference.

A "very low" risk category is used to indicate the lowest risk group for developing heart disease based on age and sex. The "low" risk category indicates that a person is taking good care of his/her cardiovascular health, but small improvements can be made (unless all of the risk points came from age and family history). "Moderate" risk shows that definite improvements in lifestyle can be made to decrease the risk for disease, and/or medical treatment may be required. A final score in the "high" or "very high" category indicates a very strong probability of developing heart disease within the next three to five years and requires immediate implementation of a per-

Table 4.1.
Maximal Number of Risk Points Assigned to the Various Coronary Heart Disease Risk Factors.

CHD Risk Factor	Maximal Risk Points
Total cholesteral/HDL- ratio	10
Stress electrocardiogram	8
Smoking	8
Personal history of heart disease	8
Blood pressure	8
Cardiovascular endurance	6
Diabetes	6
Body composition (percent fat)	4
Family history of heart disease	4
Age	4
Tension and stress	4
Resting electrocardiogram	3
Triglycerides	2
Estrogen use	2

Table 4.2.
Overall Coronary Heart Disease Risk Categories*.

Risk Category	Total Risk Points
Very Low	0-5
Low	6-15
Moderate	16-25
High	26-35
Very High	36>

*Total risk score obtained from the sum of the risk points for all the risk factors

sonal risk reduction program, including medical, nutritional, and exercise intervention indicated by professional staff.

An important concept in CHD risk management is that with the exception of age, family history of heart disease, and certain ECG abnormalities, all of the other risk factors are preventable and reversible. To aid in the implementation of lifetime risk reduction programs, the leading risk factors for coronary heart disease will now be discussed along with the general recommendations for risk reduction.

CARDIOVASCULAR ENDURANCE

Cardiovascular endurance has been defined as the ability of the heart, lungs, and blood vessels to deliver adequate amounts of oxygen and nutrients to the cells to meet the demands of prolonged physical activity. The level of cardiovascular endurance (or fitness) is most commonly given by the maximal amount of oxygen (in milliliters) that every kilogram (2.2 pounds) of body weight is able to utilize per minute of physical activity (ml/kg/min). As maximal oxygen uptake increases, so does the efficiency of the cardiovascular

system. The CHD risk points and risk categories for cardiovascular endurance are shown in Table 4.3.

Even though cardiovascular endurance is not the most significant factor in terms of the maximal number of risk points assigned (six points for a poor level of fitness, as compared to ten for a very high total cholesterol/HDL-cholesterol ratio — see Table 4.1), improving cardiovascular endurance through aerobic exercise has perhaps the greatest impact in overall heart disease risk reduction. While specific recommendations can be followed to improve each individual risk factor, engaging in a regular aerobic exercise program has shown to control most of the major risk factors that lead to heart disease. Aerobic exercise will help with all of the following: (a) increase cardiovascular endurance, (b) decrease and control blood pressure, (c) decrease body fat, (d) decrease blood lipids (cholesterol and triglycerides), (e) improve HDL-cholesterol, (f) help control diabetes, (g) increase and maintain good heart function, improving in many cases certain ECG abnormalities, (h) motivate toward smoking cessation, (i) decrease tension and stress, and (j) prevent a personal history of heart disease. In the words of Dr. Kenneth H. Cooper, pioneer of the aerobic movement in the

Table 4.3.
Cardiovascular Endurance* CHD Risk Points, Risk Categories, and Fitness Categories.

	Risk Category:	Very High	High	Moderate	Low	Very Low
	Fitness Category:	Poor	Fair	Average	Good	Excellent
	Age					
Men	>19	35-39	40-44	45-49	50-54	55+
	20-29	32-36	37-41	42-46	47-51	52+
	30-39	29-33	34-38	39-43	44-48	49+
	40-49	26-30	31-35	36-40	41-45	46+
	50-59	23-27	28-32	33-37	38-42	43+
	60>	20-24	25-29	30-34	35-39	40+
Women	<19	26-30	31-35	36-40	41-45	46+
	20-29	24-28	29-33	34-38	39-43	44+
	30-39	22-26	27-31	32-36	37-41	42+
	40-49	20-24	25-29	30-34	35-39	40+
	50-59	18-22	23-27	28-32	33-37	38+
	60>	16-20	21-25	26-30	31-35	36+
	Risk Points:	6.0-4.8	4.5-3.3	3.0-1.8	1.5-0.3	0.0

*Maximal oxygen uptake expressed in ml/kg/min

United States, the evidence of the benefits of aerobic exercise in the reduction of heart disease is "far too impressive to be ignored."

Caution should be taken, however, not to ignore the other risk factors. Although aerobically fit individuals have a lower incidence of cardiovascular disease, a regular aerobic exercise program by itself is not an absolute guarantee for a lifetime free of cardiovascular problems. Poor lifestyle habits such as smoking, eating excessive fatty/salty/sweet foods, excess body fat, and high levels of stress increase cardiovascular risk and will not always be completely eliminated through aerobic exercise. Overall risk factor management is the best guideline to minimize the risk for cardiovascular disease. Yet, aerobic exercise, if carried out properly, is one of the most important aspects in the prevention and reduction of cardiovascular problems. The basic principles for cardiovascular exercise prescription are given in Appendix C.

RESTING AND STRESS ELECTROCARDIOGRAMS

The electrocardiogram, or ECG, is a valuable record of the heart's function. It is a record of the electrical impulses that stimulate the heart to contract. In the actual reading of an ECG, five general areas are interpreted: heart rate, the heart's rhythm, the heart's axis, enlargement or hypertrophy of the heart, and myocardial infarction or heart attack.

On a standard twelve-lead ECG, ten electrodes are placed on the person's chest. From these ten electrodes, twelve "pictures" or leads of the electrical impulses as they travel through heart muscle (myocardium) are studied from twelve different positions. By looking at the tracings of an ECG, it is possible to identify abnormalities in the functioning of the heart. Based on the findings, the ECG may be interpreted as normal, equivocal, or abnormal. Since not all problems will always be identified by an ECG, a normal tracing is not an absolute problem-free guarantee, nor does an abnormal tracing necessarily mean the presence of a serious condition.

ECGs are taken at rest, during stress of exercise, and during recovery. A stress ECG is also known as a maximal exercise tolerance test. Similar to a high-speed road test on a car, a stress ECG reveals the tolerance of the heart to high-intensity exercise. It is a much better test for the discovery of coronary heart disease (as compared to a resting ECG). It is also used to determine cardiovascular fitness levels, to screen persons for preventive and cardiac rehabilitation programs, to detect abnormal blood pressure response during exercise, and to establish actual or functional maximal heart rate for exercise prescription purposes. The recovery ECG also becomes an important diagnostic tool in the monitoring of the return of the heart's activity to normal conditions. The different risk categories for a resting and stress ECG are determined according to the physician's interpretation of the ECG (see Table 4.4).

TOTAL CHOLESTEROL/HDL-CHOLESTEROL RATIO

The term "blood lipids" (fats) is mainly used in reference to cholesterol and triglycerides. These lipids are carried in the bloodstream by molecules of protein known as high-density lipoproteins, low-density lipoproteins, very low-density lipoproteins, and chylomicrons. A significant elevation in blood lipids has long been associated with heart and blood vessel disease.

Cholesterol has received considerable attention in the last few years. This fatty or lipid substance is

Table 4.4.
Resting and Stress Electrocardiogram CHD Risk Points and Risk Categories (men and women of all ages).

Risk Category	Results	Risk Points	
		Resting	Stress
Very Low	Normal	0.0	0.0
Moderate	Equivocal	1.0	4.0
Very High	Abnormal	3.0	8.0

Figure 4.2. *Left: normal electrocardiogram (P wave = atrial depolarization, QRS complex = ventricular depolarization, T wave = ventricular repolarization). Right: abnormal electrocardiogram showing a depressed S-T segment (this abnormality is commonly seen during exercise in patients with coronary disease).*

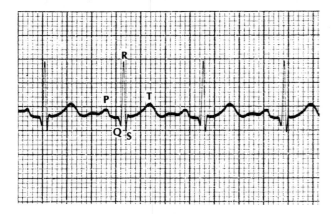

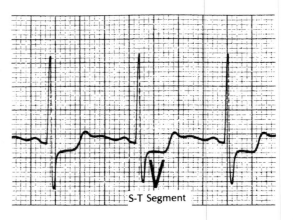

essential for certain metabolic functions in the body. However, high levels of blood cholesterol contribute to the formation of the atherosclerotic plaque, or the buildup of fatty tissue in the walls of the arteries. In the case of the heart, as the plaque builds up, it obstructs the coronary vessels. Since these arteries supply the heart muscle (myocardium) with oxygen and nutrients, when obstruction occurs, a myocardial infarction or heart attack will follow. Unfortunately, the heart disguises its problems quite effectively, and typical symptoms of heart disease, such as angina pectoris or chest pain, do not start until the arteries are about 75 percent occluded; in many cases, the first symptom is sudden death.

Only a few years ago the general recommendation was to keep total blood cholesterol levels below 200 mg/dl (milligrams per deciliter). Even though this guideline should still be followed, the crucial factor seems to be the way in which cholesterol is "packaged" or carried in the bloodstream rather than the total amount present.

Cholesterol is primarily transported in the form of high-density lipoprotein cholesterol (HDL-cholesterol) and low-density lipoprotein cholesterol (LDL-cholesterol). The high-density molecules have a high affinity for cholesterol and tend to attract cholesterol, which is then carried to the liver to be metabolized and excreted. In other words, they act as "scavengers" removing cholesterol from the body, thus preventing plaque formation in the arteries. On the other hand, LDL-cholesterol tends to release cholesterol, which

may then penetrate the lining of the arteries, enhancing the process of atherosclerosis.

From the previous discussion, it can easily be seen that the more HDL-cholesterol present, the better. HDL-cholesterol is the so-called "good cholesterol" and offers a certain degree of protection against heart disease. Many authorities now believe that the ratio of total cholesterol to HDL-cholesterol is a better indicator of potential risk for cardiovascular disease than the total value by itself. It is generally accepted that a 4.5 or lower ratio (total cholesterol/HDL-cholesterol) is excellent for men, and 4.0 or lower is best for women. For instance, 50 mg/dl of HDL-cholesterol as compared to 200 mg/dl of total cholesterol yields a ratio of 4.0 (200/50 = 4.0). The lower the ratio, the greater the protection. In another instance, a person's total cholesterol could also be 200 mg/dl, but if the HDL-cholesterol is only 20 mg/dl, the ratio could be 10.0. Such a ratio is extremely dangerous and very conducive to atherosclerosis and coronary disease (*see* Table 4.5).

Although cholesterol is found in different types of food (*see* Figure 4.3), most of the body's supply does not come from cholesterol-containing foods but is manufactured by the body from saturated fats. These fats are found primarily in meats and dairy products but are seldom found in foods of plant origin. Poultry and fish also contain less saturated fat than beef. Unsaturated fats are mainly of plant origin and cannot be converted to cholesterol. There are individual differences as to how much cholesterol can be manufactured by the

Table 4.5.
Total Cholesterol/HDL-Cholesterol Ratio CHD Risk Points and Risk Categories
(men and women of all ages).

	Risk Category				
	Very Low	Low	Moderate	High	Very High
Men	<4.5	4.6-5.5	5.6-6.5	6.6-7.7	7.8-10.0>
Women	<4.0	4.1-5.0	5.1-6.0	6.1-7.2	7.3-9.5
Risk Points	0.0	0.4-3.0	3.2-5.0	5.2-7.0	7.2-10.0

body. Some people have higher than normal intakes of saturated fats and still maintain normal blood levels, while others with a lower intake can have abnormally high levels.

If the total cholesterol HDL-cholesterol ratio is higher than ideal, certain guidelines should be followed to lower the ratio. Initially, total cholesterol levels should be lowered. This can be accomplished by lowering the LDL-cholesterol component. This type of cholesterol increases proportionally with the amount of saturated fats and cholesterol intake in the regular diet. Total fat consumption on a daily basis should not exceed 30 percent of the total caloric intake, and less than 10 percent of the total calories consumed should be in the form of saturated fats. The average intake of cholesterol should also be limited to less than 300 mg per day. LDL-cholesterol can also be lowered by losing excess body fat and using medication. As a general rule of thumb, the following dietary guidelines are recommended to lower LDL-cholesterol levels: (a) egg consumption should be limited to less than three eggs per week: (b) red meats should be eaten less than three times per week, and organ meats (e.g., liver and kidneys), sausage, bacon, hot dogs, and canned meats should be avoided; (c) low-fat milk (1 percent or less preferably) and low-fat dairy products are recommended: (d) shellfish, coconut oil, palm oil, and cocoa butter should be avoided; and (e) ideal body weight should be achieved.

The second factor involved in improving the ratio is increasing the HDL-cholesterol component. HDL-cholesterol is genetically determined and women have higher values than men. This is probably one of the reasons why heart disease is

less common among women. Research has indicated that increases in HDL-cholesterol values are almost completely dependent upon a very regular aerobic exercise program. There seems to be a linear relationship between HDL-cholesterol and aerobic exercise. The greater the amount of exercise, the higher the HDL-cholesterol. A cardiovascular exercise program, if properly prescribed, should yield positive results. A combination of adequate nutrition and aerobic exercise is the best prescription for achieving a "zero risk" ratio.

You should also be aware that several other factors can lower the HDL-cholesterol levels. Beta-blocker type medications (used in treating heart disease and hypertension), tobacco usage, and birth control pills all have a negative effect on HDL-cholesterol levels. A combination of two or three of these is even worse.

TRIGLYCERIDES

Triglycerides are also known as free fatty acids, and in combination with cholesterol, they accelerate the formation of plaque. Triglycerides are carried in the bloodstream primarily by very low-density lipoproteins (VLDL) and chylomicrons. These fatty acids are found in poultry skin, lunch meats, and shellfish. However, they are mainly manufactured in the liver from refined sugars, starches, and alcohol. High intake of alcohol and sugars (honey included) will significantly increase triglyceride levels. Thus, they can be lowered by decreasing the consumption of the above-mentioned foods along with weight reduction (if

Figure 4.3. *Cholesterol and Saturated Fat Content of Selected Foods.*

Food	Serving Size	Cholesterol (mg)	Sat. Fat (gr)
Avocado	1/8 med.	—	3.2
Bacon	2 slc.	30	2.7
Beans (all types)	any	—	—
Beef — Lean, fat trimmed off	3 oz.	75	6.0
Beef — Heart (cooked)	3 oz.	150	1.6
Beef — Liver (cooked)	3 oz.	255	1.3
Butter	1 tsp.	12	0.4
Cheese — American	2 oz.	54	11.2
Cheese — Cheddar	2 oz.	60	12.0
Cheese — Cottage (1% fat)	1 cup	10	0.4
Cheese — Cottage (4% fat)	1 cup	31	6.0
Cheese — Cream	2 oz.	62	6.0
Cheese — Muenster	2 oz.	54	10.8
Cheese — Parmesan	2 oz.	38	9.3
Cheese — Swiss	2 oz.	52	10.0
Caviar	1 oz.	85	—
Chicken (no skin)	3 oz.	45	0.4
Chicken — Liver	3 oz.	472	1.1
Chicken — Thigh, Wing	3 oz.	69	3.3
Egg (yolk)	1	250	1.8
Frankfurter	2	90	11.2
Fruits	any	—	—
Grains (all types)	any	—	—
Halibut, Flounder	3 oz.	43	0.7
Ice Cream	1/2 cup	27	4.4
Lamb	3 oz.	60	7.2
Lard	1 tsp.	5	NA*
Lobster	3 oz.	170	0.5
Margarine (all vegetable)	1 tsp.	—	0.7
Mayonnaise	1 tbsp.	10	2.1
Milk — Skim	1 cup	5	0.3
Milk — Low Fat (2%)	1 cup	18	2.9
Milk — Whole	1 cup	34	5.1
Nuts	1 oz.	—	1.0
Oysters	3 oz.	42	—
Salmon	3 oz.	30	0.8
Scallops	3 oz.	29	—
Sherbet	1/2 cup	7	1.2
Shrimp	3 oz.	128	0.1
Trout	3 oz.	45	2.1
Tuna (canned — drained)	3 oz.	55	—
Turkey — Dark Meat	3 oz.	60	0.6
Turkey — Light Meat	3 oz.	50	0.4
Vegetables (except avocado)	any	—	—

*Not available

overweight) and aerobic exercise. The various risk categories for triglycerides are shown in Table 4.6.

Individuals who have never had a blood chemistry test should probably have one done in the near future. An initial test is always useful to establish a baseline for future reference. Make sure that the test does include the HDL-cholesterol component, since many clinics and hospitals still do not include this factor in their regular analyses. While no definite guidelines have yet been given, following an initial normal baseline test, and as long as the recommended dietary and exercise guidelines are kept, a blood analysis every two or three years prior to the age of thirty-five should suffice. After the age of thirty-five, a blood lipid test should be conducted every year in conjunction with a regular preventive medicine physical examination.

DIABETES

Diabetes is a condition where the blood glucose is unable to enter the cells because of insufficient insulin production by the pancreas.

Several studies have shown that the incidence of cardiovascular disease among diabetic patients is quite high. Cardiovascular disease is also the leading cause of death among these patients.

Individuals with chronically elevated blood glucose levels may also have problems in metabolizing fats. This, in turn, can increase susceptibility to atherosclerosis, increasing the risk for coronary disease and other conditions such as vision loss and kidney damage. Fasting blood glucose levels over 120 mg/dl may be an early sign of diabetes and should be brought to the attention of a physician. Blood glucose levels around 150 to 160 mg/dl are considered by many health care practitioners as borderline diabetes. Three risk points are assigned to glucose levels over 150 mg/dl, and an additional three points are given to all diabetic patients regardless of current glucose levels (*see* Table 4.7).

Although there is a genetic predisposition to diabetes, adult-onset diabetes is closely related to obesity. In most cases, this type of condition can be corrected by following a special diet, a weight loss program, and exercise. If you have elevated blood glucose levels, you should consult your physician and let him/her decide on the best approach to treat this condition.

Table 4.6.
Triglycerides* CHD Risk Points and Risk Categories (men and women of all ages).

	Risk Category				
	Very Low	Low	Moderate	High	Very High
	<100	101-145	146-190	191-235	236-272>
Risk Points	0.0	0.1-0.5	0.6-1.0	1.1-1.5	1.6-2.0

*Expressed in mg/dl

Table 4.7.
Blood Glucose* CHD Risk Points and Risk Categories (men and women of all ages).

	Risk Categories				
	Very Low	Low	Moderate	High	Very High
	<120	121-128	129-136	137-144	145-150>
Risk Points	0.0	0.1-0.8	0.9-1.6	1.7-2.4	2.5-3.0

*Expressed in mg/dl

BLOOD PRESSURE

There are some 60,000 miles of blood vessels running through the human body. As the heart forces the blood through these vessels, the fluid is under pressure. Hence, blood pressure is but a measure of the force exerted against the walls of the vessels by the blood flowing through them. Blood pressure is measured in milliliters of mercury and is usually expressed in two numbers. Ideal blood pressure should be 120/80 or below. The higher number reflects the pressure exerted during the forceful contraction of the heart or systole (therefore, the name "systolic" pressure), and the lower pressure is taken during the heart's relaxation, or diastolic phase, when no blood is being ejected.

When Is Blood Pressure Considered Too High?

A few years ago, a systolic pressure of 100 plus your age was the acceptable standard. However, this is no longer the case. Hypertension has been viewed as the point where the pressure doubles the mortality risk. This pressure has been determined at about 160/96. Traditionally, the upper limits of normal were established at 140/90, a reading that by today's standards is considered by many as borderline hypertension. Readings between 140/90 and 160/96 (either number being in that range) were classified as mild hypertension. However, statistical evidence clearly indicates that blood pressure readings above 140/90 increase the risk of disease and premature death. Consequently, in 1986, the American Heart Association revised its standards and now considers all blood pressures over 140/90 as hypertension. The different risk categories for blood pressure are established according to current readings and are contained in Table 4.8.

While the threshold for hypertension has been set at 140/90, many experts believe that the lower the blood pressure, the better. Even if the pressure is around 90/50, as long as that person does not have any symptoms of low blood pressure or hypotension, he/she does not need to be concerned. Typical hypotension symptoms are dizziness, lightheadedness, and fainting.

Blood pressure may also fluctuate during a regular day. Many factors affect blood pressure, and one single reading may not be a true indicator of your real pressure. For example, physical activity and stress increase blood pressure, while rest and relaxation decrease it. Consequently, several measurements should be made before a diagnosis of elevated pressure is suggested.

Based on 1986 estimates by the American Heart Association, almost 55 million adults and 2.7 million children (six to seventeen years old) in the United States are hypertensive. As a disease, hypertension has been referred to as the silent killer. It does not hurt, it does not make you feel sick, and unless you check it, years may go by before you even realize that you have a problem. Elevated blood pressure is a risk factor not only for coronary heart disease, but also for congestive heart failure, strokes, and kidney failure.

Table 4.8.
Blood Pressure* CHD Risk Points and Risk Categories (men and women).

	Risk Category				
	Very Low	Low	Moderate	High	Very High
Systolic Pressure	<120	121-130	131-140	141-150	151-160>
Diastolic Pressure	<80	81-89	90-98	99-106	107-116>
Risk Points	0.0	0.1-1.0	1.1-2.0	2.1-3.0	3.1-4.0

* Expressed in mmHg

What Makes Hypertension A Killer

All inner walls of arteries are lined by a layer of smooth endothelial cells. The nature of this lining is such that blood lipids cannot penetrate it and build up unless damage is done to the cells. High blood pressure is a leading factor contributing to the destruction of this lining. As blood pressure rises, so does the risk for atherosclerosis or the development of fatty-cholesterol deposits in the walls of the arteries. The higher the pressure, the greater the damage that is done to the arterial wall, allowing a faster occlusion of the vessels, especially if serum cholesterol is also elevated. Occlusion of the coronary vessels decreases the blood supply to the heart muscle and can lead to heart attacks. When brain arteries are involved, strokes may follow.

A clear example of the role of elevated pressure in the development of atherosclerosis can be seen by comparing blood vessels in the human body. Even when significant atherosclerosis is present throughout major arteries in the body, fatty plaques are rarely seen in the pulmonary artery, which goes from the right heart to the lungs. The pressure in this artery is normally below 40 mmHg, and at such low pressure, significant deposits do not occur. This is one of the reasons why people with low blood pressure have a lower incidence of cardiovascular disease.

Constantly elevated blood pressure also causes the heart to work much harder. Initially the heart does well, but in time, this constant strain results in a pathologically enlarged heart and subsequent congestive heart failure. Furthermore, high blood pressure damages blood vessels to the kidneys and eyes, leading to eventual kidney failure and vision loss.

How Can Hypertension Be Controlled?

Ninety percent of all hypertension has no definite cause. This type of hypertension is referred to as essential hypertension and is treatable. Aerobic exercise, weight reduction, a low-sodium/high-potassium diet, stress reduction, smoking cessation, a decrease in blood lipids, a lower caffeine and alcohol intake, and anti-hypertensive medication have all been used effectively in treating essential hypertension. The other 10 percent is caused by such pathological conditions as narrowing of the kidney arteries, glomerulonephritis (a kidney disease), tumors of the adrenal glands, and narrowing of the aortic artery. With this type of hypertension, the pathological cause has to be treated first in order to correct the blood pressure problem.

Anti-hypertensive medications are many times the first choice of treatment modality, but they also produce multiple side effects, such as lethargy, somnolence, sexual difficulties, increased blood cholesterol and glucose levels, lower potassium levels, and elevated uric acid levels. Often, a physician may end up treating these side effects as much as the hypertension problem itself. Because of the multiple side effects, approximately 50 percent of the patients will stop taking the medication within the first year of treatment.

Perhaps one of the most significant factors contributing to elevated blood pressure is excessive sodium in the diet (salt is sodium chloride and contains approximately 40 percent sodium). Water retention increases with high sodium intake. As water retention increases, so does the blood volume, which, in turn, drives the pressure up. On the other hand, high intake of potassium seems to regulate water retention and therefore appears to lower the pressure slightly.

While sodium is essential for normal physiological functions, only 200 mg or one-tenth of a teaspoon of salt is required on a daily basis. Even under the most strenuous conditions, such as jobs and sports participation where heavy sweating is involved, the greatest amount of sodium required by the organism never exceeds 3,000 mg per day. Yet, in the typical American diet, sodium intake ranges between 6,000 and 20,000 mg per day! No wonder hypertension is so prevalent today.

In underdeveloped countries and Indian tribes where no salt is used in cooking or added at the table, and the only sodium consumed comes from food in its natural form, daily intake seldom exceeds 2,000 mg. Blood pressure among these people does not increase with age, and hypertension is practically unknown. These findings seem to indicate that the human body may be able to handle 2,000 mg per day, but higher intakes than that on a regular basis may cause a gradual rise in blood pressure over the years.

Many people ask themselves, where does all the sodium come from? The answer is found in Figure 4.4. Most individuals do not realize the amount of sodium contained in various foods, and the list in Table 7.4 does not include the salt

Figure 4.4. *Sodium, Potassium, Calcium, and Magnesium Levels of Selected Foods*

Food	Serving Size	Sodium (mg)	Potassium (mg)	Calcium (mg)	Magnesium (mg)
Apple	1 med.	1	182	10	6
Asparagus	1 cup	2	330	26	24
Avocado	1/2	4	680	11	NA*
Banana	1 med.	1	440	8	33
Bologna	3 oz.	1,107	133	6	12
Bouillon Cube	1	960	4	0	0
Cantaloupe	1/4	17	341	20	NA
Carrot (raw)	1	34	225	27	12
Cheese					
American	2 oz.	614	93	376	16
Cheddar	2 oz.	342	56	408	16
Muenster	2 oz.	356	77	406	16
Parmesan	2 oz.	1,056	53	672	24
Swiss	2 oz.	148	64	410	16
Chicken (light meat)	6 oz.	108	700	20	20
Corn (canned)	1/2 cup	195	80	4	NA
Corn (natural)	1/2 cup	3	136	2	29
Frankfurter	1	627	136	4	5
Haddock	6 oz.	300	594	66	41
Hamburger (reg)	1	500	321	63	25
Lamb (leg)	6 oz.	108	700	18	22
Milk (whole)	1 cup	120	351	288	33
Milk (skim)	1 cup	126	406	296	28
Orange	1 med.	1	263	54	13
Orange Juice	1 cup	1	200	26	27
Peach	1 med.	2	308	14	9
Pear	1 med.	2	130	13	9
Peas (canned)	1/2 cup	200	82	22	20
Peas (boiled-natural)	1/2 cup	2	178	18	24
Pizza (cheese - 14" diam.)	1/8	456	85	110	25
Potato	1 med.	6	763	14	75
Potato Chips	10	150	226	8	25
Potato (french fries)	10	5	427	12	40
Pork	6 oz.	96	438	17	25
Roast Beef	6 oz.	98	448	15	27
Salami	3 oz.	1,047	170	12	5
Salmon (canned)	6 oz.	198	756	262	50
Salt	1 tsp.	2,132	0	14	7
Soups					
Chicken Noodle	1 cup	979	55	17	5
Clam Chowder (New England)	1 cup	914	146	43	7
Cream of Mushroom	1 cup	955	98	191	5
Vegetable Beef	1 cup	1,046	162	12	6
Soy Sauce	1 tsp.	1,123	22	13	2
Spaghetti (tomato sauce and cheese)	6 oz.	648	276	54	20
Strawberries	1 cup	1	244	31	16
Tomato (raw)	1 med.	3	444	12	11
Tuna (drained)	3 oz.	38	255	7	0

*Not available

added at the table. Even if you do not have a blood pressure problem now, you need to be concerned about sodium intake — otherwise blood pressure may sneak up on you.

New research studies have also indicated that there may be a link between hypertension and calcium and magnesium deficiencies. The connection between calcium and hypertension isn't quite clear, but a recent national dietary survey linked calcium deficiency to high blood pressure. Magnesium supplementation has been used effectively to lower blood pressure in patients suffering from hypertensive encephalopathy and in patients affected by diuretic-induced low magnesium levels. However, no evidence at this point shows a decrease in blood pressure in patients with normal magnesium levels.

When treating high blood pressure, prior to using medication (unless elevation is extremely high), many sports medicine physicians prefer a combination of aerobic exercise, weight loss, and sodium reduction. In most instances this treatment modality will bring blood pressure under control.

The link between hypertension and obesity has been well established. Not only does blood volume increase with excess body fat, but every additional pound of fat requires an estimated extra mile of blood vessels to feed this tissue. Furthermore, blood capillaries are constricted by the adipose tissue as these vessels run through them. As a result, the heart muscle must work harder to pump the blood through a longer, constricted network of blood vessels.

The role of aerobic exercise in the treatment of hypertensive patients is becoming more important each day. On the average, cardiovascularly fit individuals have lower blood pressures than unfit people. Several well-documented studies have shown that nearly 90 percent of hypertensive patients who initiate an aerobic exercise program can expect a significant decrease in blood pressure after only a few months of training. These changes, however, are not maintained if aerobic exercise is discontinued.

The best tip, though, is to use a preventive approach. It is a lot easier to keep blood pressure under control rather than try to bring it down once it is elevated. Blood pressure should be checked regularly, regardless of whether elevation is present or not. Regular physical exercise, weight control, a low-salt diet, smoking cessation, and stress management are the basic guidelines for blood pressure control. Those who suffer from hypertension should not stop using the medication unless their personal physician so indicates. Remember — high blood pressure kills people if not treated properly. Combining the medication with the other treatment modalities may eventually lead to a reduction or complete elimination of the drug therapy.

BODY COMPOSITION

Body composition refers to the ratio of lean body weight to fat weight. If too much fat is accumulated, the person is considered to be obese. Obesity has been long recognized as a primary risk factor for coronary heart disease. But until a few years ago, experts felt that the disease was actually brought on by some of the other risk factors that usually deteriorate with increased body fat (higher cholesterol and triglycerides, hypertension, diabetes, lower level of cardiovascular fitness). Recent evidence, however, suggests that excess body fat, in and of itself, is a serious coronary risk factor. Even when all of the other risk factors are in good range, individuals with body fat percentages higher than the "ideal" standard have a higher incidence of coronary disease. The risk categories for body composition (determined by percent body fat), based on age and sex, are given in Table 4.9.

Attaining ideal body composition is not only important in decreasing cardiovascular risk, but also in achieving a better state of health and wellness. The only positive thing that can be said about excess body fat accumulation is that it can be lost through a combination of diet and exercise. Dieting by itself very seldom works. If you have a weight problem and you desire to achieve ideal weight, two things must take place: (a) an increase in the level of physical activity, and (b) a moderate reduction in caloric intake that will still provide all of the necessary nutrients to sustain normal physiological body functions. Additional recommendations for weight reduction and weight control are discussed in Chapter 6.

SMOKING

Cigarette smoking is the single largest preventable cause of illness and premature death in the United States. Smoking has been linked to cardiovascular disease, cancer, bronchitis, emphysema, and peptic ulcers. In relation to coronary disease,

Table 4.9.
Body Composition* CHD Risk Points, Risk Categories and Fitness Categories.

Risk Category:		Very Low	Low	Moderate	High	Very High
Fitness Category:		Ideal	Good	Average	Overweight	Obese
	Age					
	<19	<12	12.5-17.0	17.5-22.0	22.5-27.0	27.5-32.0>
	20-29	<13	13.5-18.0	18.5-23.0	23.5-28.0	28.5-33.0>
Men	30-39	<14	14.5-19.0	19.5-24.0	24.5-29.0	29.5-34.0>
	40-49	<15	15.5-20.0	20.5-25.0	25.5-30.0	30.5-35.0>
	50>	<16	16.5-21.0	21.5-26.0	26.5-31.0	31.5-36.0>
	<19	<17	17.5-22.0	22.5-27.0	27.5-32.0	32.5-37.0>
	20-29	<18	18.5-23.0	23.5-28.0	28.5-33.0	33.5-38.0>
Women	30-39	<19	19.5-24.0	24.5-29.0	29.5-34.0	34.5-39.0>
	40-49	<20	20.5-25.0	25.5-30.0	30.5-35.0	35.5-40.0>
	50>	<21	21.5-26.0	26.5-31.0	31.5-36.0	36.5-41.0>

*Expressed in percent of body fat

not only does it speed up the process of atherosclerosis, but there is also a threefold increase in the risk of sudden death following a myocardial infarction.

Smoking causes the release of nicotine and some other 1,200 toxic compounds into the bloodstream. Similar to hypertension, many of these substances are destructive to the inner membrane that protects the walls of the arteries. As mentioned before, once the lining is damaged, cholesterol and triglycerides can be readily deposited in the arterial wall. As the plaque builds up, blood flow is significantly decreased as obstruction of the arteries occurs. Furthermore, smoking enhances the formation of blood clots, which can completely obstruct an already narrowed artery due to atherosclerosis. In addition, carbon monoxide, a byproduct of cigarette smoke, significantly decreases the oxygen-carrying capacity of the blood. A combination of obstructed arteries, decreased oxygen, and the presence of nicotine itself in the heart muscle greatly increases the risk for a serious heart problem.

Smoking also increases heart rate, blood pressure, and the irritability of the heart, which can trigger fatal cardiac arrhythmias. Another harmful effect is a decrease in HDL-cholesterol, or the "good type" that helps control your blood lipids. There is no question that smoking actually causes a much greater risk of death from heart disease than from lung disease. Risk points and risk categories for smoking are assigned according to the type and amount of tobacco used (*see* Table 4.10).

Pipe and/or cigar smoking and chewing tobacco also increase risk for heart disease. Even if no smoke is inhaled, certain amounts of toxic substances can be absorbed through the mouth membranes and end up in the bloodstream. Individuals who use tobacco in any of these three forms also have a much greater risk for cancer of the oral cavity.

Cigarette smoking, along with a poor total cholesterol/HDL-cholesterol ratio and high blood pressure, are the three most significant risk factors for coronary disease. Nevertheless, the risk for both cardiovascular disease and cancer starts to decrease the moment you quit. The risk approaches that of a lifetime nonsmoker ten and fifteen years, respectively, following cessation. A more thorough discussion of the harmful effects of cigarette smoking, the benefits of quitting, and a complete program for smoking cessation are outlined in Chapter 8.

Table 4.10.
Smoking CHD Risk Points and Risk Categories (men and women of all ages).

Risk Category	Tobacco Use	Risk Points
Very Low	-Lifetime nonsmoker	0.0
	-Ex-smoker over one year	0.0
Low	-Ex-smoker, less than one year	1.0
	-Less than one cigarette per day	1.0
	-Pipe, cigar smoker or chew tobacco	2.0
	-Nonsmoker living and/or working	
	in smoking environment	2.0
Moderate	1-9 cigarettes per day	3.0
High	10-19 cigarettes per day	4.0
	20-29 cigarettes per day	5.0
Very High	30-39 cigarettes per day	6.0
	40+ cigarettes per day	8.0`

TENSION AND STRESS

Tension and stress have become a normal part of every person's life. Everyone has to deal with goals, objectives, responsibilities, pressures, etc. in daily life. Almost everything in life (whether positive or negative) is a source of stress. However, it is not the stressor itself that creates the health hazard, but rather the individual's response to it that may pose a health problem.

There are basically two types of behavior. Type A behavior is typical of a person who is hard-driving, high-strung, overly competitive, and easily irritated. Type B behavior, on the contrary, is characteristic of a relaxed, easy-going, casual person who sometimes even appears apathetic toward life. A person exhibiting Type A behavior (high stress) is at higher risk for coronary disease than Type B. Such individuals actually become ill due to their inability to deal with increasing quantities of stress. The tension and stress rating for the CHD risk profile is determined according to the responses given by an individual to the tension and stress surveys contained in the wellness questionnaire. The respective risk categories for tension and stress are found in Table 4.11.

The way in which the human body responds to stress is by increasing the amount of catecholamines (hormones) to prepare the body for the so-called "fight or flight" mechanism. These hormones increase heart rate, blood pressure, and blood glucose levels, preparing the individual to take action. If the person "fights or flees," the increased levels of catecholamines are metabolized and the body is able to return to a "normal" state. However, if a person is under constant stress and unable to take action (such as in the case of the death of a close relative or friend, loss of a job, trouble at work, financial security, etc.), the catecholamines will remain elevated in the bloodstream. The person cannot relax and will experience a constant low-level strain on the cardiovascular system that could manifest itself in the form of heart disease. Additionally, when a person is in a stressful situation, the coronary arteries that feed the heart muscle constrict (clamp down), reducing the oxygen supply to the heart. If significant arterial occlusion due to atherosclerosis is present, abnormal rhythms of the heart or a heart attack itself may follow.

Individuals who are mostly of the Type A behavior and feel that they are under a lot of

Table 4.11.
Tension and Stress CHD Risk Points and Risk Categories (men and women of all ages).

Risk Category	Questionnaire Results	Risk Points
Very Low	Hardly ever tense	0.0
Low	Sometimes tense	1.0
Moderate	Often tense	2.0
High	Nearly always tense	3.0
Very High	Always tense	4.0

stress, and do not cope well with it, need to begin to take appropriate measures to reduce the effects of stress in their lives. Type A behavior is mostly a learned behavior. One of the best recommendations to overcome stress is to identify the sources of stress and learn how to cope with those events. Even slight changes in behavioral responses can slide individuals along the continuum so that they become more Type B and less Type A. These people need to take control of themselves and examine and act upon the things of greatest importance in their lives. Less significant or meaningless details should be ignored.

Physical exercise has been found to be one of the best ways to relieve stress. When a person engages in physical activity, excess catecholamines are metabolized, and the body is able to return to a normal state. Exercise also increases muscular activity, which causes muscular relaxation upon completion of physical activity. Many executives in large cities are choosing the evening hours for their physical activity programs, stopping right after work at the health or fitness club. This way they are able to "burn up" the excess tension built up during the day and better enjoy the evening hours. This has proven to be one of the best stress management techniques. Additional information on several stress management techniques commonly used is presented in Chapter 7.

PERSONAL AND FAMILY HISTORY

Individuals who have suffered from cardiovascular problems are at higher risk over someone else who has never had a problem. People with such history should be strongly encouraged to maintain the other risk factors as low as possible. Since most risk factors are reversible, this practice significantly decreases the risk for future problems. The longer it has been since the incidence of the cardiovascular problem, the lower the risk for recurrence.

The genetic predisposition toward heart disease has been clearly demonstrated and seems to be gaining in importance each day. All other factors being equal, a person who has had blood relatives who suffered from heart disease prior to age sixty runs a greater risk than someone who has no such history. The younger the age at which the incident happened to the relative, the greater the risk for the disease. The various risk categories for personal and family history are given in Tables 4.12 and 4.13.

In many cases there is no way of knowing whether there is a true genetic predisposition or simply poor lifestyle habits that led to a particular problem. It is quite possible that a person may have been physically inactive, overweight, have smoked, have had bad dietary habits, etc., leading to a heart attack, and therefore all blood relatives would fall in the family history category. Since there is no definite way of telling them apart, a person with a family history should keep a close watch on all other factors and maintain them at as low a risk level as possible. In addition, an annual blood chemistry analysis is strongly recommended to make sure that blood lipids are being handled properly.

Table 4.12.
Personal History CHD Risk Points and Risk Categories (men and women of all ages).

Risk Category	History	Risk Points
Very Low	-No history of cardiovascular disease	0.0
Low	-History of cardiovascular disease over five years ago	2.0
Moderate	-History of cardiovascular disease two to five years ago	3.0
High	-History of cardiovascular disease one to two years ago	5.0
Very High	-History of cardiovascular disease within last year	8.0

Table 4.13.
Family History CHD Risk Points and Risk Categories (men and women of all ages).

Risk Category	History	Risk Points
Very Low	-No family history	0.0
Low	-Family history after the age of sixty	1.0
Moderate	-Family history between the ages of fifty and sixty	2.0
Very High	-Family history prior to the age of fifty	4.0

ESTROGEN USE

Only recently were estrogens (found in oral contraceptives and certain other drugs) added to the list of risk factors for coronary disease. Estrogens cause an increase in blood pressure, enhance the clotting mechanism of the blood, and also decrease HDL-cholesterol (the "good guys"). High blood pressure by itself will increase the susceptibility to atherosclerosis. If in addition to that, HDL-cholesterol is reduced, a greater amount of fats can be deposited in the arteries (even worse among women smokers, as this also decreases HDL-cholesterol). As plaque builds up, complete obstruction may occur from a blood clot enhanced by the use of estrogen. It is therefore recommended that women at moderate, high, or very high risk for heart disease consult their physician in this regard.

The number of risk points and risk categories for estrogen used are assessed according to the age of the person and the length of time that estrogens have been used. This information is summarized in Table 4.14.

AGE

Age has also become a risk factor because of the greater incidence of heart disease among older people. This tendency may be partly induced by an increased risk among the other factors due to changes in lifestyle as we get older (less physical activity, poor nutrition, obesity, etc.).

Young people, however, should not feel that heart disease will not affect them. The disease process begins early in life. This was clearly shown among American soldiers who died during the Korean and Vietnam conflicts. Autopsies conducted on soldiers killed at twenty-two years old and younger revealed that approximately 70 percent of them showed early stages of athero-sclerosis. Other studies have found elevated blood cholesterol levels in children as young as ten years old.

While the aging process cannot be stopped, it can certainly be slowed down. It has often been said that certain individuals in their sixties or older possess the bodies of twenty-year-olds. The opposite also holds true: twenty-year-olds often are in such poor condition and health that they almost seem to have the bodies of sixty-year-olds. Adequate risk factor management and positive lifestyle habits are the best ways to slow down the natural aging process.

Risk points for the age factor are given only after the age of twenty, and up to four points at age sixty (one-tenth of a point for each year after twenty — see Table 4.15).

A FINAL WORD ON CORONARY RISK REDUCTION

As was mentioned at the beginning of this chapter, most of the risk factors for coronary heart disease are reversible and preventable. The fact that a person has a family history of heart disease and possibly some of the other risk factors because of neglect in lifestyle does not signify by any means that this person is doomed. The objective of the first part of this chapter was to provide the guidelines and recommendations to decrease the risk of suffering from cardiovascular disease (particularly coronary heart disease). As has been

Table 4.14.
Estrogen Use CHD Risk Points and Risk Categories.

Risk Category	Estrogen Use	Risk Points
Low	-No use	0.0
Moderate	-Thirty-five years or younger and have used estrogen for less than five years	1.0
Very High	-Have used estrogen for over five years	2.0
	-Thirty-five years or older and using estrogen	2.0

Table 4.15.
Age CHD Risk Points and Risk Categories (men and women).

Risk Category	Age	Risk Points
Very Low	<20	0.0
Low	21-29	0.1-0.9
Moderate	30-39	1.0-1.9
High	40-49	2.0-2.9
Very High	50-60>	3.0-4.0

discussed, a healthier lifestyle — free of cardio-vascular problems — is something that people can pretty much control by themselves. They should be encouraged to be persistent. It requires willpower and commitment to develop positive patterns that will eventually turn into healthy habits conducive to total well-being. Only individuals themselves can act on it by taking control of their lifestyle and thereby reaping the benefits of wellness.

PHYSICAL FITNESS PROFILE INTERPRETATION

People are considered to be physically fit when they can meet the ordinary as well as the unusual demands of daily life safely and effectively without being overly fatigued, and still have energy left for leisure and recreational activities. From a health point of view, total physical fitness involves four basic components: (a) cardiovascular endurance, (b) muscular strength and endurance, (c) muscular flexibility, and (d) body composition. In addition to the four components of fitness, two other parameters frequently measured in health assessments will also be discussed in this section. These parameters are posture and pulmonary function.

CARDIOVASCULAR ENDURANCE

As a person breathes, part of the oxygen contained in ambient air is taken up in the lungs and transported in the blood to the heart. The heart is then responsible for pumping the oxygenated blood to all organs and tissues of the body. At the cellular level, oxygen is used to convert food substrates, primarily carbohydrates and fats, into energy necessary to conduct body functions and maintain a constant internal equilibrium.

During physical exertion, a greater amount of energy is needed to carry out the work. If cardiovascular endurance is defined as the ability of the heart, lungs, and blood vessels to deliver adequate amounts of oxygen to the cells to meet the demands of prolonged physical activity, an individual with a high level of cardiovascular endurance should be able to deliver the required amounts of oxygen to the tissues with relative

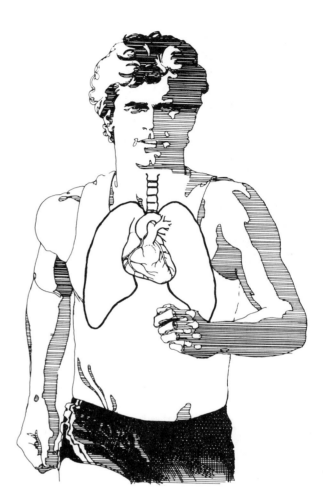

Figure 4.5. *Cardiovascular Endurance. The ability of the heart, lungs, and blood vessels to deliver adequate amounts of oxygen and nutrients to the cells to meet the demands of prolonged physical activity.*

ease. The cardiovascular system of a person with a low level of endurance would have to work much harder, since the heart has to pump more often to supply the same amount of oxygen to the tissues, and consequently would fatigue faster. Hence, a higher capacity to deliver and utilize oxygen (oxygen uptake) indicates a more efficient cardiovascular system.

The percentile ranks for cardiovascular endurance, based on maximal oxygen uptake, are given in Table 4.16. However, the cardiovascular endurance fitness category should be determined according to the maximal oxygen uptakes given in Table 4.3. For example, the "very low" risk category signifies "excellent" cardiovascular endurance. On the other hand, the "very high" risk category implies a poor cardiovascular endurance level. The reason for using criterion standards (Table 4.3) to establish fitness levels is because the percentile ranks in Table 4.16 are based on a sample population, and scientific evidence indicates that the "typical" American is not exactly a good role model when it comes to cardiovascular endurance. According to a 1986 report by the U.S. Public Health Service, only 10 to 20 percent of the adult population exercises vigorously enough to develop the cardiovascular system. However, the CHD risk (and fitness) categories in Table 4.3 were determined according to maximal oxygen uptake levels as potential predictors for heart disease. For example, the very low CHD risk (or excellent fitness) category is based on maximal oxygen uptake values that yield a low risk for heart disease and are most conducive to good health.

Cardiovascular endurance activities are also frequently referred to as "aerobic" exercises. The word "aerobic" means "with oxygen." Hence, whenever an activity is carried out where oxygen is utilized to produce energy, it is considered an aerobic exercise. Examples of cardiovascular or aerobic exercises are walking, jogging, swimming, cycling, cross-country skiing, rope skipping, aerobic dancing, etc. On the other hand, "anaerobic" activities are carried out "without oxygen." The intensity of anaerobic exercise is so high that oxygen is not utilized to produce energy. Since energy production is very limited in the absence of oxygen, these activities can only be carried out for short periods of time. The higher the intensity, the shorter the duration. Such activities as the 100, 200, and 400 meters in track and field, the 100 meters in swimming, gymnastics routines, and weight training are good examples of anaerobic activities. Only aerobic activities will help increase cardiovascular endurance. Anaerobic activities will not significantly contribute toward the development of the cardiovascular system. The basic guidelines for cardiovascular exercise prescription are given in Appendix C.

Importance of Cardiovascular Endurance

A sound cardiovascular endurance program greatly contributes toward the enhancement and maintenance of good health. Although there are four components of physical fitness, cardiovascular endurance is the single most important factor. Certain amounts of muscular strength and flexibility are necessary in daily activities to lead a normal life. However, a person can get away without large amounts of strength and flexibility but cannot do without a good cardiovascular system. Aerobic exercise is especially important in

Table 4.16.
Cardiovascular Endurance* Percentile Rankings.

	Age	\<table note: Percentile Rank\> 1-19	20-39	40-59	60-79	80-99
Men	20-29	<33.4	33.5-36.9	37.0-41.7	41.8-44.9	45.0-60.0
	30-39	<32.8	32.9-35.6	35.7-38.9	39.0-43.6	43.7-54.4
	40-49	<31.0	31.1-34.2	34.3-36.9	37.0-42.4	42.5-52.2
	50-59	<28.9	29.0-31.4	31.5-34.5	34.6-38.9	39.0-51.6
	60>	<21.7	21.8-26.1	26.2-30.9	31.0-35.5	35.6-49.5
Women	20-29	<25.2	25.3-29.5	29.6-31.4	31.5-35.6	35.7-45.0
	30-39	<24.4	24.5-28.9	29.0-31.4	31.5-34.9	35.0-43.7
	40-49	<22.6	22.7-25.2	25.3-28.9	29.0-31.4	31.5-43.7
	50-59	<20.9	21.0-23.5	23.6-26.1	26.2-30.1	30.2-42.5
	60>	<18.2	18.3-20.9	21.0-24.4	24.5-26.8	26.9-37.0

*Maximal oxygen uptake expressed in ml/kg/min.
Adapted from tables A.16 and A.17.

the prevention of coronary heart disease. A poorly conditioned heart that has to pump more often just to keep a person alive is subject to more wear-and-tear than a well-conditioned heart. In situations where strenuous demands are placed on the heart, such as doing yard work, lifting heavy objects or weights, or running to catch a train, the unconditioned heart may not be able to sustain the strain. Additionally, regular participation in cardiovascular endurance activities helps achieve and maintain ideal body weight.

Benefits of Cardiovascular Endurance Training

Every individual who initiates a cardiovascular or aerobic exercise program can expect several physiological changes as a result of training. Some of these benefits are:

1. A decrease in resting heart rate and an increase in cardiac muscle strength. During resting conditions, the heart ejects between five and six quarts of blood per minute. This amount of blood is sufficient to meet the energy demands in the resting state. As any other muscle, the heart responds to training by increasing in strength and size. As the heart gets stronger, the muscle can produce a more forceful contraction that causes a greater ejection of blood with each beat (stroke volume), yielding a decreased heart rate. This reduction in heart rate also allows the heart to rest longer between beats.

    Resting heart rates are frequently decreased by ten to twenty beats per minute (bpm) after only six to eight weeks of training. A reduction of 20 bpm would save the heart about 10,483,200 beats per year. The average heart beats between 70 and 80 bpm. However, in highly trained athletes, resting heart rates are commonly found around 40 bpm.

2. A lower heart rate at given workloads. When compared with untrained individuals, a trained person has a lower heart rate response to a given task. This is due to the increased efficiency of the cardiovascular system. Individuals are also surprised to find that following several weeks of training, a given workload (let's say a ten-minute mile) elicits a much lower heart rate as compared to the initial response when training first started.

3. A decrease in recovery time. Trained individuals enjoy a quicker recovery to resting values following an exercise bout. A fit system is able to restore at a greater speed any internal equilibrium that was disrupted during exercise.

4. An increase in the number and size of the mitochondria. All energy necessary for cell function is produced in the mitochondria. As the size and number increase, so does the potential to produce energy for muscular work.

5. An increase in the number of functional capillaries. These smaller vessels allow for the exchange of oxygen and carbon dioxide between the blood and the cells. As more vessels open up, a greater amount of gas exchange can take place, thereby decreasing the onset of fatigue during prolonged exercise. This increase in capillaries also speeds up the rate at which waste products of cell metabolism can be removed. Increased capillarization is also seen in the heart, which enhances the oxygen delivery capacity to the heart muscle itself.

6. An increase in the oxygen-carrying capacity of the blood. As a result of training, there is an increase in the red blood cell count, which contains hemoglobin that is responsible for transporting oxygen in the blood.

7. A higher oxygen uptake. The amount of oxygen that the body is able to utilize during physical activity is significantly increased. This allows the individual to exercise longer and at a higher rate before becoming fatigued.

8. A decrease in blood lipids. A regular aerobic exercise program will cause a reduction in blood fats such as cholesterol and triglycerides, both of which have been linked to the formation of the atherosclerotic plaque that obstructs the arteries. This reduction decreases the risk of cardiovascular disease.

MUSCULAR STRENGTH AND ENDURANCE

Many people are under the impression that muscular strength and endurance are only necessary for athletes and other individuals who hold jobs that require heavy muscular work. However, strength and endurance are important components of total physical fitness and have become an integral part of everyone's life.

Adequate levels of strength significantly enhance a person's health and well-being throughout life. Strength is important in daily activities such as sitting, walking, running, lifting and carrying objects, and doing housework. Strength is also of great value in improving posture, personal appearance, self-image, in developing sports skills, and in meeting certain emergencies in life where strength is necessary to cope effectively. From a health standpoint, strength helps maintain muscle tissue and a higher resting metabolism, decreases the risk for injury, helps prevent and eliminate chronic low back pain, and is an important factor in childbearing.

Perhaps one of the most significant benefits of maintaining a good strength level is its relationship to human metabolism. Metabolism is defined as all energy and material transformations that occur within living cells. A primary result of a strength training program is an increase in muscle size (lean body mass), known as muscle hypertrophy. Several studies have shown that there is a direct relationship between oxygen consumption as a result of metabolic activity and amount of lean body mass. Muscle tissue uses energy even at rest, while fatty tissue uses very little energy and may be considered metabolically inert from the point of view of caloric use. As muscle size increases, so does the resting metabolism or the amount of energy (expressed in calories) required by an individual during resting conditions to sustain proper cell function. Even small increases in muscle mass increase resting metabolism. All other factors being equal, if one takes two individuals at 150 pounds with different amounts of muscle mass, the one with the greater muscle size will have a higher resting metabolic rate, allowing this person to eat more calories to maintain the muscle tissue.

Lack of physical activity is also a reason for the decrease in metabolism as people grow older. Contrary to some beliefs, metabolism does not slow down with aging. It is not so much that *metabolism* slows down, it's that *we* slow down. Lean body mass decreases with sedentary living, which, in turn, slows down the resting metabolic rate. If people continue eating at the same rate, body fat increases. Hence, participating in a

strength training program is an important factor in the prevention and reduction of obesity.

One of the most common misconceptions about physical fitness is related to women and strength training. Due to the increase in muscle mass, many women feel that strength training programs are counterproductive because they will make them too muscular and less feminine-looking. The thought that strength training will make women less feminine is as false as to think that playing basketball will turn them into giants. Masculinity and femininity are established by genetic inheritance and not by the amount of physical activity. Variations in the degree of masculinity and femininity are determined by individual differences in hormonal secretions of androgen, estrogen, progesterone, and testosterone. Women with a bigger-than-average build are often inclined to participate in sports because of their natural physical advantage. As a result, many women have associated sports and strength participation with increased masculinity.

As the number of women who participate in sports has steadily increased in the last few years, the myth that strength training masculinizes women has gradually been disappearing. For example, per pound of body weight, women gymnasts are considered to be among the strongest athletes in the world. These athletes engage in very serious strength training programs and for their body size are most likely twice as strong as the average male. Yet, women gymnasts are among the most graceful and feminine of all women. In recent years, increased femininity has become the rule rather than the exception for women who participate in strength training programs.

Another benefit of strength training, which is accentuated even more when combined with aerobic exercise, is a decrease in adipose or fatty tissue around the muscle fibers themselves. Research has shown that in women the decrease in fatty tissue is greater than the amount of muscle hypertrophy. Therefore, it is not at all uncommon to lose inches and yet not lose body weight. However, since muscle tissue is more dense than fatty tissue, and in spite of the fact that inches are being lost, women often become discouraged because the results cannot be readily seen on the scale. This discouragement can be easily offset by regularly determining body composition to monitor changes in percent body fat as opposed to simply measuring total body weight changes.

The percentile ranks and fitness categories** for muscular strength and endurance are given in Table 4.17. The norms are based on age, sex, and the number of repetitions performed on the three strength training exercises (leg extension, bench press, and sit-up). Since muscular strength and endurance are highly specific and a high degree in one body part does not necessarily indicate a high degree in other parts, these three exercises

were selected to obtain a strength profile that would include the upper body, the lower body, and the abdominal region. An overall muscular strength/endurance rating can be determined by taking an average of the percentile ranks obtained for each exercise. The five fitness categories are established according to the average percentile rank as follows: (a) excellent, 80-99 percentile, (b) good, 60-79 percentile, (c) average, 40-59 percentile, (d) fair, 20-39 percentile, and (e) poor, 1-19 percentile. Guidelines for developing a muscular strength and/or endurance program are given in Appendix E.

** Strength and flexibility categories are determined according to normative data (instead of criterion standards) because experts do not know what constitutes an ideal or optimal level.

Table 4.17.
Muscular Strength and Endurance Standards*.

		Fitness Classification					
		Poor	Fair	Average	Good	Excellent	
	Age						
	<35	<6	7- 9	10-12	13-14	15>	
	36-49	<6	7-11	12-14	15-19	20>	Leg
	50>	<2	3- 5	6- 8	9-12	13>	Extension
	<35	<1	3- 6	7-10	11-15	16>	
Men	36-49	<5	6-11	12-19	20-26	27>	Bench
	50>	<6	7-11	12-19	20-28	29>	Press
	<35	<2	3- 7	8-11	12-16	17>	
	36-49	<2	3- 9	10-16	17-22	23>	
	50>	0	1- 5	6-10	11-16	17>	Sit-up
	<35	<4	5- 7	8- 9	10-12	13>	
	36-49	0	2- 5	6-10	11-14	15>	Leg
	50>	0	1- 3	4- 5	6-10	11>	Extension
	<35	0	1- 4	5-10	11-15	16>	
Women	36-49	<1	2- 7	8-14	15-21	22>	Bench
	50>	0	2- 5	6-12	13-19	20>	Press
	<35	0	1- 3	4- 5	6-13	14>	
	36-49	0	1- 7	8-13	14-23	24>	
	50>	<1	2- 6	7-15	16-20	21>	Sit-up
Percentile Rank		<19	20-39	40-59	60-79	80>	

*Based on the number of repetitions performed according to selected percentages of body weight (see Appendix E).
Adapted from Table A.18

FLEXIBILITY

The development and maintenance of some level of flexibility are important parts of everyone's health enhancement program, and even more so during the aging process. Sports medicine specialists have indicated that many muscular/skeletal problems and injuries, especially among adults, are related to a lack of flexibility. Approximately 80 percent of all low back problems in the United States are due to improper alignment of the vertebral column and pelvic girdle — a direct result of inflexible and weak muscles. As noted in Chapter 1, this backache syndrome cost American industry in excess of $1 billion each year in lost productivity and services alone, and an extra $225 million in Workmen's Compensation. Additionally, in daily life we are often required to make rapid or strenuous movements that we are not accustomed to make, leading to potential injury. Physical therapists have also indicated that improper body mechanics are often the result of inadequate flexibility levels.

Most experts agree that participating in a regular flexibility program will help a person maintain good joint mobility, increase resistance to muscle injury and soreness, prevent low back and other spinal column problems, improve and maintain good postural alignment, enhance proper and graceful body movement, improve personal appearance and self-image, and facilitate the development and maintenance of motor skills throughout life. Flexibility exercises have also been used successfully in the treatment of patients suffering from dysmenorrhea and general neuromuscular tension. Furthermore, stretching exercises in conjunction with calisthenics are helpful in warm-up routines to prepare the human body for more vigorous aerobic or strength training exercises, as well as subsequent cool-down routines to help the organism return to the normal resting state.

The test results for the battery of flexibility tests can be interpreted using the information contained in Tables 4.18 through 4.20. The overall flexibility rating can be determined by taking the average percentile rank of the four flexibility tests. The flexibility fitness categories are obtained in the same manner as the overall muscular strength and endurance rating (80-99 percentile = excellent, 60-79 percentile = good, 40-59 percentile = moderate, 20-39 percentile = fair, and 1-19 percentile = poor). The guidelines for developing a flexibility program are given in Appendix F.

BODY COMPOSITION

Body composition has been briefly discussed as a part of the CHD risk factor analysis. From a fitness point of view, achieving and maintaining ideal body weight (determined through body fat percentage) is a major objective of a sound program. Next to poor cardiovascular endurance, excessive body fat is the most common problem encountered in fitness and wellness assessments. Current estimates in the United States indicate that about half of the adult population has a weight problem. The evidence further shows that the

Table 4.18.
Modified Sit-and-Reach Flexibility Standards*.

		Fitness Classification				
		Poor	Fair	Average	Good	Excellent
Men	Age					
	<35	<11.5	11.6-13.4	13.5-14.9	15.0-16.9	17.0>
	36-49	<9.8	9.9-11.5	11.6-13.3	13.4-14.5	14.6>
	50>	<8.7	8.8-9.6	9.7-11.4	11.5-13.2	13.3>
Women	<35	<12.5	12.6-14.4	14.5-15.7	15.8-16.6	16.7>
	36-49	<10.9	11.0-12.7	12.8-14.4	14.5-16.1	16.2>
	50>	<8.2	8.3-10.0	10.1-12.2	12.3-14.1	14.2>
Percentile Rank		<19	20-39	40-59	60-79	80>

*Based on the total number of inches reached
Adapted from Table A.19

Table 4.19.
Trunk Rotation Flexibility Standards*.

			Fitness Classification				
		Poor	Fair	Average	Good	Excellent	
	Age						
	<35	<13.2	13.3-16.2	16.3-18.9	19.0-22.2	22.3>	
	36-49	<11.1	11.2-14.6	14.7-17.2	17.3-20.9	21.0>	
	50>	< 8.6	,8.7-11.4	11.5-14.6	14.7-16.2	16.3>	Right
	<35	<13.2	13.3-16.7	16.8-19.2	19.3-21.9	22.0>	
	36-49	<13.6	13.7-15.2	15.3-18.6	18.7-21.1	21.2>	
Men	50>	< 9.4	9.5-11.6	11.7-13.8	13.9-15.4	15.5>	Left
	<35	<13.9	14.0-15.9	16.0-17.9	18.0-20.7	20.8>	
	36-49	< 9.7	9.8-13.0	13.1-16.4	16.5-19.5	19.6>	
	50>	< 3.8	3.9-12.7	12.8-15.5	15.6-17.8	17.9>	Right
	<35	<15.1	15.2-17.1	17.2-19.2	19.3-21.4	21.5>	
	36-49	<11.5	11.6-14.7	14.8-17.6	17.7-20.1	20.2>	
Women	50>	< 6.2	6.3-13.6	13.7-15.9	16.0-19.0	19.1>	Left
Percentile Rank		<19	20-39	40-59	60-79	80>	

*Based on the total number of inches reached (see Appendix F for Trunk Rotation Flexibility Test protocols).
Adapted from A.20

Table 4.20.
Shoulder Rotation Flexibility Standards*.

			Fitness Classification			
		Poor	Fair	Average	Good	Excellent
	Age					
	<35	30.2>	30.1-25.8	25.7-23.0	22.9-18.5	<18.4
Men	36-49	33.4>	33.3-30.1	30.0-26.7	26.6-23.4	<23.3
	50>	33.2>	33.1-31.1	31.0-30.0	29.9-28.6	<28.5
	<35	26.0>	25.9-21.5	21.4-18.8	18.7-14.6	<14.5
Women	36-49	29.9>	29.8-24.5	24.4-23.2	23.1-19.3	<19.2
	50>	31.6>	31.5-28.2	28.1-25.2	25.1-22.6	<22.5
Percentile Rank		<19	20-39	40-59	60-79	80>

*Based on the final number of inches at which the shoulders rotated (see Appendix F for Shoulder Rotation Flexibility Test protocols).
Adapted from Table A.21

prevalence is still increasing. The average weight of American adults increased by about fifteen pounds in just the last decade. When Yankee stadium in New York was renovated in 1976, total seating capacity had to be reduced in order to accommodate the wider bodies of our adult population.

Although for many years people have relied on height/weight charts to determine ideal body weight, we now know that these can be highly inaccurate for many people. The proper way of determining ideal weight is through body composition, that is, by finding out what percentage of total body weight is fat, and what amount is lean tissue. Once the fat percentage is known, ideal body weight can be calculated from ideal body fat, or the recommended amount of fat where there is no detriment to human health.

In spite of the fact that different techniques used to determine percent body fat were developed several years ago, many people are still unaware of these procedures and continue to depend on height/weight charts to find out what their ideal body weight should be. The standard height/weight charts were first published in 1912 and were based on average weights (including shoes and clothing) for men and women who obtained life insurance policies between 1888 and 1905. The ideal weight on the tables is obtained according to sex, height, and frame size. Since no scientific guidelines to determine frame size are given, most people choose their size based on the column where their body weight is found.

To determine whether people are truly obese or "falsely" at ideal body weight, body composition must be established. Obesity is related to excessive body fat accumulation. If body weight is used as the only criteria, an individual can easily be overweight according to height/weight charts, and yet not be obese. This is commonly seen among football players, body builders, weight lifters, and other athletes with large muscle size. Some of these athletes in reality have very little body fat and appear to be many pounds overweight.

On the other hand, some people who weigh very little and are viewed by many as "skinny" or underweight can actually be classified as significantly overweight because of their body fat content. Not at all uncommon are cases of people weighing as little as 100 pounds who are 30 percent fat or higher (about one-third of their total body weight). Such cases are more readily observed among sedentary people and those who are constantly dieting. Both physical inactivity and constant negative caloric balance lead to a loss in lean body mass. It is clear from the previous examples that plain body weight does not always tell the true story.

Obesity by itself has been associated with several serious health problems and accounts for 15 to 20 percent of the annual mortality rate in the United States. Obesity has long been recognized as a major risk factor for diseases of the cardiovascular system, including coronary heart disease, hypertension, congestive heart failure, elevated blood lipids, atherosclerosis, strokes, thromboembolitic disease, varicose veins, and intermittent claudication.

New evidence now points toward a possible link between obesity and cancer of the colon, rectum, prostate, gallbladder, breast, uterus, and ovaries. It is interesting to note that if all deaths from cancer could be eliminated, the average life span would increase by approximately two years. If obesity was eliminated, life span could increase by as many as seven years. In addition, obesity has been associated with diabetes, osteoarthritis, ruptured intervertebral discs, gallstones, gout, respiratory insufficiency, and complications during pregnancy and delivery. Furthermore, it can lead to psychological maladjustment and increased accidental death rate. Life insurance companies are also quick to point out that there is a 150 percent greater mortality rate among overweight males as compared to the average mortality rate.

Total fat in the human body is classified into two types, essential fat and storage fat. The essential fat is needed for normal physiological functions, and without it, human health begins to deteriorate. This essential fat constitutes about 3 percent of the total fat in men and 10 to 12 percent in women. The percentage is higher in women because it includes sex-specific fat, such as found in the breast tissue, the uterus, and other sex-related fat deposits. The amount varies from 10 to 12 percent in women because of morphological (body build) differences from one woman to another.

Storage fat constitutes the fat that is stored in adipose tissue, mostly beneath the skin (subcutaneous fat) and around major organs in the body. This fat serves three basic functions: (a) as an insulator to retain body heat, (b) as energy substrate for metabolism, and (c) as padding against physical trauma to the body. The amount of storage fat does not differ between men and women, except that men tend to store fat around the waist, and women more so around the hips and thighs.

The percentile ranks for body composition (based on percent body fat) are found in Table 4.21. Similar to cardiovascular endurance (based on the fact that the typical American is not an ideal role model when it comes to body composition), body composition fitness categories are determined according to the criterion standards given in Table 4.9. The "very low" risk categories would be the equivalent of "ideal" body composition, while the "very high" risk category would imply obesity.

Once percent body fat has been established, "ideal" body weight can be easily determined using the "very low" risk guidelines contained in Table 4.9. For example, the ideal body fat percentage for a forty-year-old male is 15 percent. As noted earlier, the very low risk guidelines (or ideal fat percentage) are established at the point where the amount of fat carried by an individual does not pose a threat to his/her health. This ideal percentage does not mean that a person cannot be below this number. Many highly trained male athletes are in the range of 3 to 10 percent fat, and some female distance runners have been found around 6 percent body fat. The basic steps to compute ideal body weight based on current

percent fat and ideal percent fat are given in Appendix D.

While there is little disagreement regarding a greater mortality rate among obese people, some evidence seems to indicate that the same is true for underweight people. Being underweight and thin does not necessarily mean the same thing, though. A healthy thin person is someone with total body fat around the ideal percentage, yet an underweight person is an. individual with extremely low body fat, even to the point of compromising the essential fat. The 3 percent essential fat for men and the 10 to 12 percent for women are the lower limits for people to maintain good health. Below these percentages, normal physiologic functions can be seriously impaired. In addition, some experts point out that a little storage fat (over the essential fat) is better than none at all. As a result, the standards for ideal percent fat in Table 4.9 are set higher than the essential fat requirements, at a point that is conducive to optimal health. Additionally, because lean tissue decreases with age, one extra percentage point is allowed for every additional decade of life.

POSTURE

Posture analyses are used to detect deviations from normal body alignment. While it is most

Table 4.21.
Body Composition* Percentile Ratings.

	Age	Percentile Rank				
		1-19	20-39	40-59	60-79	80-99
Men	20-29	28.7>	28.6-22.4	22.3-18.1	18.0-14.0	13.9- 7.2
	30-39	28.1>	28.0-23.7	23.6-20.2	20.1-16.3	16.2- 7.1
	40-49	28.6>	28.5-24.7	24.6-21.6	21.5-17.7	17.6- 9.2
	50-59	29.2>	29.1-25.5	25.4-22.3	22.2-18.5	18.4- 9.0
	60>	29.0>	28.9-24.5	24.4-20.9	20.8-17.3	17.2-10.5
Women	20-29	33.4>	33.3-26.3	26.2-23.3	23.2-15.2	15.1- 7.8
	30-39	31.4>	31.3-25.6	25.5-21.6	21.5-16.8	16.7- 5.1
	40-49	31.5>	31.4-27.7	27.6-24.0	23.9-19.7	19.6- 7.3
	50-59	34.8>	34.7-30.5	30.4-27.1	27.0-22.8	22.7-10.8
	60>	34.8>	34.7-30.9	30.8-27.2	27.1-22.3	22.2- 6.8

*Expressed in percent body fat.
Adapted from Tables A.18 and A.19

desirable to conduct such analyses early in life, detection and correction of deviations from normal body alignment can be done at any age. Although certain postural deviations are more complex to correct in older people, if deviations are allowed to go uncorrected, they usually become more serious as the person grows older. Consequently, corrective exercises or other medical procedures should be used to stop or slow down postural degeneration.

Faulty posture along with weak and inelastic muscles are the leading causes for most chronic low back problems in the United States. It is estimated that 75 million Americans suffer from backache each year. About 80 percent of low back pain is caused by a combination of poor flexibility and improper postural alignment in the lower back and a weak abdominal wall. Consequently, using a battery of tests that would evaluate these areas becomes crucial in the prevention and rehabilitation of low back pain. Using the information provided by these tests, corrective exercises can be easily prescribed to correct and prevent future problems.

Adequate body mechanics also aid in the reduction of chronic low back pain. Proper body mechanics refers to the use of correct positions in all of daily life's activities, including sleeping, sitting, standing, walking, driving, working, and exercising. Due to the high incidence of low back pain, a series of corrective and preventive exercises, as well as illustrations on proper body mechanics, are shown in Appendix G.

Posture analyses can also be used to motivate people to engage in exercise as a means to improve body alignment. Most people are unaware of how faulty their posture is until they see themselves in a photograph, such as shown in Figure 3.9, Chapter 3. This type of photograph can be quite a shock for many people, and often is sufficient to motivate change. Besides engaging in the recommended exercises to improve deviations, people need to be continuously aware of the corrections that they are trying to make in order to elicit changes in postural alignment. As posture improves, people frequently become motivated to make changes in other areas of their health/fitness program (e.g., improve muscular strength and flexibility, and decrease body fat). The various posture categories are determined according to the sum of the ratings obtained for each body segment. Table 4.22 contains the different categories as determined by the "final" posture score.

PULMONARY FUNCTION

Pulmonary function is not generally related to heart disease or overall fitness levels, but it does have implications in the maintenance of good health. The types of pulmonary disease include obstructive lung disease, restrictive lung disease, and combined lung disease. Individuals with obstructive lung disease are unable to exhale maximally, primarily due to increased airway resistance caused by bronchospasm, pulmonary secretions, and/or breakdown of the bronchioles. Restrictive lung disease is seen in subjects with decreased lung compliance (distensibility) as a result of changes in lung tissue (parenchyma), the chest wall, or both. Restrictive lung disease is caused by conditions such as lung inflammation, fibrotic lung disease, kyphoscoliosis, neuromuscular diseases, and neoplasms.[24] Pulmonary function measurements through spirometry provide valuable information in screening individuals with possible obstructive lung disease. To determine

Table 4.22.
Posture Analysis Standards (men and women).

Classification	Total Points*
Excellent	45>
Good	40-44
Average	30-39
Fair	20-29
Poor	<19

restrictive lung disease, total lung capacity must be determined, which cannot be done through simple spirometry.

Research has shown that some loss of lung function is seen during the aging process; nevertheless, there are several other factors that have a much more serious effect on lung function loss. Smoking and/or living in a smoke-filled or highly polluted environment enhance the degeneration process of the lungs. Side-stream smoke can also have detrimental effects on lung function. According to one report, a nonsmoker who works in a smoking environment for eight hours a day has smoked the equivalent of four cigarettes.

Forced vital capacity (FVC), forced expiratory volume at one second (FEV1), forced mid-expiratory flow (FEF25-75%), and forced expiratory flow rate at 75 to 85 percent (FEF75-85%) are all measured through spirometry.

FVC represents the maximal amount of air that a person can forcefully exhale after a maximal inspiration. Under normal circumstances, this volume is directly related to age, height, and gender and as any of the other volumes, has no major impact on exercise potential nor does it change with exercise training. Even though the guidelines for normal values vary from one laboratory or physician to another, results over 80 percent of predicted are usually considered normal. FEV1 is the volume of air moved from the lungs during the first second of FVC. As with FVC, FEV1 should be at least 80 percent of predicted. These two volumes are used to determine the FEV1/FVC ratio, which is used as an indicator of large airway obstruction. The ratio (FEV1/FVC) should be about 75 percent. In other words, a person should be able to forcefully exhale at least 75 percent of the FVC in the first second. A lower value probably indicates large airway obstruction.

FEF25-75% represents the average flow across the middle half of the forced expiration or FVC and is significant in determining middle to small airway obstruction. Reduction below 75 percent of predicted may indicate partial obstruction. FEF75-85% measures the average flow of the latter part of the forced expiration. Significant reductions in FEF75-85%, that is, below 60 percent of predicted, are used as indicators of small airway obstruction and seem to be especially valuable in detecting early obstruction.

As noted in Chapter 3, extreme care must be taken to insure that "true" volumes are indeed obtained through spirometry. Lung function tests administered by inexperienced technicians often yield questionable results. All positive tests should

Figure 4.6. *Types of Pulmonary Diseases. Redrawn from Egan's **Fundamentals of Respiratory Therapy** by C. B. Spearman, R. L. Sheldon, and D. F. Egan. St. Louis: The C. V. Mosby Co., 1982.*

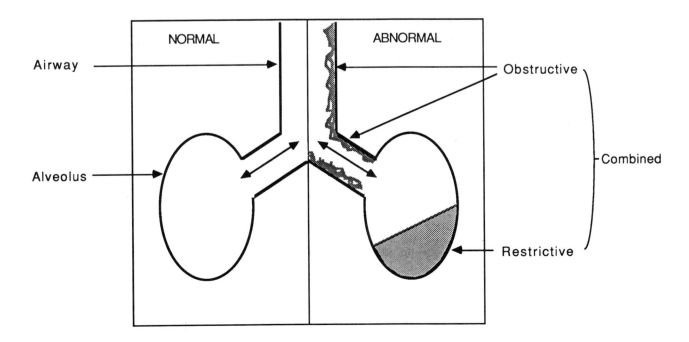

be referred to qualified medical personnel for further evaluation.

Patients with respiratory disease have a high incidence of repeated hospitalization. In addition, the inability to move air in and out of the lungs to meet physiological needs requires a constant distressful effort on the part of the patient. In this regard, serial spirometric testing is valuable in detecting early obstruction and evaluating disease progression. Since the disease process seems to be reversible at the early stages, serial testing may be helpful in detecting initial changes in lung function, and the results may be used to help motivate people to change unhealthy behavior and/or environmental conditions. Subsequent testing is useful in verifying the initial results, as well as in detecting additional changes caused by disease, reversibility of the disease process, and effectiveness of a rehabilitation protocol.

PHYSICAL FITNESS AND WELLNESS MAINTENANCE

Many present lifestyle patterns are such a serious threat to our health that they actually increase the deterioration rate of the human body and often lead to premature illness and mortality. However, scientific evidence has clearly shown that improving the quality and most likely the longevity of our lives is a matter of personal choice. As a nation, we have long recognized the value of preventive medicine, but it was not until recently that organizations began to realize that it costs less to keep people healthy than to treat them once they become ill. Consequently, many organizations have turned to health promotion programs as a means to improve the health of their employees and contain medical costs.

Nevertheless, we need to be reminded that the benefits of physical fitness and wellness can only be maintained through a regular lifetime program. Positive changes in behavior must be a lifelong commitment and not seasonal in nature. While initial changes in behavior require willpower and commitment, adhering to a fitness and wellness program long enough will cause rewarding physiological and psychological changes. Once new physical heights are reached, it becomes very difficult to regress to previous unhealthy behaviors. Although it is the duty of the health care practitioner to test, counsel, and motivate people toward a positive lifestyle, only the individual can act on it by changing negative behavior and in turn reap the benefits of wellness. Perhaps the new quality of life enjoyed by wellness program participants was best explained by Dr. George Sheehan, cardiologist and runner, when he wrote[17]:

> For every runner who tours the world running marathons, there are thousands who run to hear the leaves and listen to the rain, and look to the day when it is all suddenly as easy as a bird in flight. For them, sport is not a test but a therapy, not a trial but a reward, not a question but an answer.

The real challenge in the health promotion field is to help motivate people to get started. Initially, most people require a structured setting to enhance adherence. However, after several weeks of practicing new positive behaviors and actually experiencing the physical transformation called "wellness," it becomes easier to maintain such throughout life. But, for someone who has never experienced the feelings expressed by Dr. Sheehan or undergone this physical transformation, it is difficult to know what wellness is really like. Therein lies the importance of a good health and fitness leader: someone who can help people take control of their personal lifestyles and get them started on the road to total well-being.

REFERENCES

1. American Heart Association. *Coronary Risk Handbook: Estimating Risk of Coronary Heart Disease in Daily Practice.* Dallas, TX: The Association, 1973.
2. American Heart Association. *Heart Facts.* Dallas, TX: The Association, 1985.
3. Blair, S. N., N. N. Goodyear, L. W. Gibbons, and K. H. Cooper. "Physical Fitness and Incidence of Hypertension in Healthy Normotensive Men and Women." *JAMA* 252:487-490, 1984.
4. Blair, S. N., K. H. Cooper, L. W. Gibbons, L. R. Gettman, S. Lewis, and N. N. Goodyear. "Changes in Coronary Heart Disease Risk Factors Associated with Increased Treadmill Time in 753 Men." *American Journal of Epidemiology* 3:352-359, 1983.
5. Cooper, K. H. *Running Without Fear.* New York: Mount Evans and Co., 1985.
6. Cooper, K. H. *The Aerobics Way.* New York: Mount Evans and Co., 1977.
7. Cooper, K. H. *The Aerobics Program for Total Well-Being.* New York: Mount Evans and Co., 1982.
8. Diethrich, E. B. *The Arizona Heart Institute's Heart Test.* New York: International Heart Foundation, 1981.
9. Gibbons, L. W., S. Blair, K. H. Cooper, and M. Smith. "Association Between Coronary Heart Disease Risk Factors and Physical Fitness in Healthy Adult Women." *Circulation* 5:977-983, 1983.
10. Guss, S. B. *Heart Attack Risk Score.* Cardiac Alert, 1983.
11. Hoeger, W. W. K. *Ejercicio, Salud y Vida [Exercise, Health and Life].* Caracas, Venezuela: Editorial Arte, 1980.
12. Hoeger, W. W. K. *Lifetime Physical Fitness & Wellness: A Personalized Program.* Englewood, CO: Morton Publishing Company, 1986.
13. Hoeger, W. W. K. *U.T. Permian Basin Wellness Center: Coronary Heart Disease Risk Factor Analysis Interpretation.* Odessa, TX: U.T. Permian Basin, 1984.
14. Hoeger, W. W. K. "Self-Assessment of Cardiovascular Risk." *Corporate Fitness & Recreation* 5(6):13-16, 1986.
15. "How Good is 'Good' Cholesterol." *The Health Letter.* April 9, 1982.
16. Hubert, H. B., M. Feinleib, P. M. MacNamara, and W. P. Castelli. "Obesity as an Independent Risk Factor for Cardiovascular Disease: A 26-Year Follow-up of Participants in the Framingham Heart Study." *Circulation* 5:968-977, 1983.
17. Human Relations Media. *What is Fitness?, Dynamics of Fitness: The Body in Action.* Pleasantville, NY: The Company, 1980.
18. Johnson, L. C. *Interpreting Your Test Results.* Lake Geneva, WI: Fitness Monitoring Preventive Medicine Clinic, 1981.
19. Kannel, W. B., D. McGee, and T. Gordon. "A General Cardiovascular Risk Profile: The Framingham Study." *American Journal of Cardiology* 7:46-51, 1976.
20. Kostas, G. "Three Nutrients May Help Control Blood Pressure." *Aerobics News* 1(7):6, 1986.
21. "Multiple Risk Factor Intervention Trial," "Risk Factor Changes and Mortality Results," Multiple Risk Factor Intervention Trial Research Group. *JAMA* 248:1465-1477, 1982.
22. Neufeld, H. N., and U. Gouldbourt. "Coronary Heart Disease: Genetic Aspects." *Circulation* 5:943-954, 1983.
23. Page, L. B. "On Making Sense of Salt and Your Blood Pressure." *Executive Health.* August, 1982.
24. Spearman, C. B., R. L. Sheldon, and D. F. Egan. *Egan's Fundamentals of Respiratory Therapy.* St. Louis: The C. V. Mosby Company, 1982.
25. Van Camp, S. P. "The Fixx Tragedy: A Cardiologist's Perspective." *Physician and Sports Medicine* 12:153-155, 1984.
26. Wiley, J. A., and T. C. Camacho. "Lifestyle and Future Health: Evidence from the Alameda County Study." *Preventive Medicine* 9:1-21, 1980.

CHAPTER FIVE

Cancer Risk Management

The human body has approximately 100 trillion cells, and under normal conditions these cells reproduce themselves in an orderly manner. The growth of cells occurs so that old, worn-out tissues can be replaced and injuries can be repaired. However, in some instances certain cells grow in an uncontrolled and abnormal manner. Some cells will grow into a mass of tissue called a tumor, which can be either benign or malignant. A malignant tumor is considered to be a "cancer." Cancer cells grow for no reason and multiply uncontrollably, destroying normal tissue. The rate at which cancer cells grow varies from one type to another. Certain types grow fast, while others may take years to do so.

Over 100 types of cancer can develop in any tissue or organ of the body. Cancer probably starts with the abnormal growth of one cell, which can then multiply into billions of cancerous cells. It takes approximately one billion cells, or the equivalent of a one-centimeter tumor, before cancer can be detected. Through metastasis (the movement of bacteria or body cells from one part of the body to another), cells break away from a malignant tumor and migrate to other parts of the body where they can cause new cancer. Although most cancer cells are destroyed by the immune system, it only takes one abnormal cell to lodge elsewhere and start a new cancer. In contrast, benign tumors do not invade other tissue. They can interfere with normal body functions but rarely cause death.

CANCER INCIDENCE

The 1984 report by the National Center for Health Statistics indicated that 22.2 percent of all deaths in the United States were caused by cancer. It is the second leading cause of death in the country and the leading cause among children between the ages of three and fourteen. About 462,000 people died of the disease in 1986, and approximately 910,000 new cases were expected the same year. The 1986 statistical estimates of cancer incidence and deaths by sex and site are given in Figure 5.2 (these estimates exclude non-melanoma skin cancer and carcinoma in situ). Estimates also indicated that 67 million Americans, based on the total 1986 population, would suffer from cancer in their lifetime, striking approximately three out of every four families.

As with coronary heart disease, cancer is largely a preventable disease. As much as 80 percent of all human cancers are related to lifestyle or environmental factors (includes diet, tobacco use, excessive use of alcohol, overexposure to sunlight, and exposure to occupational hazards). Most of these cancers could be prevented through positive lifestyle habits. The proportion of cancers related to environmental factors was carefully studied in the Birmingham and West Midland region of England. The report indicated that only 6 percent of cancers in men and 2 percent in women originated in the workplace. Approximately 85 to 90 percent were lifestyle related (*see Figure 5.3*).

Figure 5.1. *How Cancer Starts and Spreads. Illustration by John Stone Quinan and Jo Ellen Murphy of the* **Washington Post** *(edited by Cancer News, American Cancer Society, Texas Division, Inc., Winter 1986). Reprinted with permission of the* **Washington Post,** *copyright 1985.*

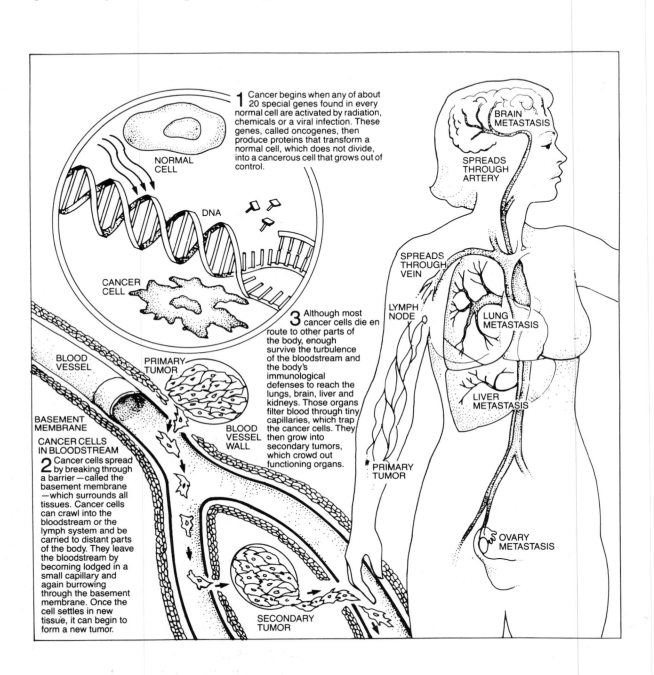

Figure 5.2. *Cancer Incidence and Deaths by Site and Sex: 1986 Estimates. From 1986 **Cancer Facts & Figures.** New York: American Cancer Society, 1986. Reproduced with permission.*

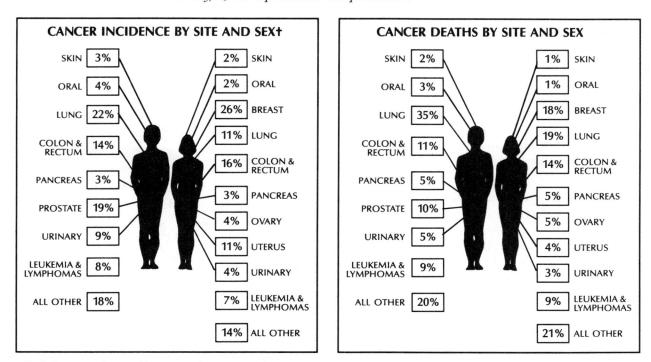

†Excluding non-melanoma skin cancer and carcinoma in situ.

Figure 5.3. *Cancer Deaths from Presumed and Environmental Factors in the Birmingham and West Midland Region of England in 1968-1972.*

Factor	Percentages of Cancer	
	Males	Females
Tobacco*	30	7
Tobacco/alcohol*	5	3
Sunlight*	10	10
Occupation*	6	2
Radiation*	1	1
Iatrogenic*	1	1
Other "Lifestyle" Factors**	30	63
Congenital**	2	2
Unknown	15	11

*Defined environmental factors.
**Presumed environmental factors.
Adapted from Higginson, J., and C. S. Muir. "Environmental Carcinogenesis: Misconceptions and Limitations to Cancer Control." *JNCL* 63(6):1291-1297, 1979.

Equally important is the fact that cancer is now viewed as the most curable of all chronic diseases. Over half of all cancers are curable. Over five million Americans were alive in 1986 who had a history of cancer. Close to three million of them were considered cured. The biggest factor in fighting cancer today is health education. People need to be informed regarding the risk factors for cancer and the guidelines for early detection.

GUIDELINES FOR CANCER PREVENTION

The most effective way to protect against cancer is by changing negative lifestyle habits and behaviors that have been practiced for years. The American Cancer Society[2] has issued the following recommendations in regard to cancer prevention:

1. **Dietary changes.** Fundamentally, a diet low in fat, high in fiber, and with ample

amounts of vitamins A and C from natural sources. Cruciferous vegetables are encouraged in the diet, alcohol should be used in moderation, and obesity should be avoided.

High fat intake has been linked primarily to breast, colon, and prostate cancers. Low fiber intake seems to increase the risk of colon cancer. Foods high in vitamins A and C may help decrease the incidence of larynx, esophagus, and lung cancers. Additionally, salt-cured, smoked, and nitrite-cured foods should be avoided. These foods have been linked to cancer of the esophagus and stomach. Vitamin C seems to help decrease the formation of nitrosamines (cancer-causing substances that are formed when cured meats are eaten). Cruciferous vegetables (cauliflower, broccoli, Brussels sprouts, and kohlrabi) should be included in the diet, since they seem to decrease the risk for the development of certain cancers.

Alcohol should be used in moderation. Alcoholism increases the risk of certain cancers, especially when combined with tobacco smoking or smokeless tobacco. In combination, they significantly increase the risk of mouth, larynx, throat, esophagus, and liver cancers. According to some research, the synergistic action of heavy use of alcohol and tobacco yield a fifteen-fold increase in cancer of the oral cavity.

Maintenance of ideal body weight is also recommended. Obesity has been associated with colon, rectum, breast, prostate, gallbladder, ovary, and uterine cancers.

2. **Abstinence from cigarette smoking.** It has been reported that 83 percent of lung cancer and 30 percent of all cancers are attributed to smoking. Smokeless tobacco also increases the risk of mouth, larynx, throat, and esophagus cancers. About 138,600 annual cancer deaths are attributed to the use of tobacco. However, cigarette smoking by itself is a major health hazard. When considering all related deaths, cigarette smoking is responsible for 350,000 unnecessary deaths per year. The average life expectancy for a chronic smoker is seven years less than for a nonsmoker.

3. **Avoid sun exposure.** Sunlight exposure is a major factor in the development of skin cancer. Almost 100 percent of the 400,000 non-melanoma skin cancer cases reported annually in the United States are related to sun exposure. Sunscreen lotion should be used at all times when the skin is going to be exposed to sunlight for extended periods of time. Tanning of the skin is the body's natural reaction to cell damage taking place as a result of excessive sun exposure.

4. **Avoid estrogen use, radiation exposure, and occupational hazard exposure.** Estrogen use has been linked to endometrial cancer but can be taken safely under careful physician supervision. Radiation exposure also increases cancer risk. Many times, however, the benefits of X-ray use outweigh the risk involved, and most medical facilities use the lowest dose possible to decrease the risk to a minimum. Occupational hazards, such as asbestos fibers, nickel and uranium dusts, chromium compounds, vinyl chloride, bis-chlormethyl ether, etc., increase cancer risk. The risk of occupational hazards is significantly magnified by the use of cigarette smoking.

The contribution of many of the other much publicized factors are not as significant as the above factors. The contribution to total cancer incidence of intentional food additives, saccharin, processing agents, pesticides, and packaging materials in current use in the United States and other developed countries appears to be minimal.

Genetics plays a role in susceptibility in only 2 percent of all cancers. Most of it is seen in early childhood years. Some cancer can be seen as a combination of genetic and environmental liability. Genetics may act to enhance environmental risks of certain types of cancers. The biggest carcinogenic exposure in the work place is cigarette smoke. However, environment means more than pollution, smoke, etc. It includes diet, lifestyle-related events, viruses, and physical agents such as X-rays and sun exposure.

Equally important is the fact that through early detection, many cancers can be controlled or cured. The real problem is the spreading of cancerous cells. Once spreading occurs, it becomes very difficult to wipe the cancer out. It is therefore crucial to practice effective prevention or at least catch cancer when the possibility of cure is greatest. Herein lies the importance of proper periodic screening for prevention and/or early detection.

The following are the seven warning signals for cancer. Every individual should become familiar with these warning signals and bring them to the attention of a physician if any of them are present:

1. Change in bowel or bladder habits

2. A sore that does not heal

3. Unusual bleeding or discharge

4. Thickening or lump in breast or elsewhere

5. Indigestion or difficulty in swallowing

6. Obvious change in wart or mole

7. Nagging cough or hoarseness

In addition to the seven warning signals, the American Medical Association has developed an "early warning signs of possible serious illness" questionnaire to help alert people to symptoms that may indicate a serious health problem. This questionnaire is given in Figure 5.4. Although in most cases there is nothing seriously wrong, if any of the described symptoms arise, a physician should be consulted as soon as possible. Furthermore, the Guidelines for Screening Recommendations by the American Cancer Society outlined in Figure 5.5 should be included in regular physical examinations as part of a cancer prevention program.

There is also growing evidence that the body's auto-immune system may play a role in preventing cancer. Studies have indicated that exercise improves the auto-immune system. On the other hand, high levels of tension and stress and/or poor coping may have a negative effect on this system and consequently reduce the body's effectiveness in dealing with the various cancers. Other recent research has indicated that moderately intense, long-term athletic participation lowers the risk for breast and reproductive system cancers. The possible link may be related to the fact that highly trained athletes possess lower estrogen levels.

Scientific evidence and testing procedures for prevention and/or early detection of cancer do change. Results of current clinical and epidemiologic studies provide constant new information about cancer prevention and detection. The purpose of cancer prevention programs is to educate and guide individuals toward a lifestyle that will aid them in the prevention and/or early detection

of malignancy. Treatment of cancer should always be left to specialized physicians and cancer clinics.

CANCER QUESTIONNAIRE: ASSESSING YOUR RISKS *

This simple self-testing questionnaire was designed by the Texas Division of the American Cancer Society to help people assess their risk for cancer. Some people may have more than the average risk of developing certain cancers. These people will be identified by risk factors for certain common types of cancer. These are the major risk factors and by no means represent the only ones that might be involved. The following are the instructions given to people who take this questionnaire:

Read each question concerning each site and its specific risk factors. Be honest in the responses. Place the number in parentheses (risk points) in the correct blank space provided to the left of each question. For example, Question #2 on lung cancer: If you are fifty-three years old (age fifty to fifty-nine), then enter five (risk points) as your score on the left. At the end of each site, total the number of points for that particular site.

Men should complete the questions for lung, colon-rectum, and skin cancer. Additionally, three major cancer sites for women are included with space to enter the score totals.

Check your own risks with the answers contained on this questionnaire. Individual numbers for specific questions are not to be interpreted as a precise measure of relative risk, but the totals for a given site should give you a general indication of your risk. An explanation of the different risk factors for each type of cancer follows the questionnaire. You are advised to discuss the results with your physician if you are at higher risk.

---

* Cancer Questionnaire: Assessing Your Risks obtained from the Texas Division of the American Cancer Society and reproduced with permission. (NOTE: This questionnaire is not available nationwide; distribution is limited to Texas residents only).

Figure 5.4. *Early Warning Signs of Possible Serious Illness.*

Many serious illnesses begin with apparently minor or localized symptoms that, if they are recognized early, can alert you to act in time for the disease to be cured or controlled. In most cases, of course, nothing is seriously wrong. If you experience any of the following symptoms, discuss the problem with your physician without delay.

1. Rapid loss of weight — more than about 4 kg (10 lbs) in 10 weeks — without apparent cause.

2. A sore, scab or ulcer, either in the mouth, or on the body, that fails to heal within a period of about three weeks.

3. A skin blemish or mole that begins to bleed or itch, or that changes color, size, or shape.

4. Severe headaches that develop for no obvious reason.

5. Sudden attacks of vomiting, without preceding nausea.

6. Fainting spells for no apparent reason.

7. Visual problems such as seeing "haloes" around lights, or intermittently blurred vision, especially in dim light.

8. Increasing difficulty with swallowing.

9. Hoarseness without apparent cause that lasts for a week or more.

10. A "smoker's" cough or any other nagging cough that has been getting worse.

11. Blood in coughed-up phlegm, or sputum.

12. Constantly swollen ankles.

13. A bluish tinge to the lips, the insides of the eyelids, or the nailbeds.

14. Extreme shortness of breath for no apparent reason.

15. Vomiting of blood or a substance that resembles coffee-grounds.

16. Persistent indigestion or abdominal pain.

17. A marked change in normal bowel habits, such as alternating attacks of diarrhea and constipation.

18. Bowel movements that look black and tarry.

19. Rectal bleeding.

20. Unusually cloudy, pink, red or smoky-looking urine.

21. In men, discomfort or difficulty when urinating.

22. In men, discharge from the tip of the penis.

23. In women, a lump or unusual thickening of a breast or any alteration in breast shape such as flattening, bulging or puckering of skin.

24. In women, bleeding or unusual discharge from the nipple.

25. In women, vaginal bleeding or "spotting" that occurs between usual menstrual periods or after menopause.

Reproduced with permission from *Family Medical Guide* by the American Medical Association. New York: Random House, 1982.

Figure 5.5. *Guidelines for Cancer Screening.*

Test	Patient age	Frequency
Breast physical examination	20-40 Over 40	Every 3 yr Annually
Breast self-examination	Over 20	Monthly
Chest X-ray	No specific recommendation	No specific recommendation
Digital rectal examination	Over 40	Annually
Endometrial tissue examination	At menopause[a]	At menopause
Mammography	35-40 40-49 Over 50	One baseline Every 1-2 yr Annually
Pap smear	20-65 and sexually active teenagers	2 consecutive yr, then every 3 yr
Pelvic examination	20-40 Over 40 At menopause	Every 3 yr Annually
Sigmoidoscopy	Over 50	2 consecutive yr, then every 3-5 yr
Sputum cytology	No specific recommendation	No specific recommendation
Stool guaiac	Over 50	Annually
Health counseling and cancer check-up[b]	Over 20 Over 40	Every 3 yr Every yr

From *Guidelines for the Cancer-Related Checkup: Recommendations and Rationale.* New York: American Cancer Society, July/August 1980. Reproduced with permission.

[a] Recommended for obese women with a history of involuntary infertility, failure of ovulation, abnormal uterine bleeding, or estrogen therapy.

[b] To include examinations for cancers of the thyroid, testicles, prostate, ovaries, lymph nodes, oral region, and skin.

Lung Cancer

_____ 1. **Sex**
   a. Male (2)
   b. Female (1)

_____ 2. **Age**
   a. 39 or less (1)
   b. 40 - 49 (2)
   c. 50 - 59 (5)
   d. 60 + (7)

_____ 3. **Smoking status**
   a. Smoker (8)
   b. Nonsmoker (1)

_____ 4. **Type of smoking**
   a. Current cigarettes or little cigars (10)
   b. Pipe and/or cigar, but not cigarettes (3)
   c. Ex-cigarette smoker (2)

_____ 5. **Amount of cigarettes smoked per day**
   a. 0 (1)
   b. Less than ½ pack per day (5)
   c. ½ - 1 pack (9)
   d. 1 - 2 packs (15)
   e. 2 + packs (20)

_____ 6. **Type of cigarette**
   a. High tar/nicotine (10)*
   b. Medium T/N (9)
   c. Low T/N (7)
   d. Nonsmoker (1)

_____ 7. **Duration of smoking**
   a. Never smoked (1)
   b. Ex-smoker (3)
   c. Up to 15 years (5)
   d. 15 - 25 years (10)
   e. 25 + years (20)

_____ 8. **Type of industrial work**
   a. Mining (3)
   b. Asbestos (7)
   c. Uranium & radioactive products (5)

Total _____

*High T/N   20 mg + Tar/1.3 + mg. nicotine
 Medium T/N 16 - 19 mg. Tar/1.1 - 1.2 nicotine
 Low T/N   15 mg. or less Tar/1.0 mg. or less
                      nicotine

Colon-Rectum Cancer

_____ 1. **Age**
   a. 39 or less (10)
   b. 40 - 59 (20)
   c. 60 + (50)

_____ 2. **Has anyone in your immediate family ever had:**
   a. Colon cancer (20)
   b. One or more polyps of the colon (10)
   c. Neither (1)

_____ 3. **Have you ever had:**
   a. Colon cancer (100)
   b. One or more polyps of the colon (40)
   c. Ulcerative colitis (20)
   d. Cancer of the breast or uterus (10)
   e. None (1)

_____ 4. **Bleeding from the rectum** (other than obvious hemorrhoids or piles)
   a. Yes (75)
   b. No (1)

Total _____

Skin Cancer

_____ 1. **Frequent work or play in the sun:**
   a. Yes (10)
   b. No (1)

_____ 2. **Work in mines, around coal tars, or around radioactivity:**
   a. Yes (10)
   b. No (1)

_____ 3. **Complexion** - Fair and/or light skin:
   a. Yes (10)
   b. No (1)

Total _____

Breast Cancer

_____ 1. **Age group**
   a. 20 - 34 (10)
   b. 35 - 49 (40)
   c. 50 + (90)

_____ 2. **Race group**
   a. Oriental (5)
   b. Black (20)
   c. White (25)
   d. Mexican American (10)

_____ 3. **Family history**
   a. Mother, sister, aunt, or grandmother with breast cancer (30)
   b. None (10)

_____ 4. **Your history**
   a. Previous lumps or cysts (25)
   b. No breast disease (10)
   c. Previous breast cancer (100)

_____ 5. **Maternity**
    a. 1st pregnancy before 25 (10)
    b. 1st pregnancy after 25 (15)
    c. No pregnancies (20)

Total _____

Cervical Cancer

(Lower Portion of Uterus. These questions would not apply to a woman who has had a total hysterectomy.)

_____ 1. **Age group**
    a. Less than 25 (10)
    b. 25 - 39 (20)
    c. 40 - 54 (30)
    d. 55+ (30)

_____ 2. **Race**
    a. Oriental (10)
    b. Puerto Rican (20)
    c. Black (20)
    d. White (10)
    e. Mexican American (20)

_____ 3. **Number of pregnancies**
    a. 0 (10)
    b. 1 to 3 (20)
    c. 4 and over (30)

_____ 4. **Viral infections**
    a. Herpes and other viral infections or ulcer formations on the vagina (10)
    b. Never (1)

_____ 5. **Age at first intercourse**
    a. Before 15 (40)
    b. 15 - 19 (30)
    c. 20 - 24 (20)
    d. 25 and over (10)
    e. Never (5)

_____ 6. **Bleeding between periods or after intercourse**
    a. Yes (40)
    b. No (1)

Total _____

Endometrial Cancer

(Body of Uterus. These questions would not apply to a woman who has had a total hysterectomy.)

_____ 1. **Age group**
    a. 39 or less (5)
    b. 40 - 49 (20)
    c. 50 + (60)

_____ 2. **Race**
    a. Oriental (10)
    b. Black (10)
    c. White (20)
    d. Mexican American (10)

_____ 3. **Births**
    a. None (15)
    b. 1 to 4 (7)
    c. 5 or more (5)

_____ 4. **Weight**
    a. 50 or more pounds overweight (50)
    b. 20 - 49 pounds overweight (15)
    c. Underweight for height (10)
    d. Normal (10)

_____ 5. **Diabetes** (elevated blood sugar)
    a. Yes (3)
    b. No (1)

_____ 6. **Estrogen hormone intake**
    a. Yes, regularly (15)
    b. Yes, occasionally (12)
    c. None (10)

_____ 7. **Abnormal uterine bleeding**
    a. Yes (40)
    b. No (1)

_____ 8. **Hypertension** (high blood pressure)
    a. Yes (3)
    b. No (1)

Total _____

CANCER QUESTIONNAIRE INTERPRETATION

The following interpretation of the cancer questionnaire is to summarize, explain new evidence, and provide valuable information on the individual risk that a person may have for each type of cancer. Potential cancer risk is based on individual lifestyle and medical history.

LUNG CANCER

1. **Sex.** Men have a higher risk of getting lung cancer than do women, equating them for type, amount, and duration of smoking. Since more women are smoking cigarettes for a longer duration than previously, their incidence of lung and upper respiratory tract (mouth, tongue, and larynx) cancer is increasing.

2. **Age.** The occurrence of lung and upper respiratory tract cancer increases with age.

3. **Smoking status.** Cigarette smokers have up to twenty times or even greater risk than nonsmokers. However, the rates of ex-smokers who have not smoked for ten years approach those of nonsmokers.

4. **Type of smoking.** Pipe and cigar smokers are at a higher risk for lung cancer than nonsmokers. Cigarette smokers are at a much higher risk than nonsmokers or pipe and cigar smokers. All forms of tobacco, including chewing, markedly increase the user's risk of developing cancer of the mouth.

5. **Amount of cigarettes smoked per day.** Male smokers of less than one-half pack per day have five times higher lung cancer rates than nonsmokers. Male smokers of one to two packs per day have fifteen times higher lung cancer rates than nonsmokers. Smokers of more than two packs per day are twenty times more likely to develop lung cancer than nonsmokers.

6. **Type of cigarette.** Smokers of low-tar/nicotine cigarettes have slightly lower lung cancer rates.

7. **Duration of smoking.** The frequency of lung and upper respiratory tract cancer increases with the duration of smoking.

8. **Type of industrial work.** Exposures to materials used in the industries mentioned in the questionnaire have been demonstrated to be associated with lung cancer. Smokers who work in these industries may have greatly increased risks. Exposures to materials in other industries may also carry a higher risk.

Total Risk

24 or less ... You have a low risk for lung cancer (low risk category).

25 - 49 ...... You may be a light smoker and would have a good chance of kicking the habit (light risk).

50 - 74 ...... As a moderate smoker, your risks of lung and upper respiratory tract cancer are increased. If you stop smoking now, these risks will decrease (moderate risk).

75 - over .... As a heavy cigarette smoker, your chances of getting lung and upper respiratory tract cancer are greatly increased. Your best bet is to stop smoking now — for the health of it. See your doctor if you have a nagging cough, hoarseness, persistent pain, or a sore in the mouth or throat (high risk).

COLON-RECTUM CANCER

1. **Age.** Colon cancer occurs more frequently after the age of fifty.

2. **Family predisposition.** Colon cancer is more common in families with a previous history of this disease.

3. **Personal history.** Polyps and bowel diseases are associated with colon cancer.

4. **Rectal bleeding.** Rectal bleeding may be a sign of colorectal cancer.

Total Risk

29 or less ... You are at a low risk for colon-rectum cancer.

30 - 69 ...... This is a moderate risk category. Testing by your physician may be indicated.

70 - over . . . . This is a high-risk category. You should see your physician for the following tests: digital rectal exam, guaiac slide test, and protoscopic exam.

In addition to the risk factors mentioned in the questionnaire, a diet high in fat and low in fiber, as well as a history of breast or endometrial cancer, also increase the risk for colon-rectum cancer.

SKIN CANCER

1. **Sun exposure.** Excessive ultraviolet light causes cancer of the skin. Protect yourself with a sunscreen medication.

2. **Work environment.** Working in mines, around coal tar, or around radioactive materials can cause cancer of the skin.

3. **Complexion.** Persons with light complexions need more protection than others.

Total Risk

Numerical risks for skin cancer are difficult to state. For instance, a person with a dark complexion can work longer in the sun and be less likely to develop cancer than a light-complected person. Furthermore, a person wearing a long-sleeve shirt and wide-brimmed hat may work in the sun and be less at risk than a person who wears a bathing suit for only a short period. The risk greatly increases with age.

If you answer "yes" to any question, you need to protect your skin from the sun or any other toxic material. Changes in moles, warts, or skin sores are very important and need to be seen by your doctor.

BREAST CANCER

1. **Age.** The risk for breast cancer significantly increases after age fifty.

2. **Race.** Breast cancer occurs more frequently in white women than any other groups.

3. **Family history.** The risk for breast cancer is higher in women with a family history of this type of cancer. The risk is even higher if more than one family member has developed breast cancer, and is also enhanced by the closeness

in terms of immediacy, e.g., mother, sister, aunt, or grandmother.

4. **Personal history.** A previous history of breast or ovarian cancer would indicate a greater risk.

5. **Maternity.** The risk is greater in women who have never had children and in women who bear children after age thirty.

Total Risk

Under 100 . . . . . . Low-risk women should practice monthly breast self-examination (BSE) and have their breasts examined by a doctor as a part of a cancer-related checkup.

100 - 199 . . . . Moderate-risk women should practice BSE and have their breasts examined by a doctor as part of a cancer-related checkup. Periodic breast X-rays should be included as your doctor may advise.

200 - over . . . . High-risk women should practice monthly BSE and have the above examinations more often. See your doctor for the recommended (frequency of breast physical examinations and X-ray) examinations related to you.

Other possible risk factors for breast cancer not listed in the questionnaire are a diet high in fat, onset of menstruation prior to age thirteen, chronic cystic disease, and ionizing radiation.

CERVICAL CANCER

1. **Age.** The highest occurrence is in the forty and over age group. The numbers represent the relative rates of cancer for different age groups. A forty-five-year-old woman has a risk three times higher than a twenty-year-old.

2. **Race.** Puerto Ricans, Blacks, and Mexican Americans have higher rates of cervical cancer.

3. **Number of pregnancies.** Women who have delivered more children have a higher occurrence.

4. **Viral infections.** Viral infections of the cervix and vagina are associated with cervical cancer.

5. **Age at first intercourse.** Women with earlier intercourse and with more sexual partners are at a higher risk.

6. **Bleeding.** Irregular bleeding may be a sign of uterine cancer.

Total Risk

40 - 69 . . . . This is a low-risk group. Ask your doctor for a pap test. You will be advised how often you should be tested after your first test.

70 - 99 . . . . In this moderate-risk group, more frequent pap tests may be required.

100 - over . . . . . . You are in a high-risk group and should have a pap test (and pelvic exam) as advised by your doctor.

ENDOMETRIAL CANCER

1. **Age.** Endometrial cancer is seen in older age groups. The numbers by the age groups represent relative rates of endometrial cancer at different ages. A fifty-year-old woman has a risk twelve times higher than a thirty-five-year-old woman.

2. **Race.** Caucasians have a higher occurrence.

3. **Births.** The fewer children one has delivered, the greater the risk of endometrial cancer.

4. **Weight.** Women who are overweight are at greater risk.

5. **Diabetes.** Cancer of the endometrium is associated with diabetes.

6. **Estrogen use.** Cancer of the endometrium may be associated with prolonged continuous estrogen hormone intake. This occurs in only

a small number of women. You should consult your physician before starting or stopping any estrogen medication.

7. **Abnormal bleeding.** Women who do not have cyclic regular menstrual periods are at greater risk.

8. **Hypertension.** Cancer of the endometrium is associated with high blood pressure.

Total Risk

45 - 59 . . . . You are at low risk for developing endometrial cancer.

60 - 99 . . . . Your risks are slightly higher (moderate risk). Report any abnormal bleeding immediately to your doctor. Tissue sampling at menopause is recommended.

100 - over . . . . . . Your risks are much greater (high risk). See your doctor for tests as appropriate.

Additional risk factors that may be associated with endometrial cancer, not included in the questionnaire, are infertility, a prolonged history of failure to ovulate, and menopause after age fifty-five.

OTHER CANCER SITES

Risk factors and prevention techniques for other types of cancer not contained in the cancer questionnaire have also been outlined in the American Cancer Society *Cancer Book* and in a series of pamphlets on "Facts on Cancer" (one each for selected cancer sites). These types of cancer are listed next, along with the risk factors associated with each type and preventive techniques to help decrease risk. Unlike the previous questionnaire, no numeric weights for the different risk factors have been assigned.

PROSTATE CANCER

The prostate gland is actually a cluster of smaller glands that encircles the top section of the urethra (urinary channel) at the point where it leaves the bladder. The function of the prostate is not quite clear, but the muscles of these small glands help squeeze prostatic secretions into the urethra.

Risk Factors

1. The highest incidence of prostate cancer is found in men over fifty-five. The incidence is also higher among Blacks than Whites, and more married than single men develop this type of cancer.

2. A history of venereal disease. Herpes Simplex Virus Type 2 and Cytomegalovirus (herpes virus) have been linked to prostate cancer.

3. A history of prostate infections (more than two).

4. A diet high in fat may also increase risk.

Prevention and Warning Signals

Prostate cancer is difficult to control because the causes are not known. Death rates can be decreased through early detection and awareness of the warning signals. Detection is made by a rectal exam of the gland and should be conducted once a year after the age of forty. Possible warning signals include: difficulties in urination (especially at night), painful urination, blood in the urine, and constant pain in the lower back or hip area.

TESTICULAR CANCER

Testicular cancer accounts for only 1 percent of all male cancers. However, it is the most common type of cancer seen in men between the ages of twenty-five and thirty-five. The incidence is slightly higher in Caucasians as compared to Blacks, and it is rarely seen in middle-aged and older men. The malignancy rate of testicular tumors is 96 percent, but this type of cancer is highly curable if it is diagnosed early.

Risk Factors

1. An undescended testicle not corrected before age six.

2. Atrophy of the testicle following mumps or virus infection.

3. A family history of testicular cancer.

4. Recurrent injury to the testicle.

5. Abnormalities of the endocrine system (e.g., high hormone levels of pituitary gonadotropin or androgens).

6. Incomplete testicular development.

Prevention and Warning Signals

The incidence of testicular cancer is quite high in males born with an undescended testicle. Therefore, this condition should be corrected early in life. Parents of infant males need to make sure that the child is checked by a physician to insure that the testes have descended into the scrotum. Testicular self-examination (TSE) once a month following a warm bath or shower (when the scrotal skin is relaxed) is recommended. Each testicle is gently examined by rolling it between the thumb and fingers. The individual should feel for a firm lump about the size of a pea. While most lumps are noncancerous, if detected, a physician should be promptly consulted.

Some of the warning signs associated with testicular cancer are: a small lump found on the testicle, slight enlargement (usually painless) and change in consistency of the testis, sudden buildup of blood or fluid in the scrotum, groin and lower abdominal pain or discomfort accompanied by a sensation of dragging and heaviness, breast enlargement or tenderness, and enlarged lymph glands.

Early diagnosis of testicular cancer is essential since this type of cancer spreads rapidly to other parts of the body. Because in most cases no early symptoms or pain are associated with testicular cancer, most people do not see a physician for months following the discovery of a lump or a slightly enlarged testis. Unfortunately, this delay allows almost 90 percent of testicular cancers to metastasize before a diagnosis is made.

PANCREATIC CANCER

The pancreas is a thin gland that lies behind the stomach. This gland releases insulin and pancreatic juice. Insulin regulates blood sugar and pancreatic juice contains enzymes that aid in food digestion.

Possible Risk Factors

1. The incidence increases between the ages of thirty-five and seventy but is significantly higher around the age of fifty-five.

2. Cigarette smoking.

3. High cholesterol diet.

4. Exposure to unspecified environmental agents.

Prevention and Warning Signals

Detection of pancreatic cancer is difficult because (a) no symptoms are evoked in the early disease process, and (b) advanced disease symptoms are similar to those of other diseases. Warning signals that may be related to pancreatic cancer include pain in the abdomen or lower back, jaundice, loss of weight and appetite, nausea, weakness, agitated depression, loss of energy and feeling weary, dizziness, chills, muscle spasms, double vision, and coma.

KIDNEY AND BLADDER CANCER

The kidneys are the organs that filter the urine, and the bladder stores and empties the urine. The majority of these two types of cancers are caused by environmental factors. Bladder cancer occurs most frequently between the ages of fifty and seventy. Eighty percent of bladder cancers are seen in men, and the incidence is twice as high in White males as compared to Black males.

Risk Factors

1. Congenital abnormalities of either organ (these conditions are detected by a physician).

2. Exposure to certain chemical compounds such as aniline dyes, naphthalenes, or benzidines.

3. Heavy cigarette smoking.

4. A history of schistosomiasis (a parasitic bladder infection).

5. Frequent urinary tract infections, particularly after the age of fifty.

Prevention and Warning Signals

Avoidance of cigarette smoking and occupational exposure to cancer-causing chemicals are important to decrease risk. Bloody urine, especially repeated occurrences, is always an important warning sign and requires immediate evaluation.

ORAL CANCER

Oral cancer includes the mouth, lips, tongue, salivary glands, pharynx, larynx, and floor of the mouth. Most of these cancers seem to be related to cigarette smoking and excessive alcohol consumption.

Risk Factors

1. Heavy smoking and/or drinking.

2. Broken or ill-fitting dentures.

3. A broken tooth that irritates the inside of the mouth.

4. Chewing and dipping tobacco.

5. Excessive sun exposure (lip cancer).

Prevention and Warning Signals

Regular examinations and good dental hygiene help in the prevention and early detection of oral cancer. Warning signals may include the following: a nonhealing sore or white patch in the mouth, the presence of a lump, problems with chewing and swallowing, and a constant feeling of having "something" in the throat. A person with any of the previous conditions should be evaluated by a physician or dentist. A tissue biopsy is normally conducted to diagnose the presence of cancer.

ESOPHAGEAL AND STOMACH CANCER

The incidence of gastric cancer in the United States has decreased by about 40 percent in the last thirty years. Cancer experts attribute this drastic decrease to changes in dietary habits and increased use of refrigeration. This type of cancer is more common in men, and the incidence is also higher among Black males as compared to Whites.

Risk Factors

1. A diet high in starch and low in fresh fruits and vegetables.

2. Increased consumption of salt-cured, smoked, and nitrate-cured foods.

3. Stomach acid imbalance.

4. A history of pernicious anemia.

5. Chronic gastritis or gastric polyps.

6. A family history of these types of cancer.

Prevention and Warning Signals

Prevention is primarily accomplished by increasing dietary intake of complex carbohydrates and fiber and decreasing the intake of salt-cured, smoked, and nitrate-cured foods. In addition, regular guaiac testing for occult blood (hemoccult test) is recommended. Warning signals for this type of cancer include: indigestion for over two weeks or longer, blood in the stools, vomiting, and rapid weight loss.

OVARIAN CANCER

The ovaries are part of the female reproductive system which produces and releases the egg and the hormone estrogen. Ovarian cancer develops more frequently after menopause, and the highest incidence is seen between the ages of fifty-five and sixty-four.

Risk Factors

1. Women over fifty years old are at higher risk.

2. A history of ovarian problems.

3. Extensive history of menstrual irregularities.

4. A family history of ovarian cancer.

5. A personal history of breast, bowel, or endometrial cancer.

6. Nulliparity (not having given birth to a child).

Prevention and Warning Signals

In most cases, there are no signs or symptoms related to ovarian cancer. Therefore, regular pelvic examinations to detect signs of enlargement or other abnormalities are highly recommended.

Some warning signals that may occur with ovarian cancer are: an enlarged abdomen, abnormal vaginal bleeding, unexplained digestive disturbances in women over forty, and normal-sized ovaries (premenopause size) after menopause has occurred.

THYROID CANCER

The thyroid gland is located in the lower portion of the front of the neck and helps regulate growth and metabolism. Thyroid cancer among women occurs almost twice as often as in men, and the incidence is also higher in Whites as compared to Blacks.

Risk Factors

1. Risk increases with age.

2. Radiation therapy of the head and neck region received in childhood or adolescence.

3. A family history of thyroid cancer.

Prevention and Warning Signals

Regular inspection for thyroid tumors is done by palpation of the gland and surrounding areas during a physical examination. Thyroid cancer is a slow-growing process; therefore, this malignancy is highly treatable. However, any unusual lumps in front of the neck should be promptly reported to a physician. Although thyroid cancer is quite asymptomatic, warning signals (besides a lump) may include: difficulty in swallowing, choking, labored breathing, and persistent hoarseness.

LIVER CANCER

The incidence of liver cancer in the United States is very low. Men are more prone to liver cancer, and the disease is more common after the age of sixty.

Risk Factors

1. A history of cirrhosis of the liver.

2. A history of hepatitis B virus.

3. Exposure to vinyl chloride (industrial gas used when plastics are manufactured) and aflotoxin (natural food contaminant).

4. Heavy alcohol consumption.

Prevention and Warning Signals

Prevention is primarily accomplished by avoidance of the risk factors and awareness of warning signals. Possible signs and symptoms are a lump or pain in the upper right abdomen (which may radiate into the back and the shoulder), fever, nausea, rapid deteriorating health, jaundice, and liver tenderness.

LEUKEMIA

Leukemia is a type of cancer that interferes with blood-forming tissues (bone marrow, lymph nodes, and spleen), bringing about the production of two many immature white blood cells. Consequently, people afflicted by leukemia cannot fight infection effectively. For the most part, the causes of leukemia are unknown, although suspected risk factors have been identified.

Risk Factors

1. Inherited susceptibility, but not directly transmitted from parent to child.

2. An increased incidence is observed among children with Down's syndrome (mongolism) and a few other genetic abnormalities.

3. Excessive exposure to ionizing radiation.

4. Environmental exposure to chemicals such as benzene.

Prevention and Warning Signals

Detection is not easy because early symptoms may be attributed to less serious ailments. Early warning signals may include fatigue, pallor, weight loss, easy bruising, nosebleeds, paleness, loss of appetite, repeated infections, hemorrhages, night sweats, bone and joint pain, and fever. At a more advanced stage, fatigue increases, hemorrhages become more severe, pain and high fever continue, and swelling of the gums and various skin disorders occur.

LYMPHOMAS

Lymphomas are cancers that afflict the lymphatic system. The lymphatic system consists of lymph nodes found throughout the body and a connecting network of vessels that link these nodes. The lymphatic system participates in the body's immune reaction to foreign cells, substances, and infectious agents.

Risk Factors

As with leukemia, the causes for lymphomas are unknown at this time. Some researchers suspect that a particular form of herpes virus, referred to as Epstein-Barr virus, is active in the initial stages of lymphosarcomas. Other researchers hypothesize that certain external factors may alter the immune system, making it more susceptible to the development and multiplication of cancer cells.

Prevention and Warning Signals

Prevention of lymphomas is limited because little is known regarding its causes. Enlargement of a lymph node or cluster of lymph nodes is the initial sign of lymphoma. Other signs and symptoms may be an enlarged spleen or liver, weakness, fever, back or abdominal pain, nausea and/or vomiting, unexplained weight loss, unexplained itching and sweating, or fever at night that lasts for a prolonged period of time.

A FINAL WORD ON CANCER RISK MANAGEMENT

Individuals who are at high risk for any of the cancer sites are advised to discuss any particular problems with a physician. An ounce of prevention is worth a pound of cure! Although cardiovascular disease is the number one killer in the United States, cancer is the number one fear. Keep in mind that 60 to 80 percent of all cancers are preventable and about 50 percent are curable. Since most cancers are lifestyle related, awareness of the risk factors and implementation of the screening guidelines (Figure 5.5), along with the basic recommendations for cancer prevention, will significantly decrease cancer risk.

REFERENCES

1. American Cancer Society, Texas Division. *Cancer: Assessing Your Risks* Dallas, TX: The Society, 1982.
2. American Cancer Society. *1986 Cancer Facts and Figures*. New York: The Society, 1986.
3. American Cancer Society. *Cancer Book*. New York: The Society, 1986.
4. American Cancer Society. *Guidelines for the Cancer-Related Checkup: Recommendations and Rationale*. New York: The Society, 1980.
5. American Cancer Society. Pamphlets on *Facts on "Selected" Cancer Sites*. New York: The Society, pamphlets published between 1978 and 1983.
6. Greenwald, P. "Assessment of Risk Factors for Cancer." *Preventive Medicine* 9:260-263, 1980.
7. Hammond, E. C., and H. Seidman. "Smoking and Cancer in the United States." *Preventive Medicine* 9:169-173, 1980.
8. Higginson, J. "Proportion of Cancers Due to Occupation." *Preventive Medicine* 9:180-188, 1980
9. Rothman, K. J. "The Proportion of Cancer Attributable to Alcohol Consumption." *Preventive Medicine* 9:174-179, 1980.
10. Weisburger, J. H., D. M. Hegsted, G. B. Gori, and B. Lewis. "Extending the Prudent Diet to Cancer Prevention." *Preventive Medicine* 9:297-304, 1980.
11. Williams, C. L. "Primary Prevention of Cancer Beginning in Childhood." *Preventive Medicine* 9:275-280, 1980.
12. Williams, P. A. "A Productive History and Physical Examination in the Prevention and Early Detection of Cancer." *Cancer* 47:1146-1150, 1981.

C H A P T E R S I X

Nutrition For Weight Control and Wellness

The science of nutrition studies the relationship of foods to optimal health and performance. Ample scientific evidence has long linked good nutrition to overall health and well-being. Proper nutrition signifies that a person's diet is supplying all of the essential nutrients to carry out normal tissue growth, repair, and maintenance. It also implies that the diet will provide sufficient substrates to obtain the energy necessary for work, physical activity, and relaxation. Unfortunately, the typical American diet is too high in calories, sugars, fats, and sodium and not high enough in fiber — none of which is conducive to good health.

NUTRIENTS

The essential nutrients required by the human body are carbohydrates, fats, protein, vitamins, minerals, and water. The first three have been referred to as fuel nutrients because they are the only substances used to supply the energy necessary for work and normal body functions. Vitamins, minerals, and water have no caloric value but are still essential for normal body functions and maintenance of good health. In addition, many nutritionists like to add a seventh nutrient to this list that has received a great deal of attention recently — dietary fiber.

Carbohydrates are the major source of calories used by the body to provide energy for work, cell maintenance, and heat. They also play a crucial role in the digestion and regulation of fat and protein metabolism. Each gram of carbohydrates provides the human body with approximately four calories. Carbohydrates are found primarily in breads, cereals, fruits, and vegetables.

Carbohydrates are classified into two types. Simple carbohydrates (frequently denoted as sugar) are formed by simple or double sugar units with little nutritive value (e.g. candy, ice cream, pop, cakes, etc.). Eating too many simple carbohydrates can take the place of more nutritive foods in the diet. Complex carbohydrates are formed by complex sugar chains and not only provide many valuable nutrients to the body, but can also be an excellent source of fiber or roughage.

Fats or lipids are also used as a source of energy in the human body. They are the most concentrated source of energy. Each gram of fat supplies nine calories to the body. Fats are also a part of the cell structure. They are used as stored energy and as an insulator for body heat preservation. They provide shock absorption, supply essential fatty acids, and carry the fat-soluble vitamins A, D, E, and K. The basic sources of fat are milk, dairy products, and meats and alternates.

Depending on the source, fats can be classified into saturated and polyunsaturated (or unsaturated) fats. The saturated fats are those that do not melt at room temperature (e.g. meats, cheese, butter). Polyunsaturated fats are in liquid form at room temperature. In general, saturated fats increase the blood cholesterol level, while polyunsaturated fats decrease the cholesterol content (the role of cholesterol in health and disease was discussed in Chapter 4).

Proteins are the main substances used to build and repair tissues such as muscles, blood, internal organs, skin, hair, nails, and bones. They are a part of hormones, enzymes, and antibodies and help maintain normal body fluid balance. Proteins can also be used as a source of energy, but only if there are not enough carbohydrates and fats available. Each gram of protein yields about four calories of energy, and the primary sources are meats and alternates, milk, dairy products, and some breads and cereals.

Vitamins are organic substances essential for normal metabolism, growth, and development of the body. They are classified into two types based on their solubility: fat-soluble vitamins (A, D, E, and K), and water-soluble vitamins (B complex and C). Vitamins cannot be manufactured by the body; hence, they can only be obtained through a well-balanced diet. A description of the functions of each vitamin is presented in Figure 6.1.

Minerals are inorganic elements found in the body and in food. They serve several important functions. Minerals are constituents of all cells, especially those found in hard parts of the body (bones, nails, teeth). They are crucial in the maintenance of water balance and the acid-base balance. They are essential components of respiratory pigments, enzymes, and enzyme systems, and they regulate muscular and nervous tissue excitability. The specific functions of some of the most important minerals are contained in Figure 6.2.

Approximately 70 percent of total body weight is water. It is the most important nutrient and is involved in almost every vital body process. Water is used in digestion and absorption of food, in the circulatory process, in removing waste products, in building and rebuilding cells, and in the transport of other nutrients. Water is contained in almost all foods, but primarily in liquid foods, fruits, and vegetables. Besides the natural content in foods, it is recommended that every person drink at least eight to ten glasses of fluids a day.

Dietary fiber is basically a type of complex carbohydrate made up of plant material that cannot be digested by the human body. It is mainly present in leaves, skins, roots, and seeds. Processing and refining foods removes almost all of the natural fiber. In our daily diets, the main surces of dietary fiber are whole grain cereals and breads, fruits, and vegetables.

Fiber is important in the diet because it binds water, yielding a softer stool that decreases transit time of food residues in the intestinal tract. Many researchers feel that speeding up the passage of food residues through the intestines decreases the risk for colon cancer, primarily because of the decreased time that cancer-causing agents remain in contact with the intestinal wall. The increased water content of the stool may also dilute the cancer-causing agents, decreasing the potency of these substances.

The risk for coronary disease also decreases with increased fiber intake. This decreased risk can be attributed to two factors. First, all too often saturated fats take the place of dietary fiber in the diet, thereby increasing cholesterol absorption and/or formation. Second, some specific water-soluble fibers such as pectin and guar gum found in beans, oats, corns, and fruits seem to bind cholesterol in the intestines, thereby preventing its absorption. In addition, several other health disorders have been linked to low fiber intake, including constipation, diverticulitis, hemorrhoids, ulcerative colitis, gallbladder disease, appendicitis, and obesity.

Determining the amount of fiber in the diet can be confusing at times, because it can be measured either as crude fiber or dietary fiber. Crude fiber is the smaller portion of the dietary fiber that actually remains after chemical extraction in the digestive tract. The recommended amount of dietary fiber is about twenty-five grams per day, or the equivalent of seven grams of crude fiber. On the other hand, be aware that too much fiber consumption can be detrimental to health, since excessive amounts can lead to increased loss of calcium, phosphorus, and iron, not to mention increased gastrointestinal discomfort. It is also important to increase fluid intake when fiber consumption is increased, since too little fluid can lead to dehydration and/or constipation.

THE BALANCED DIET

Most people would like to live life to its fullest, maintain good health, and lead a productive life. One of the fundamental ways to accomplish this

Figure 6.1 *Major Functions of Vitamins.*

NUTRIENT	GOOD SOURCES	MAJOR FUNCTIONS	DEFICIENCY SYMPTOMS
Vitamin A	Milk, cheese, eggs, liver, and yellow/dark green fruits and vegetables	Required for healthy bones, teeth, skin, gums, and hair. Maintenance of inner mucous membranes, thus increasing resistance to infection. Adequate vision in dim light	Night blindness, decreased growth, decreased resistance to infection, rough-dry skin
Vitamin D	Fortified milk, cod, liver oil, salmon, tuna, egg yolk	Necessary for bones and teeth. Needed for calcium and phosphorus absorption	Rickets (bone softening), fractures and muscle spasms
Vitamin E	Vegetable oils, yellow and green leafy vegetables, margarine, wheat germ, whole grain breads and cereals	Related to oxydation and normal muscle and red blood cell chemistry	Leg cramps, red blood cell breakdown
Vitamin K	Green leafy vegetables, cauliflower, cabbage, eggs, peas, and potatoes	Essential for normal blood clotting	Hemorrhaging
Vitamin B$_1$ (Thiamin)	Whole grain or enriched bread, lean meats and poultry, fish, liver, pork, poultry, organ meats, legumes, nuts, and dried yeast	Assists in proper use of carbohydrates. Normal functioning of nervous system. Maintenance of good appetite	Loss of appetite, nausea, confusion, cardiac abnormalities, muscle spasms
Vitamin B$_2$ (Riboflavin)	Eggs, milk, leafy green vegetables, whole grains, lean meats, dried beans and peas	Contributes to energy release from carbohydrates, fats, and proteins. Needed for normal growth and development, good vision and healthy skin	Cracking of the corners of the mouth, inflammation of the skin, impaired vision
Vitamin B$_6$ (Pyridoxine)	Vegetables, meats, whole grain cereals, soybeans, peanuts, and potatoes	Necessary for protein and fatty acids metabolism, and normal red blood cell formation	Depression, irritability, muscle spasms, nausea
Vitamin B$_{12}$	Meat, poultry, fish, liver, organ meats, eggs, shellfish, milk, and cheese	Required for normal growth, red blood cell formation, nervous system and digestive tract functioning	Impaired balance, weakness, drop in red blood cell count
Niacin	Liver and organ meats, meat, fish, poultry, whole grains, enriched breads, nuts, green leafy vegetables, and dried beans and peas	Contribute to energy release from carbohydrates, fats, and proteins. Normal growth and development, and formation of hormones and nerve-regulating substances	Confusion, depression, weakness, weight loss
Biotin	Liver, kidney, eggs, yeast, legumes, milk, nuts, dark green vegetables	Essential for carbohydrate metabolism and fatty acid synthesis	Inflamed skin, muscle pain, depression, weight loss
Folic Acid	Leafy green vegetables, organ meats, whole grains and cereals, and dried beans	Needed for cell growth and reproduction and red blood cell formation	Decreased resistance to infection
Pantothenic Acid	All natural foods, especially liver, kidney, eggs, nuts, yeast milk, dried peas and beans, and green leafy vegetables	Related to carbohydrate and fat metabolism	Depression, low blood sugar, leg cramps, nausea, headaches
Vitamin C (Ascorbic Acid)	Fruits and vegetables	Helps protect against infection. Formation of collagenous tissue. Normal blood vessels, teeth and bones	Slow healing wounds, loose teeth, hemorrhaging, rough-scaly skin, irritability

Figure 6.2 *Major Functions of Minerals.*

NUTRIENT	GOOD SOURCES	MAJOR FUNCTIONS	DEFICIENCY SYMPTOMS
Calcium	Milk, yogurt, cheese, green leafy vegetables, dried beans, sardines, and salmon	Required for strong teeth and bone formation. Maintenance of good muscle tone, heart beat, and nerve function	Bone pain and fractures, periodontal disease, muscle cramps
Iron	Organ meats, lean meats, seafoods, eggs, dried peas and beans, nuts, whole and enriched grains, and green leafy vegetables	Major component of hemoglobin. Aids in energy utilization	Nutritional anemia, and overall weakness
Phosphorus	Meats, fish, milk, eggs, dried beans and peas, whole grains, and processed foods	Required for bone and teeth formation. Energy release regulation	Bone pain and fracture, weight loss, and weakness
Zinc	Milk, meat, seafood, whole grains, nuts, eggs, and dried beans	Essential component of hormones, insulin, and enzymes. Used in normal growth and development	Loss of appetite, slow healing wounds, and skin problems
Magnesium	Green leafy vegetables, whole grains, nuts, soybeans, seafood, and legumes	Needed for bone growth and maintenance. Carbohydrate and protein utilization. Nerve function. Temperature regulation	Irregular heartbeat, weakness, muscle spasms, and sleeplessness
Sodium	Table salt, processed foods, and meat	Body fluid regulation. Transmission of nerve impulse. Heart action	Rarely seen
Potassium	Legumes, whole grains, bananas, orange juice, dried fruits, and potatoes	Heart action. Bone formation and maintenance. Regulation of energy release. Acid-base regulation	Irregular heartbeat, nausea, weakness

goal is eating a well-balanced diet. Generally, the daily caloric intake should be distributed in such a way that 50 to 60 percent of the calories come from carbohydrates, 25 to 30 percent from fat, and 15 to 20 percent from protein. Less than 10 percent of the total caloric intake should come from saturated fats. In addition, all of the vitamins, minerals, and water must be provided.

Achieving and maintaining a balanced diet is not as difficult as most people think. The difficult part is retraining individuals to eat the right type of foods and avoid those that have little or no nutritive value. Yet, most people are not willing to change their eating patterns. Even when faced with such conditions as obesity, elevated blood lipids, hypertension, etc., people still do not change. The motivating factor seems to be when a major health breakdown actually occurs (e.g. a heart attack, a stroke, cancer). By this time the damage has already been done. In many cases it is irreversible and, for some, fatal.

Figure 6.3. *Crude Fiber Content of Selected Foods.*

Food	Serving Size	Crude Fiber (gr)
Almonds	½ cup	1.9
Apple	1 medium	1.5
Banana	1 medium	0.3
Beans (cooked)		
Kidney	½ cup	1.4
Lima	½ cup	1.3
White	½ cup	1.4
Blackberries	½ cup	3.0
Beets (cooked)	½ cup	0.7
Bran	2 tbsp.	0.9
Brazil nuts	½ cup	2.1
Broccoli (cooked)	½ cup	1.2
Brown rice (cooked)	½ cup	0.3
Carrots (cooked)	½ cup	0.8
Cashew nuts	½ cup	1.0
Cauliflower (cooked)	½ cup	0.6
Corn (cooked)	½ cup	0.6
Eggplant (cooked)	½ cup	0.9
Graham Crackers	2	0.4
Lettuce	3 leafs	0.3
Orange	1 medium	0.9
Parsnips (cooked)	½ cup	1.5
Peanuts (roasted)	½ cup	1.7
Pear	1 medium	2.2
Peas (cooked)	½ cup	1.5
Popcorn	3 cups	0.4
Potato (cooked)	1 medium	0.9
Rye Wafers	2	0.3
Strawberries	½ cup	0.9
Stringbeans (cooked)	½ cup	0.8
Summer squash (cooked)	½ cup	0.6
Watermelon	1 cup	0.4
Zucchini (cooked)	½ cup	0.7

Source: Calculated from Composition of Foods, Agriculture Handbook No. 8 and Nutritive Value of American Foods in Common Units, Agriculture Handbook No. 456. U.S. Dept. of Agriculture.

Nutritional Analysis

To evaluate a person's diet, a complete nutritional analysis must be conducted. This analysis can be an educational experience, because most people do not realize how detrimental and non-nutritious many common foods are. The instructions and necessary information to conduct the analysis are provided in Appendix J. To rate the person's diet, the results of the analysis should be compared against the Recommended Dietary Allowances (RDA), also contained in Appendix J. By comparing the results against the RDAs, a good indication of areas of strength and deficiency in the person's diet are obtained. The nutritional analysis can be simplified by using the computer software for this analysis, available through Morton Publishing Company in Englewood, Colorado.

Achieving A Balanced Diet

An individual who has completed a nutritional analysis and has given careful consideration to Figures 6.1 and 6.2 (Vitamins and Minerals) would probably realize that in order to have a well-balanced diet, a variety of foods must be consumed, along with a decreased daily intake in fats and sweets. Although achieving a balanced diet may seem very complex, simple guidelines to achieve an optimal diet are given in Figure 6.4. The basic rules of this "New American Eating Guide" are: (a) to eat the minimum number of servings required for each one of the four basic food groups, and (b) obtain a final positive ("+") score at the end of each day. If these two simple principles are met, the diet will most likely have all of the required nutrients for proper body functions.

To aid a person in balancing the diet, the log given at the end of Appendix J (Figure J.3) can be used to record daily food intake. This record sheet is much easier to keep than the complete dietary analysis. First, the person should make a copy of Figure 6.4 and post it somewhere visible in the kitchen or keep it accessible at all times. Figure J.3 can then be used. Whenever food is consumed, the person must record the code for the food (from Appendix J) and the "+", "NP" (no points), or "–" characters (*see* Figure 6.4: "New American Eating Guide") in the corresponding spaces provided for each day. Individuals on a weight reduction program should also record the caloric content of each food. This information can be obtained from Appendix J, the food container itself, or some of the references given at the end of the Appendix. The information should be recorded immediately after each meal, since it will be easier to keep track of foods and the amount eaten. If twice the amount of a particular serving is eaten, the calories must be doubled and two "+", "–"or "NP" characters should also be recorded. At the end of the day, the diet is evaluated by checking whether the minimum required servings for each food group were

Figure 6.4. *The New American Eating Guide.*

NEW AMERICAN EATING GUIDE

Instructions

Eating can be a real joy, especially when you know that your diet is keeping you healthy. Eat foods from each of the four groups every day. Each food group contains different nutrients that your body needs. But each group has some foods that are better than others. This figure will help you pick the foods that best contribute to good health. A good diet consists of vegetalbes, fruits, whole wheat bread and grains, potatoes, beans, lean meat, fish, poultry, and low-fat dairy products. This diet is high in nutrients and low in fat, sugar, salt and cholesterol. Pick plenty of ANYTIME foods— they should be the backbone of your diet. They are low in fat (less than 30% of a food's calories) and low in sugar and salt. Grain foods are mostly unrefined, whole grains, and therefore high in fiber and trace minerals. Next best are the IN MODERATION foods. They contain moderate amounts of either saturated fats [1] or unsaturated fats [2]. Some items contain large amounts of fat, but mostly mono-unsaturated or polyunsaturated [3]. (The small numbers listed after items in the chart denote a food's drawbacks.) Eat small portions of NOW & THEN foods and eat them less often than the other foods. They are usually high in fat, with large amounts of saturated fats [4], or they are very high in added sugar [5], salt [6], or cholesterol [7]. Foods that are sometimes high in salt, depending on the manufacturer or recipe, are designated [6]. Try to eat only two NOW & THEN foods a day. Foods that contain low to moderate amounts of fat but are high in sugar, salt, cholesterol, or refined grains [8], are usually moved one or sometimes two categories to the right. You can make a game out of rating your diet by keeping track of the foods you eat for one or several days. ANYTIME foods get one point; IN MODERATION foods do not get any points; and NOW & THEN foods lose one point. If you have a "+" score, congratulations! If you have a "-" score, shape up! BON APPETIT!

1—moderate fat, saturated   2—moderate fat, unsaturated   3—high fat, unsaturated   4—high fat, saturated   5—high in added sugar

6—high in salt or sodium   (6)—may be high in salt or sodium   7—high in cholesteral   8—refined grains

	Anytime	In Moderation	Now & Then
group 1 **Beans, Grains & Nuts** FOUR OR MORE SERVINGS/DAY	bread & rolls (whole grain) bulghur dried beans & peas (legumes) lentils oatmeal pasta, whole wheat rice, brown rye bread sprouts whole grain hot & cold cereals whole wheat matzoh	cornbread - 8 flour tortilla - 8 granola cereals - 1 or 2 hominy grits - 8 macaroni and cheese - 1, (6), 8 matzoh - 8 nuts - 3 pasta, except whole wheat - 8 peanut butter - 3 pizza - 6, 8 refined, unsweetened cereals - 8 refined beans, commercial - 1, or homemade in oil - 2 seeds - 3 soybeans - 2 tofu - 2 waffles or pancakes with syrup - 5, (6), 8 white bread and rolls - 8 white rice - 8	croissant - 4, 8 doughnut (yeast-leavened) - 3 or 4, 5, 8 presweetened breakfast cereals - 5, 8 sticky buns - 1 or 2, 5, 8 stuffing (made with butter) - 4, (6), 8
group 2 **Fruits & Vegetables** FOUR OR MORE SERVINGS/DAY	all fruits and vegetables except those listed at right applesauce (unsweetened) unsweetened fruit juices unsalted vegetable juices potatoes, white or sweet	avocado - 3 cole slaw - 3 cranberry sauce (canned) - 5 dried fruit french fries, homemade in vegetable oil - 2, commercial - 1 fried eggplant (vegetable oil) - 2 fruits canned in syrup - 5 gazpacho - 2, (6) glazed carrots - 5, (6) guacamole - 3 potatoes au gratin - 1, (6) salted vegetable juices - 6 sweetened fruit juices - 5 vegetables canned with salt - 6	coconut - 4 pickles - 6

Figure 6.4. *The New American Eating Guide (continued)*

group 3 Milk Products

CHILDREN: 3 TO 4 SERVINGS/DAY

ADULTS: 2 SERVINGS/DAY

ANYTIME	IN MODERATION	NOW AND THEN
buttermilk made from skim milk	cocoa made with skim milk - 5	cheesecake - 4, 5
lassi (low-fat yogurt & fruit juice drink)	cottage cheese, regular, 4% milkfat - 5	cheese fondue - 4, (6)
low-fat cottage cheese	frozen lowfat yogurt - 5	cheese souffle - 4, (6), 7
low-fat milk, 1% milkfat	ice milk - 5	egg nog - 1, 5, 7
low-fat yogurt	low-fat milk, 2% milkfat - 1	hard cheeses: bleu, brick, camembert, cheddar, muenster, swiss - 4, (6)
non-fat dry milk	low-fat yogurt, sweetened - 5	ice cream - 4, 5
skim milk cheeses - (6)	mozzarella cheese, part-skim type only - 1, (6)	processed cheeses - 4, 6
skim milk		whole milk - 4
skim milk & banana shake		whole milk yogurt - 4

group 4 Poultry, Fish, Meat & Eggs

TWO SERVINGS/DAY

VEGETARIANS: Nutrients in these foods can be obtained by eating more foods in Groups 1, 2 & 3

ANYTIME	IN MODERATION	NOW AND THEN
FISH	FISH *(drained well, if canned)*	POULTRY
cod	fried fish - 1 or 2	fried chicken, commercially prepared - 4
flounder	herring - 3, 6	
gefilte fish - (6)	mackerel, canned - 2, (6)	EGG
haddock	salmon, pink, canned - 2, (6)	cheese omelet - 4, 7
halibut	sardines - 2, (6)	egg yolk or whole egg (about 3/week) - 3, 7
perch	shrimp - 7	
pollock	tuna, oil-packed - 2, (6)	RED MEATS
rockfish	POULTRY	bacon - 4, (6)
shellfish, except shrimp	chicken liver, baked or broiled - 7, (just one!)	beef liver, fried - 1, 7
sole	fried chicken, homemade in vegetable oil - 3	bologna - 4, 6
tuna, water-packed - (6)	chicken or turkey, broiled, baked, or roasted (with skin) - 2	corned beef - 4, 6
EGG PRODUCTS	RED MEATS *(trimmed of all outside fat!)*	ground beef - 4
egg whites **only**	flank steak - 1	ham, trimmed well - 1, 6
POULTRY	leg or loin of lamb - 1	hot dogs - 4, 6
chicken or turkey boiled, baked or roasted (no skin)	pork shoulder or loin, lean - 1	liverwurst - 4, 6
	round steak or ground round - 1	pig's feet - 4
	rump roast - 1	salami - 4, 6
	sirloin steak, lean - 1	sausage - 4, 6
	veal - 1	spareribs - 4
		untrimmed red meats - 4

Sweets

Adding a teaspoon of sugar to your food or eating occasional sweets will not cause any problems. Sugar becomes a problem when foods high in sugar are eaten frequently, particularly between meals. Refined sugars now make up almost one-fifth of the average diet, three times as much as a hundred years ago. This sugar promotes tooth decay and obesity. Also, sugar's "empty calories" squeeze more nutritious foods out of the diet.

Fats added to food

Fats, oils and shortening—like the fat that occurs in meat, dairy products, and other foods—add calories to the diet and can help make you fat. Even more importantly, eating too much *saturated* fat greatly increases the risk of heart disease. Use as little fat as you can. The better fats are mayonnaise, margarine, and vegetable oils (except coconut and palm), but even these can be overdone. The fats to avoid are those richest in saturated fat: butter, sour cream, cream cheese, lard and coconut and palm oils. Fats used commercially (restaurants, baked goods, etc.) often are high in saturated fat.

Snacks

Snacking is fine, as long as the snacks are healthful and do not spoil your appetite for meals. Fruit, plain popcorn, raw vegetables, banana/skim milk shakes and some of the foods in the ANYTIME column all make fine snacks. Chocolate, doughnuts, ice cream, pies and pastries are among the worst snacks, because they are high in both sugar and fat. When a sweet tooth strikes, and you are out of fruit, choose blueberry muffins, gingerbread, ice milk, sherbet, animal crackers and graham crackers, which are high in sugar, but at least low in fat. Drink water, fruit or vegetable juice, or low-fat milk instead of soda pop and imitation fruit drinks. Good snacks usually lead to good teeth.

Reprinted from **New American Eating Guide** poster which is available from the **Center for Science in the Public Interest**, 1501 16th Street, N.W., Washington, D.C., for $3.95. copyright 1982.
One serving equals: Group 1 = 1 slice of bread, 1 cup ready-to-eat cereal, ½ cup cooked cereal/pasta/grits, or equivalent; **Group 2** = ½ cup cooked or juice, or 1 medium size fruit; **Group 3** = 1 cup milk/yogurt, 1½ oz. cheese, 1 cup pudding/ice cream, 2 cups cottage cheese, or equivalent; **Group 4** = 2 oz. cooked lean meat/fish/poultry, 2 eggs, or equivalent.

consumed, and by adding up the "+" and "–" points accumulated. If the required servings have been met and the person ends up with a positive score, a well-balanced diet has been achieved.

PHYSIOLOGY OF WEIGHT CONTROL

Achieving and maintaining ideal body weight (ideal body fat percentage) is a major objective of a good physical fitness and wellness program. Next to poor cardiovascular fitness, obesity is the most common problem encountered in fitness and wellness assessments. Estimates indicate that only 5 to 10 percent of all the people who ever initiate a traditional weight loss program are able to lose the desired weight, and worse yet, only one in 200 is able to keep the weight off for a significant period of time. You may ask why the traditional diets have failed. The answer is simply because very few diets teach the importance of lifetime changes in food selection and the role of exercise as the keys to successful weight loss. The diet industry is a multimillion-dollar industry that tries to capitalize on the idea that weight can be lost quickly, without taking into consideration the long-term consequences of fast weight loss.

Fad Dieting

There are several reasons why fad diets continue to deceive people and can claim that weight will indeed be lost if "all" instructions are followed. Most diets are low in calories and/or deprive the body of certain nutrients, creating a metabolic imbalance that can even cause death. Under such conditions, a lot of the weight loss is in the form of water and protein and not fat. On a crash diet, close to 50 percent of the weight loss is in lean (protein) tissue. When the body uses protein instead of a combination of fats and carbohydrates as a source of energy, weight is lost as much as ten times faster. A gram of protein yields half the amount of energy that fat does. In the case of muscle protein, one-fifth of protein is mixed with four-fifths water. In other words, each pound of muscle yields only one-tenth the amount of energy of a pound of fat. As a result, most of the weight loss is in the form of water, which on the scale, of course, looks good. Nevertheless, when regular eating habits are resumed, most of the lost weight comes right back.

Some diets only allow the consumption of certain foods. If people would only realize that there are no "magic" foods that will provide all of the necessary nutrients, and that a person has to eat a variety of foods to be well-nourished, the diet industry would not be as successful. The unfortunate thing about most of these diets is that they create a nutritional deficiency which at times can be fatal. The reason why some of these diets succeed is because in due time people get tired of eating the same thing day in and day out and eventually start eating less. If they happen to achieve the lower weight, once they go back to old eating habits without implementing permanent dietary changes, weight is quickly gained back again.

A few diets recommend exercise along with caloric restrictions, which, of course, is the best method for weight reduction. A lot of the weight lost is due to exercise; hence, the diet has achieved its purpose. Unfortunately, if no permanent changes in food selection and activity level take place, once dieting and exercise are discontinued, the weight is quickly gained back.

Although only a few years ago the principles that govern a weight loss and maintenance program seemed to be pretty clear, we now know that the final answers are not yet in. The traditional concepts related to weight control have been centered around three assumptions: (1) that balancing food intake against output allows a person to achieve ideal weight, (2) that fat people just eat too much, and (3) that it really does not matter to the human body how much (or little) fat is stored. While there may be some truth to these statements, they are still open to much debate and research.

The Energy-Balancing Equation

The energy-balancing equation basically states that as long as caloric input equals caloric output, the person will not gain or lose weight. If caloric intake exceeds the output, the individual will gain weight. When output exceeds input, weight is lost. This principle is simple, and if daily energy requirements could be accurately determined, it seems reasonable that the conscious mind could be used to balance caloric intake versus output.

Unfortunately, this is not always the case, because there are large individual differences, genetic and lifestyle-related, which determine the number of calories required to maintain or lose body weight. Some general guidelines for estimating daily caloric intake according to lifestyle patterns are given in Figure 6.5. But remember that this is only an estimated figure and, as will be discussed later on in this chapter, it only serves as a starting point from whence individual adjustments will have to be made.

Perhaps some examples may help explain this. It is well known that one pound of fat equals 3,500 calories. Assuming that the basic daily caloric expenditure for a given person is 2,500 calories, if this person decreased the daily intake by 500 calories per day, one pound of fat should be lost in seven days (500 x 7 = 3,500). Research has shown, however, and many dieters have probably experienced, that even when caloric input is carefully balanced against caloric output, weight loss does not always come as predicted. Furthermore, two people with similar measured caloric intake and output will not necessarily lose weight at the same rate.

The most common explanation given by many in the past regarding individual differences in weight loss or weight gain was variations in human metabolism from one person to the other. We have all seen people who can eat all day long and yet not gain an ounce of weight, while others cannot even "dream" about food without gaining weight. Since many experts did not believe that such extreme differences could be accounted to human metabolism alone, several theories have been developed that may better explain these individual variations.

Setpoint Theory

Recent scientific research has indicated that there is a weight-regulating mechanism (WRM) located in the hypothalamus of the brain that regulates how much the body should weigh. This mechanism has a setpoint that controls both appetite and the amount of fat stored. It is hypothesized that the setpoint works like a thermostat for body fat, maintaining body weight fairly constant because it knows at all times the exact amount of adipose tissue stored in the fat cells. Some people have high settings, and others are low. If body weight decreases (as in dieting), this change is sensed by the setpoint which, in turn, triggers the WRM to increase the person's appetite or make the body conserve energy to maintain the "set" weight. The opposite may also be true. Some people who consciously try to gain weight have an extremely difficult time in doing so. In this case, the WRM decreases appetite or causes the body to waste energy to maintain the lower weight.

Dieting Makes People Fat!

Every person has his/her own certain body fat percentage (as established by the setpoint) that the body attempts to maintain. The genetic instinct to survive tells the body that fat storage is vital, and therefore it sets an inherently acceptable fat level. This level of fat remains pretty constant or may gradually climb due to poor lifestyle habits. For instance, under strict caloric reductions, the body may make extreme metabolic adjustments in an effort to maintain its setpoint for fat. The basal metabolic rate may drop dramatically against a consistent negative caloric balance, and a person may be on a plateau for days or even weeks without losing much weight. Dietary restriction alone will not lower the setpoint even though weight and fat may be lost. When the dieter goes back to the normal or even below normal caloric intake, at which the weight may have been stable for a long period of time, the fat loss is quickly regained as the body strives to regain a comfortable fat store.

Let's use a practical illustration. A person would like to lose some body fat and assumes that a stable body weight has been reached at an average daily caloric intake of 1,800 calories (no weight gain or loss occurs at this daily intake). This person now starts a strict low-calorie diet, or even worse, a near-fasting diet in an attempt to achieve rapid weight loss. Immediately the body activates its survival mechanism and readjusts its metabolism to a lower caloric balance. After a few weeks of dieting at less than 400 to 600 calories per day, the body can now maintain its normal functions at 1,000 calories per day. Having lost the desired weight, the person terminates the diet but realizes that the original caloric intake of 1,800 calories per day will need to be decreased to maintain the new lower weight. Therefore, to adjust to the new lower body weight, the intake is restricted to about 1,500 calories per day, but the individual is surprised to find out that even at this lower daily intake (300 fewer calories), weight is gained back at a rate of one pound every one to two weeks. This new lowered metabolic rate, as pointed out in a Swedish study, may take a year or more after terminating the diet to kick back up to its normal level.

From this explanation, it is clear that individuals should never go on very low-calorie diets. Not only will this practice decrease resting metabolic rate, but it will also deprive the body of the basic daily nutrients required for normal physiological functions. Under no circumstances should a person ever engage in diets below 1,200 and 1,500 calories for women and men, respectively. Remember that weight (fat) is gained over a period of months and years and not overnight. Equally, weight loss should be accomplished gradually and not abruptly. Daily caloric intakes of 1,200 to 1,500 calories will still provide the necessary nutrients if properly distributed over the four basic food groups (meeting the daily required servings from each group). Of course, the individual will have to learn which foods meet the requirements, and yet are low in fat and sugar. This can be easily learned after only a few days of following the "New American Eating Guide."

Setpoint and Nutrition

Other researchers feel that a second way in which the setpoint may work is by keeping track of the nutrients and calories that are consumed on a daily basis. The body, like a cash register, records the daily food intake, and the brain will not feel satisfied until the calories and nutrients have been "registered."

For some people this setpoint for calories and nutrients seems to work regardless of the amount of physical activity that they do, as long as it is not too exhausting. Numerous studies have shown that hunger does not increase with moderate physical activity. In such cases, people can choose to lose weight by either going hungry or by increasing daily physical (aerobic) activity. The increased number of calories burned through exercise will help decrease body fat.

The most common question that individuals seem to have regarding the setpoint is how can it

be lowered so that the body will feel comfortable at a lower fat percentage. Several factors seem to have a direct effect on the setpoint. Aerobic exercise and a diet high in complex carbohydrates, nicotine, and amphetamines all have been shown to decrease this fat thermostat. The last two, however, are more destructive than the overfatness, thereby eliminating themselves as reasonable alternatives (it has been said that as far as the extra strain on the heart is concerned, smoking one pack of cigarettes per day is the equivalent of carrying fifty to seventy-five pounds of excess body fat). On the other hand, a diet high in fats and refined carbohydrates, near-fasting diets, and even artificial sweeteners seem to increase the setpoint. Therefore, it looks as though the only practical and effective way to lower the setpoint and lose fat weight is through a combination of aerobic exercise and a diet high in complex carbohydrates and low in fat and sugar.

Because of the effects of proper food management on the body's setpoint, many nutritionists now believe that the total number of calories should not be a concern in a weight control program, but rather the source of those calories. In this regard, most of the effort is spent in retraining eating habits, increasing the intake of complex carbohydrates and high-fiber foods and decreasing the use of refined carbohydrates (sugars) and fats. In addition, a "diet" is no longer viewed as a temporary tool to aid in weight loss, but rather as a permanent change in eating behaviors to insure adequate weight management and health enhancement. The role of increased physical activity must also be considered, because successful weight loss, maintenance, and ideal body composition are seldom achieved without a regular exercise program.

Yellow Fat Versus Brown Fat

For years it has been known that there are two different types of fat, yellow and brown. The proportion of yellow to brown could be another factor that influences weight regulation. The average ratio is about 99 percent yellow fat to 1 percent brown fat. The difference between the two is that yellow fat simply stores energy in the form of fat, while brown fat has a high amount of the iron-containing hemoglobin pigment found in red blood cells. The brown cells do not store fat, but rather have the capacity to produce body heat by burning the fat. Under resting conditions, brown fat produces an estimated 25 percent of the total body heat, and, according to Dr. George A. Bray of the Los Angeles Medical Center at Harbour University of California, the brown fat can actually produce as much heat as the entire rest of the body.

The fact that brown fat converts food energy to heat may also explain why some individuals simply do not gain weight. Even though the amount of brown fat is genetically determined and cannot be changed throughout life, people with only slightly higher levels may have an advantage when it comes to weight control. It is also possible that some individuals may have active brown cells that generate more heat. Perhaps you have come across thin people who are warm even when everyone else seems comfortable. On the contrary, since one of the basic functions of fat is body heat preservation, obese people who are successful in losing weight but have a lower proportion of less active brown fat may feel cold when it is actually pleasantly warm.

Diet and Metabolism

Fat can be lost using proper food selection, aerobic exercise, and/or caloric restrictions. However, when weight loss is pursued by means of dietary restrictions alone, there will always be a decrease in lean body mass (muscle protein, along with vital organ protein). The amount of lean body mass lost depends exclusively on the caloric restriction of your diet. In near-fasting diets, up to 50 percent of the weight loss can be lean body mass, and the other 50 percent will be actual fat loss. When diet is combined with exercise, 98 percent of the weight loss will be in the form of fat, and there may actually be an increase in lean tissue. Lean body mass loss is never desirable because it weakens the organs and muscles and slows down the metabolism.

Contrary to some beliefs, metabolism does not decrease with age. It has been shown that basal metabolism is directly related to lean body weight. The greater the lean tissue, the higher the metabolic rate. What happens is that as a result of sedentary living and less physical activity, the lean component decreases and fat tissue increases. The organism, though, continues to use the same amount of oxygen per pound of lean body mass. Since fat is considered metabolically inert from the point of view of caloric use, the lean tissue uses most of the oxygen even at rest. Consequently, as muscle and organ mass decreases, the energy requirements at rest also decrease.

Decreases in lean body mass are commonly seen with aging (due to physical inactivity) and severely restricted diets. The loss of lean body mass may also account for the lower metabolic rate described under "dieting makes people fat" and the lengthy period of time that it takes to kick back up. There are no diets with caloric intakes below 1,200 to 1,500 calories that can insure no loss of lean body mass. Even at this intake, there is some loss unless the diet is combined with exercise. Many diets have claimed that the lean component is unaltered with their particular diet, but the simple truth is that regardless of what nutrients may be added to the diet, if caloric restrictions are too severe, there will always be a loss of lean tissue.

Unfortunately, too many people constantly engage in low-calorie diets, and every time they do so, the metabolic rate keeps slowing down as more lean tissue is lost. It is not uncommon to find individuals in the forties or older who weigh the same as they did when they were twenty and feel that they are at ideal body weight. Nevertheless, during this span of twenty years or more, they have "dieted" all too many times without engaging in physical activity. The weight is regained shortly after terminating each diet, but most of that gain is in fat. Perhaps at age twenty they weighed 150 pounds and were only 15 to 16 percent fat. Now at age forty, even though they still weigh 150 pounds, they may be 30 to 40 percent fat. They may feel that they are at ideal body weight and wonder why it is that they are eating very little and still have a difficult time maintaining weight.

Exercise: The Key to Successful Weight Loss and Weight Maintenance

Based on the preceding discussion on weight control, it can be easily concluded that exercise is the key to weight loss. Not only will exercise maintain lean tissue, but advocates of the setpoint theory also indicate that it resets the fat thermostat to a new lower level. For a lot of people this change occurs rapidly, but in some instances it may take time. There are overweight individuals who have faithfully exercised on an almost daily basis, sixty minutes at a time, for a whole year before significant weight changes started to occur. Individuals who have a very "sticky" setpoint will need to be patient and persistent.

For individuals who are trying to lose weight, a combination of aerobic and strength training exercises works best. Aerobic exercise is the key to offset the setpoint, and because of the continuity and duration of these types of activities, many calories are burned in the process. On the other hand, strength training exercises have their greatest impact in increasing lean body mass. Strength training is especially recommended for individuals who feel that they are at optimal body weight, but yet the body fat percentage is higher than ideal. Nevertheless, the number of calories burned during an "average" hour of strength training is significantly less than during an hour of aerobic exercise. Due to the high intensity of weight training, frequent rest intervals are required to recover from each set of exercise. The average individual only engages in actual lifting a total of twelve minutes out of every hour of exercise. Weight loss can occur with a regular weight training program but at a much slower rate. The guidelines for developing aerobic and strength training programs are given in Appendices C and D.

It is also important to clarify that just doing several sets of daily sit-ups will not help to get rid of fat in the midsection of the body. Research has shown that there is no such thing as spot reducing. When fat comes off, it does so from throughout the entire body, and not just the exercised area. The greatest proportion of fat may come off the largest fat deposits, but the caloric output of a few sets of sit-ups is practically nil to have a real effect on total body fat reduction. The amount of exercise has to be much longer to have a real impact on weight reduction.

Although we now know that a negative caloric balance of 3,500 calories will not always result in an exact loss of one pound of fat, the role of exercise in achieving a negative balance by burning additional calories is significant in weight reduction and maintenance programs. Sadly, some individuals claim that the amount of calories burned during exercise is hardly worth the effort. These individuals feel that it is easier to cut the daily intake by some 200 calories, rather than

participate in some sort of physical activity that would burn the equivalent amount of calories. The only problem is that the willpower to cut those 200 calories only lasts a few weeks, and then it is right back to the old eating patterns. If a person gets into the habit of exercising regularly, say three times per week, running three miles per exercise session (about 300 calories burned), this would represent 900 calories in one week, 3,600 in one month, or 43,200 calories per year. This apparently insignificant amount of exercise could mean as many as twelve extra pounds of fat in one year, twenty-four in two, and so on. We tend to forget that our weight creeps up gradually over the years, and not just overnight. Hardly worth the effort? And we have not even taken into consideration the increase in lean tissue, the possible resetting of the setpoint, the benefits to the cardiovascular system, and most important, the improved quality of life! There is very little argument that the fundamental reasons for over-fatness and obesity are physical inactivity and sedentary living.

LOSING WEIGHT THE SOUND AND SENSIBLE WAY

Dieting has never been fun and never will be. Individuals who have a weight problem and are serious about losing weight will have to make exercise a regular part of their daily life, along with proper food management, and perhaps even sensible adjustments in caloric intake. Some precautions are necessary, since excessive body fat is a risk factor for cardiovascular disease. Depending on the extent of the weight problem, a stress ECG may be required prior to initiating the exercise program. A physician should be consulted in this regard.

Significantly overweight individuals may also have to choose activities where they will not have to support their own body weight, but that will still be effective in burning calories. Joint and muscle injuries are very common among overweight individuals who participate in weight-bearing exercises such as walking, jogging, and aerobic dancing. Swimming may not be a good exercise either. The increased body fat makes the person more buoyant, and most people do not have the skill level to swim fast enough to get an optimal training effect. The tendency is to just "float" along, limiting the amount of calories burned as well as the benefits to the cardiovascular system. Some better alternatives are riding a bicycle (either road or stationary), walking in a shallow pool, or running in place in deep water (treading water). The last exercise is quickly gaining in popularity and has proven to be effective in achieving weight reduction without the "pain" and fear of injuries.

How long should each exercise session last? To develop and maintain cardiovascular fitness, twenty to thirty minutes of exercise at the ideal target rate, three to five times per week is sufficient. For weight loss purposes, many experts recommend exercising for an hour at a time, five to six times per week. Nevertheless, a person should not try to increase the duration and frequency of exercise too fast. It is recommended that unconditioned beginners start with about fifteen minutes three times per week, and then gradually increase the duration by approximately five minutes each week and the frequency by one day per week during the next three to four weeks. Exercising for sixty minutes an average of five to six times per week will not only insure a high caloric output, but due to the prolonged duration of exercise, will also keep the metabolic rate at a higher level long after the individual has finished the exercise session. In other words, extra calories are still being burned even though the person is done exercising. The longer the duration of exercise in the appropriate cardiovascular target zone, the longer it will take the body to return to the basal rate.

One final benefit of exercise as related to weight control is that fat can be burned more efficiently. Since both carbohydrates and fats are sources of energy, when the glucose levels begin to decrease during prolonged exercise, more fat is used as energy substrate. Equally important is the fact that fat-burning enzymes increase with aerobic training. The role of these enzymes is significant, because fat can only be lost by burning it in muscle. As the concentration of the enzymes increase, so does the ability to burn fat.

In addition to exercise and adequate food management, many experts still recommend that individuals take a look at their daily caloric intake and compare it against the estimated daily requirement. The daily caloric intake is determined through the nutritional analysis (*see* Appendix J). While this intake may not be as crucial if proper food management and exercise are incorporated into the person's lifestyle, it is still beneficial in certain circumstances. All too often the nutritional analysis reveals that "faithful" dieters are not consuming enough calories and actually need to increase the daily caloric intake (combined with an exercise program) in order to get the metabolism to kick back up to a normal level. The estimated caloric requirement based on gender, body weight, and lifestyle patterns can be determined using Figure 6.5.

There are other cases where knowledge of the daily caloric requirement is needed for successful weight control. The reasons for prescribing a certain caloric figure to either maintain or lose weight are: (a) it takes time to develop new behaviors and some individuals have difficulty in changing and adjusting to the new eating habits; (b) many individuals are in such poor physical condition that it takes them a long time to increase their activity level so as to have a significant impact in offsetting the setpoint and in burning enough calories to aid in body fat loss; (c) some dieters find it difficult to succeed unless they can count calories; and (d) some individuals will simply not alter their food selection. All of these people can benefit from a caloric intake guideline, and in many instances a sensible caloric decrease

Figure 6.5. *Average Caloric Requirement Per Pound of Body Weight Based on Lifestyle Patterns and Sex.*

	Calories per pound	
Activity Rating	**Men**	**Women**[a]
Sedentary — Limited physical activity	13.0	12.0
Moderate physical activity	15.0	13.5
Hard labor — Strenuous physical effort	17.0	15.0

[a]Pregnant or lactating women add three calories to these figures.

is helpful in the early stages of the weight reduction program. For the latter group, that is, those who will not alter their food selection, a significant increase in physical activity, a negative caloric balance, or a combination of both are the only solutions for successful weight loss.

An estimated caloric requirement can be determined by using Figures 6.5 and 6.6. Keep in mind that this is only an estimated value, and individual adjustments related to many of the factors discussed in this chapter may be required to establish a more precise value. Nevertheless, the estimated value will provide an initial guideline for weight control and/or reduction.

The average daily caloric requirement without exercise is based on typical lifestyle patterns, total body weight, and gender. Individuals who hold jobs that require heavy manual labor burn more calories during the day as opposed to those who hold sedentary jobs (such as working behind a desk). To determine the activity level, refer to Figure 6.5 and rate the person accordingly. Since the number given in Figure 6.5 is per pound of body weight, multiply the person's current weight by that number. For example, the typical caloric requirement to maintain body weight for a moderately active male who weighs 160 pounds would be 2,400 calories (160 lbs. x 15 cal/lb.).

The second step is to determine the average number of calories that are burned on a daily basis as a result of exercise. To obtain this number, you will need to figure out the total number of

Figure 6.6. *Caloric Expenditure of Selected Physical Activities (expressed in calories per pound per minute of physical activity).*

Activity	Cal/min/lb	Activity	Cal/min/lb
Archery	0.030	Rowing (vigorous)	0.090
Badminton		Running	
Recreation	0.038	11.0 min/mile	0.070
Competition	0.065	8.5 min/mile	0.090
Baseball	0.031	7.0 min/mile	0.102
Basketball		6.0 min/mile	0.114
Moderate	0.046	Deep water[a]	0.100
Competition	0.063	Skating (moderate)	0.038
Cycling (level)		Skiing	
5.5 mph	0.033	Downhill	0.060
10.0 mph	0.050	Level (5 mph)	0.078
13.0 mph	0.071	Soccer	0.059
Bowling	0.030	Swimming (crawl)	
Calisthenics	0.033	20 yrds/min	0.031
Dance		25 yrds/min	0.040
Moderate	0.030	45 yrds/min	0.057
Vigorous	0.055	50 yrds/min	0.070
Golf	0.030	Table Tennis	0.030
Gymnastics		Tennis	
Light	0.030	Moderate	0.045
Heavy	0.056	Competition	0.064
Handball	0.064	Volleyball	0.030
Hiking	0.040	Walking	
Judo/Karate	0.086	4.5 mph	0.045
Racquetball	0.065	Shallow pool	0.090
Rope Jumping	0.060	Wrestling	0.085

[a]Treading water (estimated value)

Adapted from:
  Allsen, P. E., J. M. Harrison, B. Vance. *Fitness for Life: An Individualized Approach.* Dubuque, IA: Wm. C. Brown, 1984.
  Bucher, C. A., and W. E. Prentice. *Fitness for College and Life.* St. Louis: Times Mirror/Mosby College Publishing, 1985.
  Consolazio, C. F., R. E. Johnson, and L. J. Pecora. *Physiological Measurements of Metabolic Functions in Man.* New York: McGraw-Hill Book Company, 1963.
  Hockey, R. V. *Physical Fitness: The Pathway to Healthful Living.* St. Louis: Times Mirror/Mosby College Publishing, 1985.

minutes in which the individual engages in physical activity on a weekly basis, and then determine the daily average exercise time. For instance, a person cycling at thirteen miles per hour, five times per week, for thirty minutes each time, exercises a total 150 minutes per week (5 x 30). The average daily exercise time would be twenty-one minutes (150 ÷ 7 and round off to the lowest unit). Next, using Figure 6.6, determine the energy requirement for the activity (or activities) that have been chosen for the exercise program. In the case of cycling (thirteen miles per hour), the requirement is .071 calories per minute of activity per pound of body weight (cal/min/lb). With a body weight of 160 pounds, each minute this man would burn 11.4 calories (body weight x .071 or 160 x .071). In twenty-one minutes, he would burn approximately 240 calories (21 x 11.4).

The third step is to determine the estimated total caloric requirement, with exercise, needed to maintain body weight. This value is obtained by adding the typical daily requirement (without exercise) and the average calories burned through exercise. In our example, it would be 2,640 calories (2,400 + 240).

If a negative caloric balance is recommended to lose weight, this person would have to consume less than 2,640 daily calories to achieve the objective. Because of the many different factors that play a role in weight control, the previous value is only an estimated daily requirement. Furthermore, to lose weight, it would be difficult to say that exactly one pound of fat would be lost in one week if daily intake was reduced by 500 calories (500 x 7 = 3,500 calories, or the equivalent of one pound of fat). Nevertheless, the estimated daily caloric figure will provide a target guideline for weight control. Periodic readjustments are necessary because there can be significant differences among individuals, and the estimated daily cost will change as you lose weight and modify your exercise habits.

The recommended number of calories to be subtracted from the daily intake to obtain a negative caloric balance depends on the typical daily requirement. At this point, the best recommendation is to moderately decrease the daily intake, never below 1,200 calories for women and 1,500 for men. A good rule to follow is to restrict the intake by no more than 500 calories if the daily requirement is below 3,000 calories. For caloric requirements in excess of 3,000, as many as 1,000 calories per day may be subtracted from the total intake. Remember also that the daily distribution should be approximately 60 percent carbohydrates (mostly complex carbohydrates), 25 percent fat, and 15 percent protein.

The time of the day when food is consumed may also play a role in weight reduction. A study conducted at the Aerobics Research Center in Dallas, Texas, indicated that when on a diet, weight is lost most effectively if the majority of the calories are consumed before 1:00 p.m. and not during the evening meal. The recommendation made at this center is that when attempting to lose weight, a minimum of 25 percent of the total daily calories should be consumed for breakfast, 50 percent for lunch, and 25 percent or less at dinner. Other experts have indicated that if most of your daily calories are consumed during one meal, the body may perceive that something is wrong and will slow down your metabolism so that it can store a greater amount of calories in the form of fat. Also, eating most of the calories in one meal causes you to go hungry most of the day, making it more difficult to adhere to the diet.

The principle of consuming most of the calories earlier in the day not only seems to be helpful in losing weight, but also in the management of atherosclerosis. According to one research study, the time of the day when most of the fats and cholesterol are consumed can have an impact on blood lipids and coronary heart disease. Peak digestion time following a heavy meal takes place about seven hours after that meal. If most lipids are consumed during the evening meal, digestion peaks while the person is sound asleep, at a time when the metabolism is at its lowest rate. Consequently, the body may not be able to metabolize fats and cholesterol as effectively, leading to higher blood lipids and increasing the risk for atherosclerosis and coronary heart disease.

To monitor daily progress, a form similar to Figure J.3 (Appendix J) may be used. Meeting the basic requirements from each food group should be given top priority. The caloric content for each food is found in the Nutritive Value of Selected Foods list in Appendix J. The information should be recorded immediately after each meal to obtain a more precise record. According to the person's progress, adjustments can be made in the typical daily requirement and/or the exercise program.

TIPS TO HELP CHANGE BEHAVIOR AND ADHERE TO A LIFETIME WEIGHT MANAGEMENT PROGRAM

Achieving and maintaining ideal body composition is by no means an impossible task, but it does require desire and commitment. If adequate weight management is to become a priority in life, people must realize that some retraining in behavior is crucial for success. Modifying old habits and developing new positive behaviors take time.

The following list of management techniques has been successfully used by individuals to change detrimental behavior and adhere to a positive lifetime weight control program. People are not expected to use all of the strategies listed, but they should check the ones that would apply and help in developing a retraining program.

1. Commitment to change. The first ingredient to modify behavior is the desire to do so. The reasons for change must be more important than those for carrying on with present lifestyle patterns. People must accept the fact that there is a problem and decide by themselves whether they really want to change. If a sincere commitment is there, the chances for success are already enhanced.

2. Set realistic goals. Most people with a weight problem would like to lose weight in a relatively short period of time but fail to realize that the weight problem developed over a span of several years. A sound weight reduction and maintenance program can only be accomplished by establishing new lifetime eating and exercise habits, both of which take time to develop.

   In setting a realistic long-term goal, short-term objectives should also be planned. The long-term goal may be a decrease in body fat to 20 percent of total body weight. The short-term objective may be a 1 percent decrease in body fat each month. Such objectives allow for regular evaluation and help maintain motivation and renewed commitment to achieve the long-term goal.

3. Incorporate exercise into the program. Selecting enjoyable activities, places, times, equipment, and people to work with enhances exercise adherence. Details on developing a complete exercise program are found in Appendices C (cardiovascular), E (strength), and F (flexibility).

4. Develop a healthy eating pattern. Plan on eating three regular meals per day consistent with the body's nutritional requirements. Learn to differentiate between hunger and appetite. Hunger is the actual physical need for food. Appetite is a desire for food, usually triggered by factors such as stress, habit, boredom, depression, food availability, or just the thought of food itself. Eating only when there is a physical need is wise weight management. In this regard, developing and sticking to a regular meal pattern helps control hunger.

5. Avoid automatic eating. Many people associate certain daily activities with eating. For example, people eat while cooking, watching television, reading, talking on the telephone, or visiting with neighbors. Most of the time the type of foods consumed in such situations lack nutritional value or are high in sugar and fats.

6. Stay busy. People tend to eat more when they sit around and do nothing. Keeping the mind and body occupied with activities not associated with eating helps decrease the desire to eat. Try walking, cycling, playing sports, gardening, sewing, or visiting a library, a museum, a park, etc. Develop other skills and interests or try something new and exciting to break the routine of life.

7. Plan your meals ahead of time. Wise shopping is required to accomplish this objective (by the way, when shopping, do so on a full stomach since such practice will decrease impulsive buying of unhealthy foods — and then snacking on them on the way home). Include whole-grain breads and cereals, fruits and vegetables, low-fat milk and dairy products, lean meats, fish, and poultry.

8. Cook wisely. Decrease the use of fat and refined foods in food preparation. Trim all visible fat off meats and remove skin off poultry prior to cooking. Skim the fat off gravies and soups. Bake, broil, and boil instead of frying. Use butter, cream, mayonnaise, and salad dressings sparingly. Avoid

shellfish, coconut oil, palm oil, and cocoa butter. Prepare plenty of bulky foods. Add whole-grain breads and cereals, vegetables, and legumes to most meals. Try fruits for dessert. Beware of soda pop, fruit juices, and fruit-flavored drinks. Drink plenty of water, at least six glasses a day.

9. Do not serve more food than can or should be eaten. Measure the food portions and keep serving dishes away from the table. In this manner less food is consumed, seconds are more difficult to obtain, and appetite is decreased because food is not visible. People should not be forced to eat when they are satisfied (including children after they have already had a healthy, nutritious serving).

10. Learn to eat slowly and at the table only. Eating is one of the pleasures of life, and we need to take time to enjoy it. Eating on the run is detrimental because the body is not given sufficient time to "register" nutritive and caloric consumption, and overeating usually occurs before the fullness signal is perceived. Always eating at the table also forces people to take time out to eat and will decrease snacking in between meals, primarily because of the extra time and effort that are required to sit down and eat. When done eating, do not sit around the table. Clean up and put the food away to avoid unnecessary snacking.

11. Avoid social binges. Social gatherings are a common place for self-defeating behavior. Do not feel pressured to eat or drink, nor rationalize in these situations. Choose low-calorie foods and entertain yourself with other activities such as dancing and talking.

12. Beware of raids on the refrigerator and the cookie jar. When such occur, attempt to take control of the situation. Stop and think what is taking place. For those who have difficulty in avoiding such raids, environment management is recommended. Do not bring high-calorie, high-sugar, and/or high-fat foods into the house. If they are brought into the house, they ought to be stored in places where they are difficult to get to or are less visible. If unseen or not readily available, there will be less temptation. Keeping them in places like the garage and basement may be sufficient to discourage many people from taking the time and effort to go get them. By no means should treats be completely eliminated, but all things should be done in moderation.

13. Practice adequate stress management techniques. Many people snack and increase food consumption when confronted with stressful situations. Eating is not a stress-releasing activity and can in reality aggravate the problem if weight control is an issue. Several stress management techniques are discussed in Chapter 7.

14. Monitor changes and reward accomplishments. Feedback on fat loss, lean tissue gain, and/or weight loss is a reward in itself. Awareness of changes in body composition also helps reinforce new behaviors. Furthermore, being able to exercise uninterruptedly for fifteen, twenty, thirty, sixty minutes, or swimming a certain distance, running a mile, etc., are all accomplishments that deserve recognition. When certain objectives are met, rewards that are not related to eating are encouraged. Buy new clothing, a bicycle, exercise shoes, or something else that is special and would have not been acquired otherwise.

15. Think positive. Avoid negative thoughts on how difficult it might be to change past behaviors. Instead, think of the benefits that will be reaped, such as feeling, looking, and functioning better, plus enjoying better health and improving the quality of life. Attempt to stay away from negative environments and people who will not be supportive. Those who do not have the same desires and/or encourage self-defeating behaviors should be avoided.

IN CONCLUSION

There is no simple and quick way to take off excessive body fat and keep it off for good. Weight management is accomplished through a lifetime commitment to physical activity and adequate food selection. When engaged in a weight (fat) reduction program, people may also have to moderately decrease caloric intake and implement appropriate strategies to modify unhealthy eating behaviors.

During the process of behavior modification, it is almost inevitable to relapse and engage in past negative behaviors. Nevertheless, making mistakes is human and does not necessarily mean failure. Failure comes to those who give up and do not use previous experiences to build upon and, in turn, develop appropriate skills that will prevent self-defeating behaviors in the future. "If there is a will, there is a way," and those who persist will reap the rewards.

References

1. Adams, T.D., et al. *Fitness for Life.* Salt Lake City, UT: Intermountain Health Care, Inc., 1983.
2. Bennett, W., and J. Gurin. "Do Diets Really Work?" *Science* 42-50, March 1982.
3. "Brown Fat is Good Fat." *The Health Letter.* December 11, 1981.
4. "Brown Fat/White Fat." *Aviation Medical Bulletin.* June 1981.
5. Cumming, C., and V. Newman. *Eater's Guide: Nutrition Basis for Busy People.* Englewood Cliffs, NJ: Prentice-Hall, 1981.
6. "Dangerous Dieting." *The Health Letter.* July 25, 1980.
7. Girdano, D. A., D. Dusek, and G. S. Everly. *Experiencing Health.* Englewood Cliffs, NJ: Prentice-Hall, 1985.
8. "How to Balance Your Diet." *Fit* 46-47, April 1983.
9. *Interpreting Your Nutritional Analysis.* Lake Geneva, WI: Fitness Monitoring Preventive Medicine Clinic, 1984.
10. Kirschmann, J. D. *Nutrition Almanac.* New York: McGraw-Hill Book Company, 1984.
11. Morgan, B.L.G. *The Lifelong Nutrition Guide.* Englewood Cliffs, NJ: Prentice-Hall, 1983.
12. "Obesity Not Necessarily Related to Overeating." *Aviation Medical Bulletin.* June 1981.
13. Remington, D., A. G. Fisher, and E. A. Parent. *How to Lower Your Fat Thermostat.* Provo, UT: Vitality House International, Inc., 1983.
14. Shephard, R. J. *Alive Man: The Physiology of Physical Activity.* Springfield, IL: Charles C. Thomas Publisher, 1972.
15. "Use a Variety of Fibers." *The Health Letter.* March 1982.
16. "Vitamin Information for Patients." *Medical Times* 35, November 1982.

Stress Management Techniques

Learning to live and get ahead today is practically impossible without stress. To work under pressure has become the rule rather than the exception for most people to succeed in an unpredictable world that changes with every new day. As a result, stress has become one of the most common problems that we face. According to 1986 estimates, the annual cost of stress and stress-related diseases in the United States exceeds $100 billion, a direct result of health care costs, lost productivity, and absenteeism. While excessive stress is one of the factors related to twentieth-century patterns of life that is detrimental to human health, it is also a factor that can be self-controlled. Most people have accepted stress as a normal part of their daily life, and even though everyone has to deal with it, few seem to understand it and know how to cope effectively. On the other hand, stress should not be completely avoided, since a certain amount is necessary for an optimal level of health and performance and well-being. It is difficult to succeed and have fun in life without "hits, runs, and errors."

Just what is stress? Dr. Hans Selye, one of the foremost authorities on stress, defined stress as the nonspecific response of the human organism to any demand that is placed upon it. The term "nonspecific" indicates that the body will react in a similar fashion, regardless of the nature of the event that led to the stress response. In simpler terms, stress is the mental, emotional, and physiological response of the body to any situation that is new, threatening, frightening, or exciting.

The response of the human body to stress has been the same ever since man was first put on the earth. Stress prepares the organism to react to the stress-causing event (also referred to as stressor). The problem, though, is the manner in which we react to stress. Many people thrive under stress, while others under similar circumstances are unable to handle it. The individual's reaction to the particular stress-causing agent will determine whether stress is positive or negative.

The way in which we react to stress has been defined by Dr. Selye as either "eustress" or "distress." In both cases, the nonspecific response is almost the same. In the case of eustress, health and performance continue to improve, even as stress increases. Distress, on the other hand, refers to the unpleasant or harmful stress under which health and performance began to deteriorate. This relationship between stress and performance is illustrated in Figure 7.1.
in Figure 7.1.

But stress is a fact of modern life, and every person does need an optimal level of stress that is most conducive to adequate health and performance. However, when stress levels reach the mental, emotional, and physiological limits, stress becomes distress and the person no longer functions effectively. Chronic distress increases the risk for many health disorders, including coronary heart disease, hypertension, eating disorders, ulcers, diabetes, asthma, depression, migraine headaches, sleep disorders, and chronic fatigue and may even play a role in the development of certain types of cancers. Recognizing this turning point, and overcoming the problem quickly and efficiently, are crucial in maintaining emotional and physiological stability.

SOURCES OF STRESS

During recent years, several instruments have been developed to assess sources of stress in life. One of the most common instruments used is the Life Experiences Survey, which has been included in the wellness questionnaire (Appendix B) under the Tension and Stress section. This survey identifies life changes within the last twelve months that may have an impact on a person's physical and psychological well-being. The survey is divided into two sections. Section 1 is to be completed by all respondents. This section contains a list of forty-seven life events, plus three blank spaces for other events experienced that are not listed in the survey. Section 2 contains an additional ten questions designed for students only (students should fill out both sections).

The format of the survey requires the subjects to rate the extent to which the life events that they experienced had a positive or negative impact on their life at the time they occurred. The ratings are on a seven-point scale. A rating of negative three (-3) indicates an extremely undesirable impact. A rating of zero (0) suggests neither a positive nor a negative impact. A rating of positive three (+3) indicates an extremely desirable impact. After determining the life events that have taken place, the negative and the positive points are added together separately. Both scores should be expressed as positive numbers (e.g. positive ratings: 2, 1, 3, 3, = 9 points positive score; negative ratings: -3, -2, -2, -1, -2 = 10 points negative

score). A final "total life change" score can be obtained by adding both the positive score and negative score together as positive numbers (e.g. total life change score: 9 + 10 = 19 points).

Since negative as well as positive changes can produce a nonspecific response, the total life change score gives a good indication of total life stress. However, most research in this area indicates that the negative change score is a better predictor for potential physical and/or psychological illness than the total change score. More research is necessary before the role of total change and the role of the ratio of positive to negative stress can be established. Therefore, only the negative score is used as a part of the stress profile. To obtain a stress rating, refer to Table 7.1, which presents the various stress categories based on the survey's results.

Behavior Patterns

Common life events are not the only source of stress in life. All too often, stress is brought on by the individual as a result of behavior patterns. In Chapter 4 it was briefly mentioned that individuals can be categorized as having one of two types of behavior patterns: Type A or Type B. Each type has several characteristics that are used in classifying people into one of these behavior patterns. Even though several attempts have been made to develop an objective scale to properly identify the Type A individuals, these questionnaires are not as valid and reliable as researchers would like

Figure 7.1. *Relationship Between Stress and Health and Performance.*

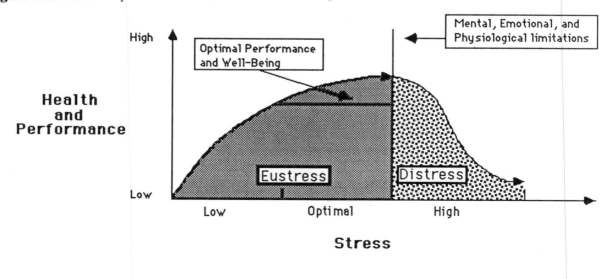

Table 7.1.
Stress Ratings for the Life Experiences Survey.*

Category	Negative Score				Total Score			
	Men		Women		Men		Women	
	I**	II	I	II	I	II	I	II
Poor	9+	13+	12+	15+	20+	27+	21+	27+
Fair	6-8	7-12	7-11	8-14	13-19	17-26	13-20	18-26
Average	5	6	6	7	12	16	12	17
Good	1-4	1-5	1-5	1-6	5-11	5-15	5-11	7-16
Excellent	0	0	0	0	0-4	0-4	0-4	0-6

* Adapted from Sarason, I. G. et al. "Assessing the Impact of Life Changes: Development of the Life Experiences Survey." *Journal of Consulting and Clinical Psychology* 46: 932-946, 1978. Data based on 345 students enrolled in introductory psychology courses at the University of Washington.

** I = refers to Section 1 of the survey to be completed by all respondents (first 47 events plus three blank spaces for other events experienced not listed in the survey). II = refers to Section 1 and Section 2 (Section 2 contains an additional ten events designed primarily for use with students).

them to be. Consequently, the primary assessment tool used to determine behavior type has been the Structured Interview method.

During the Structured Interview, a person is asked to reply to different questions that describe Type A and Type B behavior patterns. The interviewer notes not only the responses to the questions, but also mental, emotional, and physical behaviors exhibited as the individual replies to each question. Based on the answers and the behaviors exhibited, the interviewer actually rates the person along a continuum, ranging from Type A to Type B. Along this continuum, behavior patterns are classified into five categories: A-1, A-2, X (a mix of Type A and Type B), B-3, and B-4. The Type A-1 exhibits all of the Type A characteristics, while a relative absence of the Type A behaviors is observed in the Type B-4. The Type A-2 does not exhibit a complete Type A pattern, and the Type B-3 only exhibits a few Type A characteristics.

The Type A behavior is primarily characteristic of a hard-driving, overambitious, aggressive, at times hostile, and overly competitive person. These individuals often set their own goals, are self-motivated, try to accomplish many tasks at the same time, are excessively achievement-oriented, and have a high degree of time urgency. In contrast, the Type B behavior is characteristic of a calmed, casual, relaxed, and easy-going individual. The Type B person takes one thing at a time, does not feel pressured or hurried, and seldom sets his/her own deadlines.

Over the years, research studies have indicated that individuals classified as Type A are under much more stress and have a significantly higher incidence of coronary heart disease. Based on these findings, Type A individuals have been counseled to decrease their stress level by modifying many of their Type A behaviors. Most experts agree that Type A behavior is learned. Consequently, if people can learn to identify the sources of stress and make changes in behavioral responses, they can move down along the continuum and respond more like the Type B. The debate, however, has been centered around which Type A behaviors should be changed, since not all of them are undesirable.

Although experts have known that individuals exhibiting the Type A behavior were more coronary prone and that behavioral changes were needed to decrease the risk for disease, new scientific evidence indicates that not all of the typical Type A people are at a higher risk for disease. It seems that mainly the Type A individual who commonly exhibits behaviors of anger and hostility is at higher risk for disease. Therefore, many behavioral modification counselors now work primarily on changing the latter behaviors to prevent the incidence of disease.

For years it has also been known that many individuals perform well under pressure. They are typically classified as Type A but never exhibit any of the detrimental effects of stress. These people have recently been referred to by Drs. Robert and

Marilyn Kriegel as exhibiting Type C behavior. The Type C individuals are just as highly stressed as the Type A but do not seem to be at higher risk for disease than the Type B. The keys to successful Type C performance seem to be commitment, confidence, and control. These people are highly committed to what they are doing, have a great deal of confidence in their ability to do their work, and can be in constant control of their actions. In addition, Type C people love and enjoy their work and maintain themselves in top physical condition to be able to meet the mental and physical demands of their work.

STRESS VULNERABILITY

Researchers have now been able to identify a number of factors that can affect the way in which people handle stress. How they deal with these factors can actually increase or decrease their vulnerability to stress. A Stress Vulnerability survey, also found in the Tension and Stress section of the wellness questionnaire, contains a list of several of these factors and has been designed to help people determine their vulnerability quotient. This survey also helps identify particular areas where improvements can be made to cope more efficiently, and, as you may have noticed, most of the items describe situations and behaviors that are within a person's own control. On the survey, individuals rate themselves on a scale from 1 (almost always) to 5 (never), according to how each particular statement applies to them. The final stress vulnerability rating is obtained by totalling the individual ratings and subtracting 20 from the total score. The interpretation of the final score is given in Table 7.2. To decrease the vulnerability to stress, an individual should modify

Table 7.2.
Stress Vulnerability Rating.*

Category	Final Score
Poor	51-80 Points
Fair	31-50 Points
Good	11-30 Points
Excellent	0-10 Points

* From "Vulnerability Scale." *Stress Audit*, developed by Lyle H. Miller and Alma Dell Smith. Boston University Medical Center. Copyright 1983. Biobehavioral Associates. Reproduced with permission.

the behaviors on which a rating of 3 or higher was obtained. It is also recommended that they start by modifying behaviors that are easiest to change before undertaking some of the most difficult ones.

COPING WITH STRESS

Based on the previous introduction to stress, it is obvious that the way in which people perceive and cope with stress seems to be more important in the development of disease than the amount and type of stress itself. For individuals who perceive stress as a definite problem in their lives, that is, when it interferes with their optimal level of health and performance, several excellent stress management techniques have been developed to help them cope more effectively.

The initial step, of course, is to recognize that there is a problem. Many people either do not want to accept the fact that they are under too much stress and/or fail to recognize some of the typical symptoms of distress. Noting some of the stress-related symptoms will help a person respond more objectively and initiate an adequate coping response. A list of different symptoms that people experience when stress becomes distress is given in Figure 7.2. By going through this list, most of us will probably recognize some of our own bodily responses when confronted with a stressful event.

When people experience stress-related symptoms, initially they should try to identify and remove the stressor or stress-causing agent. This is not as simple as it may seem, because in some situations elimination of the stressor is impossible, or a person may not even know the exact causing agent. If the cause is unknown, it may be helpful to keep a log of the time and days when the symptoms occur, as well as the events that transpire before and after the onset of symptoms. For instance, a couple had noted that every afternoon around six o'clock, the wife became very nauseated and experienced a significant amount of abdominal pain. After seeking professional help, the couple was instructed to keep a log of daily events. It soon became clear that the symptoms did not occur on weekends, but always started just before the husband came home from work. Following some personal interviews with the couple, it was determined that the wife felt a lack of attention from her husband and subconsciously

Figure 7.2. *Common Symptoms of Stress.*

- Headaches
- Muscular aches (mainly neck, shoulders, and back)
- Grinding teeth
- Nervous tick, finger tapping, toe tapping
- Increased sweating
- Increase or loss of appetite
- Insomnia
- Nightmares
- Fatigue
- Dry Mouth
- Stuttering
- High blood pressure
- Tightness or pain in the chest
- Impotence
- Hives

- Dizziness
- Depression
- Irritation
- Anger
- Frustration
- Hostility
- Fear, panic, anxiety
- Stomach pain, flutters
- Nausea
- Cold, clammy hands
- Poor concentration
- Pacing
- Restlessness
- Rapid heart rate
- Low-grade infection
- Loss of sex drive
- Rash or acne

responded by becoming ill to the point where it required personal care and affection from her husband. Once the stressor is identified, appropriate changes in behavior can be initiated to correct the situation.

However, there are many instances where the stressor cannot be removed. For example, the death of a close family member, first year on the job, an intolerable boss, a change in work responsibility, etc. are all situations in which very little or nothing can be done to eliminate the stress-causing agent. Nevertheless, stress can still be managed through the use of adequate relaxation techniques.

The body responds to stress by activating the "fight or flight" mechanism, which prepares a person to take action by stimulating the vital defense systems. This stimulation originates in the hypothalamus and the pituitary gland in the brain. The hypothalamus activates the sympathetic nervous system and the pituitary activates the release of catecholamines (hormones) from the adrenal glands. These changes increase heart rate, blood pressure, blood flow to active muscles and the brain, glucose levels, oxygen consumption, and strength — all necessary for the body to "fight or flee." For the body to relax, action must take place. If the person "fights or flees", the body relaxes and stress is dissipated. If the person is unable to take action, tension and tightening of the muscles increases. As noted earlier, this increased tension and tightening can be effectively dissipated with the aid of coping techniques.

Several relaxation techniques will now be discussed. Although benefits are reaped immediately after performing a given technique, several months of regular practice may be necessary for complete mastery. Keep in mind that relaxation exercises are not a cure-all panacea. If the exercises outlined in this chapter do not prove effective, a more specialized textbook or professional help should be obtained. It is also possible that in some instances the symptoms that a person is experiencing may not be caused by stress, but rather related to a different medical disorder.

Biofeedback

The clinical application of biofeedback in the treatment of different medical disorders has become popular in the last few years. Besides its successful application in stress management, it is commonly used in the treatment of such medical disorders as essential hypertension, asthma, heart rhythm and rate disturbance, cardiac neurosis, eczematous dermititis, fecal incontinence, insomnia and stuttering. Biofeedback as a treatment modality has been defined as follows:[2]

A process in which a person learns to reliably influence physiological responses of two kinds: either responses which are not ordinarily under voluntary control or responses which ordinarily are easily regulated but for which regulation has broken down due to trauma or disease.

Figure 7.3. *Physiological Response to Stress: Fight or Flight Mechanism.*

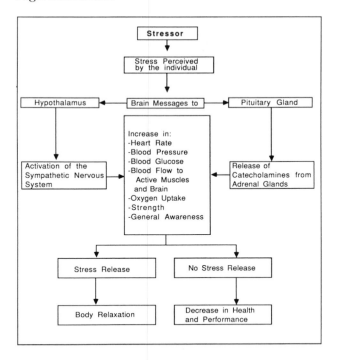

In simpler terms, biofeedback is the interaction with the interior self.[4] This interaction allows a person to learn the relationship between the mind and the biological response. The individual can actually "feel" how the thought process influences biological responses (e.g., heart rate, blood pressure, body temperature, muscle tension), and how biological responses also influence the thought process. An illustration of this process could be the association between a strange noise in the middle of a dark, quiet night and the heart rate response. Initially, the heart rate shoots up because of the stress induced by the unknown noise. The individual may even feel the heart palpitating in the chest, and while still uncertain about the noise, an attempt is made not to panic in order to prevent a larger increase in heart rate. Upon realization that all is well, the person can take control and influence the heart rate to come down, or the mind is now able to exert almost complete control over the biological response.

Complex electronic instruments are usually required to conduct the process of biofeedback. The process itself involves a three-stage closed-loop feedback system: (a) a biological response to a stressor is detected and amplified; (b) the response is processed; and (c) the results of the

response are immediately fed back to the individual. The person then uses this new input and attempts to voluntarily change the physiological response, which is, in turn, detected, amplified, and processed. The results are then fed back to the subject. The process continues with the intent of teaching the person to reliably influence for the better the physiological response.[1] The most common methods used to measure physiological responses are heart rate, finger temperature, blood pressure equipment, electromyograms, and electroencephalograms.

Although biofeedback has significant applications in the treatment of various medical disorders, including stress, it also requires adequately trained personnel and in many cases costly equipment. Therefore, several alternate methods that yield similar results are frequently used. For example, research has shown that physical exercise and progressive muscle relaxation, used successfully in stress management, seem to be just as effective as biofeedback in treating essential hypertension.

Figure 7.4. *Biofeedback Mechanism.*

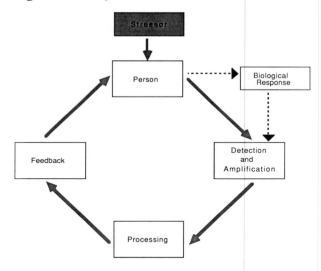

Physical Exercise as a Means for Stress Reduction

Physical exercise is one of the simplest tools used to control stress. The value of exercise in reducing stress is related to several factors. The principal factor is a decrease in muscular tension. For example, a person can be distressed because he/she had a miserable day at work, and the job required eight hours of work in a smoke-filled room with an intolerable boss. To make matters worse, it is late and on the way home the car in front is going much slower than the speed limit. The "fight-or-flight" mechanism is activated, catecholamines are on the rise, heart rate and blood pressure shoot up, breathing quickens and deepens, muscles tense up, and all systems say "go." But no action can be initiated, nor stress dissipated, because you just cannot hit your boss or the car in front of you. However, a person could surely take action by "hitting" the tennis ball, the weights, the swimming pool, or the jogging trail. By engaging in physical activity, a person is able to reduce the muscle tension and metabolize the increased catecholamines that brought about the physiological changes that triggered the "fight-or-flight" mechanism. Although exercise did not solve the problems at work or take care of the slow driver on the road, it certainly helped the person cope with stress, preventing it from becoming a chronic problem.

A point of interest is that the early evening hours are becoming the most popular time to exercise for a lot of highly stressed executives. On the way home from work, they will stop at the health club or the fitness center. Exercising at this hour helps them dissipate the excessive stress accumulated during the day. Most people can relate to exercise as a means for stress management by remembering how good they felt the last time they concluded a good strenuous exercise session after a difficult, long day at the office. A fatigued muscle is definitely a relaxed muscle. For this reason, many individuals have said that "the best part of exercise is the shower afterwards." Not only will exercise help get rid of the stress, but it will also provide an opportunity to enjoy a better evening. At home, the family will appreciate the fact that Dad or Mom comes home more relaxed (leaving work problems behind), and that all energy can be dedicated to family activities.

Research has also shown that physical exercise which requires continuous and rhythmic muscular activity, such as aerobic exercise, stimulates alpha-wave activity in the brain. These are the same wave patterns commonly seen during periods of meditation and relaxation. Furthermore, during vigorous aerobic exercise lasting thirty minutes or longer, morphine-like substances referred to as endorphins are released from the pituitary gland in the brain. These substances have been known to act not only as painkillers, but also seem to induce the soothing, calming effect often associated with aerobic exercise.

Another way that exercise helps in reducing stress is by deliberately diverting stress to various body systems. Dr. Hans Selye explains in his book *Stress Without Distress* that when the accomplishment of one specific task becomes difficult, a change in activity can be as good or better than rest itself. For example, if a person is having a difficult time with a certain task, and does not seem to be getting anywhere, it is better to go jogging or swimming for a while, rather than sitting around and getting frustrated. In this manner, the mental strain is diverted to the working muscles, and the one system helps the other relax. Another psychologist, Dr. William James, has indicated that when muscular tension is removed from the emotional strain, the emotional strain disappears. In many cases, the change of activity will suddenly clear the mind and help put the pieces together.

Other researchers have found that physical exercise gives people a psychological boost because exercise: (a) reduces feelings of anxiety, depression, frustration, aggression, anger, and hostility; (b) decreases insomnia; (c) provides an opportunity to meet social needs and develop new friendships; (d) allows the person to share common interests and problems, (e) develops discipline; and (f) provides the opportunity to do something enjoyable and constructive that will lead to better health and total well-being.

Beyond the short-term benefits of exercise in reducing stress, another important benefit of a regular aerobic exercise program is the actual strengthening of the cardiovascular system itself. Since the cardiovascular system seems to be most seriously affected by stress, a stronger system should be able to cope more effectively. For instance, good cardiovascular endurance has been shown to decrease resting heart rate and blood pressure. Since both heart rate and blood pressure rise in stressful situations, initiating the stress response at a lower baseline will decrease the negative effects of stress. There is little argument that cardiovascularly fit individuals can cope more effectively and are less affected by the stresses of daily living.

Progressive Muscle Relaxation

Progressive muscle relaxation was developed by Dr. Edmund Jacobsen in the 1930s. This technique enables individuals to relearn the sensation of deep relaxation. The technique involves progressive contraction and relaxation of muscle groups throughout the body. Since chronic stress leads to high levels of muscular tension, being closely aware of how it feels to progressively tighten and relax the muscles will release the tension on the muscles and teach the body to relax at will. Being aware of the tension felt during the exercises also helps the person be more alert to signs of distress, since similar feelings are experienced in stressful situations. In everyday life, such feelings can be used as a cue to implement adequate relaxation exercises.

Relaxation exercises should be conducted in a quiet, warm, and well-ventilated room. The recommended exercises and the duration of the routine vary from one author to the next. However, the important consideration is that the individual pays attention to the sensation felt each time the muscles are tensed up and relaxed. The exercises should include all muscle groups of the body. An example of a sequence of progressive muscle relaxation exercises is given below. The instructions outlined for these exercises can be either read to the person, memorized, or recorded on a tape. At least twenty minutes should be set aside to perform the entire sequence. Doing them any faster will defeat the purpose of the exercises. Ideally, the sequence should be performed twice a day.

Instructions: The individual performing the exercises must stretch out comfortably on the floor, face up, with a pillow under the knees, and should assume a passive attitude allowing the body to relax as much as possible. Each muscle group is contracted in sequence, taking care to avoid any strain. Muscles should only be tightened to about 70 percent of the total possible tension to avoid cramping or some type of injury to the muscle itself. Paying attention to the sensation of tensing up and relaxing is most crucial to produce the relaxation effects. Each contraction is held for about five seconds, and then the muscles must be allowed to go totally limp. Sufficient time should be taken to allow for contraction and relaxation before the next statement is given. The following list of statements given to the participant is an example of a complete progressive muscle relaxation sequence:

1. Point your feet, curling the toes downward, and study the tension in the arches and the top of the feet. Hold it and continue to note the tension, then relax. Repeat a second time.

2. Flex the feet upward toward the face and note the tension in your feet and calves. Hold it . . ., and relax . . . Repeat again.

3. Push your heels down against the floor as if burying them in the sand. Hold it and note the tension on the back of the thigh; relax. Repeat one more time.

4. Contract the right thigh by straightening the leg, gently raising the leg off the floor. Hold it and study the tension; relax . . . Repeat with the left leg, hold and relax. Repeat both legs again.

5. Tense the buttocks by raising your hips ever so slightly off the floor. Hold it and note the tension, and relax . . . Repeat again.

6. Contract the abdominal muscles. Hold them tight and note the tension; relax . . . Repeat one more time.

7. Suck in your stomach — try to make it reach your spine. Flatten your lower back to the floor; hold it and feel the tension in the stomach and lower back; relax . . . Repeat again.

8. Take a deep breath and hold it . . ., and exhale. Repeat again. Note your breathing becoming slower and more relaxed.

9. Place your arms on the side of your body and clench both fists. Hold it . . ., study the tension, and relax . . . Repeat a second time.

10. Flex the elbow by bringing both hands to the shoulders. Hold it tight and study the tension in the biceps; relax . . . Repeat again.

11. Place your arms flat on the floor, palms up, and push the forearm hard against the floor. Note the tension on the triceps; hold it . . ., and relax . . . Repeat the exercise.

12. Shrug your shoulders, raising them as high as possible. Hold it and note the tension; relax . . . Repeat again.

13. Gently push your head backward; note the tension in the back of the neck. Hold it . . ., relax . . . Repeat one more time.

14. Gently bring the head against the chest, push forward, hold, and note the tension in the neck. Relax . . . Repeat a second time.

15. Press your tongue toward the roof of your mouth. Hold it . . ., study the tension; relax . . . Repeat again.

16. Press your teeth together. Hold it and study the tension; relax . . . Repeat again.

17. Close your eyes tightly. Hold them closed and note the tension. Relax, leaving your eyes closed. Repeat again.

18. Wrinkle your forehead. Note the tension; hold it . . ., and relax . . . Repeat one more time.

In instances during the daily routine when time is a factor and an individual is not able to go through the entire sequence, only the exercises specific to the area where muscle tension is felt may be performed. Just performing a few exercises is better than none at all. Nevertheless, completion of the entire sequence yields the best results.

Breathing Techniques For Relaxation

Breathing exercises can also be used as an antidote to stress. Such exercises have been used for centuries in the Orient and India as a means to develop better mental, physical, and emotional stamina. In breathing exercises, the person concentrates on "breathing away" the tension and inhaling fresh oxygen to the entire body.

Breathing exercises can be learned in only a few minutes and require considerably less time than the progressive muscle relaxation exercises. As with any other relaxation technique, a quiet, pleasant, and well-ventilated room should be used to perform the exercise. Three examples of breathing exercises will now be presented. Any of these exercises may be performed whenever tension is felt due to stress. The following are the instructions given to the person:

1. **Deep breathing:** Lie with your back flat against the floor, place a pillow under your knees, feet slightly separated, and toes pointing outward (the exercise may also be conducted sitting up in a chair or standing straight up). Place one hand on your abdomen and the other one on your chest. Slowly breathe in and out so that the hand on your abdomen rises when you inhale and falls as you exhale. The hand on the chest should not move much at all. Repeat the exercise about ten times. Next, scan your body for tension, and compare your present tension with that felt at the beginning of the exercise. Repeat the entire process once or twice more.

2. **Sighing:** Using the abdominal breathing technique, breathe in through your nose to a specific count (i.e., 4, 5, 6, etc.). Now exhale through pursed lips to double the intake count (i.e., 8, 10, 12, etc.). Repeat the exercise eight to ten times whenever you feel tense.

3. **Complete natural breathing:** Sit in an upright position or stand straight up. Breathe through your nose and gradually fill up your lungs from the bottom up. Hold your breath for several seconds. Now exhale slowly by allowing complete relaxation of the chest and abdomen. Repeat the exercise eight to ten times.

Autogenic Training

Autogenic training is basically a form of self-suggestion, where an individual is able to place him/herself in an autohypnotic state by repeating and concentrating on feelings of heaviness and warmth in the extremities. This technique was developed by Johannes H. Schultz, a German psychiatrist who noted that hypnotized individuals developed sensations of warmth and heaviness in the limbs and torso. The sensation of warmth is caused by dilation of blood vessels, which increases blood flow to the limbs. The heaviness is felt as a result of muscle relaxation.

When using this technique, the person lies down or sits down in a comfortable position with eyes closed and progressively concentrates on six fundamental stages:

1. **Heaviness**
   My right (left) arm is heavy
   Both arms are heavy
   My right (left) leg is heavy
   Both legs are heavy
   My arms and legs are heavy

2. **Warmth**
   My right (left) arm is warm
   Both arms are warm
   My right (left) leg is warm
   Both legs are warm
   My arms and legs are warm

3. **Heart**
   My heartbeat is calm and regular
   (repeat four or five times)

4. **Respiration**
   My body breathes itself
   (repeat four or five times)

5. **Abdomen**
   My abdomen is warm
   (repeat four or five times)

6. **Forehead**
   My forehead is cool
   (repeat four or five times)

The autogenic training technique is more difficult to master than any of those previously mentioned. The individual should not move too fast through the entire exercise, since this practice may actually interfere with the learning and relaxation process. Each stage must be mastered before proceeding to the next one.

Meditation

Meditation is a mental exercise that can bring about psychological and physical benefits. The objective of meditation is to gain control over your attention, clearing the mind and blocking out the stressor(s) responsible for the increased tension. This technique can also be learned rather quickly and be used frequently during periods of increased tension and stress.

Initially, the person who is trying to learn to meditate should choose a room that is comfortable, quiet, and free of all disturbances (including telephones). Nevertheless, once the technique is learned, the person will be able to meditate just about anywhere. Approximately fifteen minutes, twice a day, are needed to meditate. The following is an example of the instructions for a meditation exercise:

1. Sit in a chair in an upright position with the hands resting either in your lap or on the arms of the chair. Close your eyes and focus on your breathing. Allow your body to relax as much as possible. Do not try to consciously relax, since trying means work. Rather, assume a passive attitude and concentrate on your breathing.

2. Allow the body to breathe regularly, at its own rhythm, and repeat in your mind the word "one" everytime you inhale, and the word "two" everytime you exhale. Paying attention to these two words keeps distressing thoughts from entering into your mind.

3. Continue to breathe for about fifteen minutes. Since the objective of meditating is to bring about a hypometabolic state, leading to body relaxation, do not use an alarm clock to remind you that the fifteen minutes have expired. The alarm will only trigger your stress response again, defeating the purpose of the exercise. It is fine to open your eyes once in a while to keep track of the time. But remember not to "rush" or anticipate the end of the fifteen minutes. This time has been set aside for meditation and you need to relax, take your time, and enjoy the exercise.

Which Technique is Best

Each person reacts to stress in a different way. Therefore, the coping strategy used will depend mostly on the individual. It does not really matter which technique is used, as long as it works. An individual may want to experiment with all of them to find out which works best, or may also use a combination of two or more. All of the coping strategies discussed help block out the stressor(s), and lead to mental and physical relaxation by diverting the attention to a different, nonthreatening action. Some of the techniques are easier to learn and may take less time per session. Regardless of which technique is selected, when stress becomes a significant problem in life, the time spent performing stress management exercises is well worth the effort. People need to learn to "relax" and take time out for themselves. As noted earlier, it is not stress that makes people ill, but rather the way in which they react to the particular stress-causing agent. Individuals who learn to be diligent and start taking control of themselves find out that they can enjoy a better, happier, and healthier life.

REFERENCES

1. Andrasik, F., D. Coleman, and L. H. Epstein. "Biofeedback: Clinical and Research Considerations." In *Behavioral Medicine: Assessment and Treatment Strategies.* Edited by D. M. Doleys, R. L. Meredith, and A. R. Ciminero. New York: Plenum Press, 1982.

2. Blanchard, E. B., and L. H. Epstein. *A Biofeedback Primer.* Reading, Mass.: Addison-Wesley, 1978.

3. Blue Cross Association. *Stress.* Chicago: The Association, 1974.

4. Brown, B. *New Mind, New Body.* New York: Harper & Row, 1974.

5. Chesney, M. A., J. R. Eagleston, and R. H. Roseman. "Type A Assessment and Intervention." In *Medical Psychology: Contributions to Behavioral Medicine.* Edited by C. K. Prokop and L. A. Bradley. New York: Academic Press, 1981.

6. Gauron, E. F. *Mental Training for Peak Performance.* Lansing, NY: Sport Science Associates, 1984.

7. Girdano, D., and G. Everly. *Controlling Stress and Tension: A Holistic Approach.* Englewood Cliffs, NJ: Prentice-Hall, Inc., 1986.

8. Greenberg, J. S. *Comprehensive Stress Management.* Dubuque, IA: Wm. C. Brown Company Publishers, 1983.

9. Kriegel, R. J., and M. H. Kriegel. *The C Zone: Peak Performance Under Stress.* Garden City, NY: Anchor Press/Doubleday, 1984.

10. Luthe, W. "Autogenic Training: Method, Research and Applications in Medicine." *American Journal of Psychotherapy* 17:174-195, 1963.

11. McKay, M., M. Davis, and P. Fanning. *Thoughts and Feelings: The Act of Cognitive Stress Intervention:* Richmond, CA: New Harbinger Publications, 1981.

12. Miller, L. H., and A. D. Smith. "Vulnerability Scale." Stress Audit, 1983.

13. Sarason, I. G., J. H. Johnson, and J. M. Siegel. "Assessing the Impact of Life Changes: Development of the Life Experiences Survey." *Journal of Consulting and Clinical Psychology* 46:932-946, 1978.

14. Selye, H. *Stress Without Distress.* New York: Signet, 1974.

15. Selye, H. *The Stress of Life.* New York: McGraw-Hill Book Co., 1978.

16. Staff. "How Running Relieves Stress." *The Runner* 8(11):38-43, 82, 1986.

17. Turk, D. C., and R. D. Kerns. "Assessment in Health Psychology: A Cognitive-Behavioral Perspective." In *Measurement Strategies in Health Psychology.* Edited by P. Karoly. New York: John Wiley & Sons, 1985.

CHAPTER EIGHT

Smoking Cessation

Tobacco has been used throughout the world for hundreds of years. Prior to the eighteenth century, it was smoked primarily in the form of pipes or cigars. Cigarette smoking per se did not become popular until the mid-1800s, and its use started to increase dramatically at the turn of the century. In 1915, 18 billion cigarettes were consumed in the United States, as compared to 640 billion in 1981. There are now more than 53 million Americans over the age of seventeen who smoke an average of one and one-half packs of cigarettes per day.

The harmful effects of cigarette smoking and tobacco usage in general were not exactly known until the early 1960s, when researchers began to show a positive link between tobacco use and disease. In 1964, the United States Surgeon General issued the first major report presenting scientific evidence that cigarettes were indeed a major health hazard in our society.

The use of tobacco in all forms is now considered a significant threat to life. Cigarette smoking is the largest preventable cause of illness and premature death in the United States. When considering all related deaths, smoking is responsible for over 350,000 unnecessary deaths each year. There is a definite increase in death rates from heart disease, cancer, stroke, aortic aneurysm, chronic bronchitis, emphysema, and peptic ulcers. Maternal cigarette smoking has been linked to retarded fetal growth, increased risk for spontaneous abortion, and prenatal death. Smoking is also the most common cause of fire deaths and injuries. The average life expectancy for a chronic smoker is seven years less than a nonsmoker, and the death rate among chronic smokers during the most productive years of life, between the ages of twenty-five and sixty-five, is twice that of the national average.

In spite of the length of time elapsed since the 1964 report by the Surgeon General on the detrimental effects of smoking on health, the Federal Trade Commission reported in 1986 that 40 percent of Americans still did not know that smoking caused lung cancer, and 20 percent were unaware that it caused any type of cancer at all. This same report indicated that 30 percent of the population did not know that smoking increased the risk for heart disease, and approximately half of all women in the country did not know that smoking during pregnancy increased the risk for miscarriage and spontaneous abortion.

According to American Heart Association estimates, over 30 percent, or 120,000 fatal heart attacks annually, are due to smoking. Heart attack risk is 50 to 100 percent greater for smokers as compared to nonsmokers. There is also an increased mortality rate following heart attacks, since they are usually more severe and the risk for deadly arrhythmias is much greater. Cigarette smoking affects the cardiovascular system by increasing heart rate, blood pressure, susceptibility to atherosclerosis, and blood clots. Evidence also indicates that it decreases high-density lipoprotein cholesterol, or the so-called "good" cholesterol, which decreases the risk for heart disease. Finally, carbon monoxide found in smoke decreases the oxygen delivery capacity of the blood to the tissues of the body.

Also known is the fact that the biggest carcinogenic exposure in the workplace is cigarette smoke. The American Cancer Society reports that 83 percent of lung cancer and 30 percent of all cancers are due to smoking. It kills about 138,000 people each year. Lung cancer is the leading cancer killer and is responsible for 35 percent of all cancer deaths. While it is encouraging to note that over 50 percent of all cancers are now curable, the five-year survival rate for lung cancer is less than 10 percent. Tobacco use also increases cancer risk of the oral cavity, larynx, esophagus, bladder, pancreas, and kidneys.

While many tobacco users are aware of the health consequences of cigarette smoking, many fail to realize the risk of pipe smoking, cigar smoking, and chewing tobacco. As a group in general, the risk for heart disease and lung cancer is lower than for cigarette smokers. However, blood nicotine levels in pipe and cigar smokers have been shown to approach those of cigarette smokers, since nicotine is still absorbed through the mouth membranes. Therefore, there is still a higher risk for heart disease as compared to nonsmokers. Cigarette smokers who substitute pipe or cigar smoking for cigarettes usually continue to inhale the smoke, which actually results in a greater amount of nicotine and tar being brought into the lungs. Consequently, the risk for disease is even greater if pipe or cigar smoke is inhaled. The risk and mortality rates for lip, mouth, and larynx cancer for pipe smoking, cigar smoking, or chewing tobacco are actually higher than for cigarette smokers.

The economical impact of cigarette smoking among American business and industry is also staggering. Companies pay in excess of $16 billion each year as a direct result of smoking at the workplace and another $37 billion in lost productivity and earnings because of illness, disability, and death. Heavy smokers have been shown to use the health care system, especially hospitals, over 50 percent more than nonsmokers. The yearly cost to a given company has been estimated between $624 and $4,611 per smoking employee. These costs include employee health care, absenteeism, additional health insurance, morbidity/disability and early mortality, on-the-job lost time, property damage/maintenance and depreciation, Workmen's Compensation, and involuntary smoking impact.

In spite of the fact that the ill effects of tobacco have been well documented, not enough is being done to decrease and eradicate its use. Consider the following example. In the summer of 1985, over 1,500 people died around the world in major airplane accidents. These accidents resulted in a tremendous amount of worldwide media attention, and planes were grounded for safety reasons. Now imagine what the coverage and concern would be if 350,000 people each year died in the United States alone because of airplane accidents. People would not even consider flying anymore. Most individuals would think of it as a form of suicide.

Similarly, think of the public outrage if over 350,000 Americans were to die annually in a meaningless war, or if a single nonprescription drug would cause over 138,000 cancer deaths and 120,000 fatal heart attacks. The American public would never tolerate such situations. We would probably mount a very intense fight to prevent these deaths. Yet, are we not committing a form of slow suicide by smoking cigarettes? Isn't tobacco a nonprescription drug available to most anyone who wishes to smoke, killing in excess of 350,000 people each year?

We may ask ourselves, why isn't there a greater campaign against all forms of tobacco use? There are primarily two reasons. First, it is extremely difficult to fight an industry that has as great a financial and political influence in a country as the tobacco industry has in the United States. The tobacco industry produces 2.5 percent of the gross national product and has cleverly influenced elections by emphasizing the individual's right to smoke, avoiding the fact that so many people die because of its use. Second, tobacco had been socially accepted for so many years that many people just learned to live with it. However, for the first time, in the 1980s, cigarette smoking is no longer acceptable in many social circles. Nonsmokers and ex-smokers alike are fighting for their right to clean air and health. Estimates have indicated that if every smoker gave up cigarettes, in one year alone, sick time would be decreased by approximately 90 million days, there would be 280,000 fewer heart conditions and 1 million fewer cases of chronic bronchitis and emphysema, and total death rates from cardiovascular disease, cancer, and peptic ulcers would drastically decrease.

It is also interesting to note that many smokers are really unaware or simply do not care to realize how much cigarette smoke bothers nonsmokers. These smokers feel that it is not really that bad, and if they can put up with it, it should not bother nonsmokers that much. In most instances, they think that blowing the smoke off to the side is sufficient to get it out of the way. As a matter of fact, it is not enough. Smokers do not comprehend this until they quit and later find themselves in such situations. At times, ex-smokers are even bothered by someone else smoking several yards away and all of a sudden come to realize why cigarette smoke is so unpleasant and undesirable to most people.

WHY DO PEOPLE SMOKE?

In most instances, people begin to smoke without realizing the detrimental effects of tobacco on their health and life in general. While there are many different reasons why people start to smoke, the three fundamental causes are peer pressure, to appear "grown up," and rebellion against authority. Unfortunately, it only takes three packs of cigarettes to develop the physiological addiction, turning it into a "nasty" habit that has become the most widespread example of drug dependency in the country.

When tobacco leaves are burned, hot air and gases containing nicotine and tar (chemical compounds) are released in the smoke. Over 1,200 toxic chemicals have been found in tobacco smoke. Tar contains about thirty chemical compounds that are proven carcinogens. The drug nicotine has strong addictive properties. Within seconds of inhalation, nicotine affects the central nervous system and can act both as a tranquilizer and a stimulant. The stimulating effect produces strong physiological and psychological dependency. The addiction to nicotine is six to eight times greater than alcohol and most likely greater than some of the hard drugs currently used around the world. The psychological dependency is developed over a longer period of time. Not only do people smoke to help them relax, but there is also a certain amount of pleasure involved with the ritual of smoking. There are many activities in daily life that smokers automatically associate with cigarettes. Events such as drinking coffee, drinking alcohol, social gatherings, after a meal, talking on the telephone, driving, reading, watching television, etc. make habitual smokers crave cigarettes. In many cases, the social rituals of smoking are the most difficult to eliminate. This psychological dependency is so strong that even years after individuals have stopped smoking, they still crave cigarettes when engaged in some of the aforementioned activities.

Most people smoke for a variety of reasons. To find out why people smoke, a simple test was developed by the National Clearinghouse for Smoking and Health (Figure 8.1). The scores obtained on this test will give an indication on each of six factors that describe people's feelings when they smoke. The first three factors point out the positive feelings people get from smoking. The fourth factor aids them in tension reduction and relaxation. The fifth shows their dependence on cigarettes. The last factor indicates habit smoking or purely automatic smoking.

WHY DO YOU SMOKE TEST

In the test contained in Figure 8.1 are some statements made by people to describe what they get out of smoking cigarettes. Smokers should indicate how often they experience the feelings described in each statement when smoking by circling one number for each statement. It is important that they answer every question. This test, as well as much of the remaining information in this chapter, is presented in the same format as it is given to smokers.

INTERPRETING THE RESULTS OF THE WHY DO YOU SMOKE TEST

In this test that examines reasons why you smoke, a score of eleven or above on any factor indicates that it is an important source of satisfaction for you. The higher you score (fifteen is the highest), the more important a particular factor is in your smoking and the more useful the discussion of that factor can be in your attempt to quit.

If you do not score high on any of the six factors, chances are that you do not smoke very much or have not been smoking for very many years. If so, giving up smoking — and staying off — should be easy.

1. Stimulation. If you score high or fairly high on this factor, it means that you are one of those

Figure 8.1. *Why-Do-You-Smoke Test.*

	Always	Fre-quently	Occa-sionally	Seldom	Never
A. I smoke cigarettes in order to keep myself from slowing down.	5	4	3	2	1
B. Handling a cigarette is part of the enjoyment of smoking it.	5	4	3	2	1
C. Smoking cigarettes is pleasant and relaxing.	5	4	3	2	1
D. I light up a cigarette when I feel angry about something.	5	4	3	2	1
E. When I have run out of cigarettes I find it almost unbearable until I can get them.	5	4	3	2	1
F. I smoke cigarettes automatically without even being aware of it.	5	4	3	2	1
G. I smoke cigarettes to stimulate me, to perk myself up.	5	4	3	2	1
H. Part of the enjoyment of smoking a cigarette comes from the steps I take to light up.	5	4	3	2	1
I. I find cigarettes pleasurable.	5	4	3	2	1
J. When I feel uncomfortable or upset about something, I light up a cigarette.	5	4	3	2	1
K. I am very much aware of the fact when I am not smoking a cigarette.	5	4	3	2	1
L. I light up a cigarette without realizing I still have one burning in the ashtray.	5	4	3	2	1
M. I smoke cigarettes to give me a "lift."	5	4	3	2	1
N. When I smoke a cigarette, part of the enjoyment is watching the smoke as I exhale it.	5	4	3	2	1
O. I want a cigarette most when I am comfortable and relaxed.	5	4	3	2	1
P. When I feel "blue" or want to take my mind off cares and worries, I smoke cigarettes.	5	4	3	2	1
Q. I get a real gnawing hunger for a cigarette when I haven't smoked for a while.	5	4	3	2	1
R. I've found a cigarette in my mouth and didn't remember putting it there.	5	4	3	2	1

Scoring Your Test:

Enter the numbers you have circled on the test questions in the spaces provided below, putting the number you have circled to question A on line A, to question B on line B, etc. Add the three scores on each line to get a total for each factor. For example, the sum of you scores over lines A, G, and M gives you your score on "Stimulation," lines B, H, and N give the score on "Handling," etc. Scores can vary from 3 to 15. Any score 11 and above is high; any score 7 and below is low.

A _____	+ G _____	+ M _____	= _____	Stimulation
B _____	+ H _____	+ N _____	= _____	Handling
C _____	+ I _____	+ O _____	= _____	Pleasure Relaxation
D _____	+ J _____	+ P _____	= _____	Crutch: Tension Reduction
E _____	+ K _____	+ Q _____	= _____	Craving: Psychological Addiction
F _____	+ L _____	+ R _____	= _____	Habit

From *A Self-Test for Smokers.* U.S. Department of Health and Human Services, 1983.

smokers who is stimulated by the cigarette — you feel that it helps wake you up, organize your energies, and keep you going. If you try to give up smoking, you may want a safe substitute — a brisk walk or moderate exercise, for example — whenever you feel the urge to smoke.

2. Handling. Handling things can be satisfying, but there are many ways to keep your hands busy without lighting up or playing with a cigarette. Why not toy with a pen or pencil? Or try doodling. Or play with a coin, a piece of jewelry, or some other harmless object.

3. Accentuation of pleasure — pleasurable relaxation. It is not always easy to find out whether you use the cigarette to feel good, that is, get real, honest pleasure out of smoking (Factor 3) or to keep from feeling bad (Factor 4). About two-thirds of smokers score high or fairly high on accentuation of pleasure, and about half of those also score as high or higher on reduction of negative feelings.

   Those who do get real pleasure out of smoking often find that an honest consideration of the harmful effects of their habit is enough to help them quit. They substitute social and physical activities and find that they do not seriously miss their cigarettes.

4. Reduction of negative feelings, or "crutch." Many smokers use the cigarette as a kind of crutch in moments of stress or discomfort. But the heavy smoker, the person who tries to handle severe personal problems by smoking many times a day, is apt to discover that cigarettes do not help in dealing with problems effectively.

   When it comes to quitting, this kind of smoker may find it easy to stop when everything is going well but may be tempted to start again in a time of crisis. Again, physical exertion or social activity may serve as useful substitutes for cigarettes, even in times of tension.

5. "Craving" or dependence. Quitting smoking is difficult for the person who scores high on this factor, that of dependence. For the addicted smoker, the craving for a cigarette begins to build up the moment the cigarette is put out, so tapering off is not likely to work. This smoker must go "cold turkey."

If you are dependent on cigarettes, it may be helpful for you to smoke more than usual for a day or two, so that the taste for cigarettes is spoiled, and then isolate yourself completely from cigarettes until the craving is gone.

6. Habit. If you are smoking out of habit, you no longer get much satisfaction from your cigarettes. You just light them frequently without even realizing you are doing so. You may find it easy to quit and stay off if you can break the habit patterns that you have built up. Cutting down gradually may be effective if there is a change in the way the cigarettes are smoked and the conditions under which they are smoked. The key to success is becoming aware of each cigarette you smoke. This can be done by asking yourself, "Do I really want this cigarette?" You may be surprised at how many you do not want.

SMOKING CESSATION

Quitting cigarette smoking is no easy task. Only about 20 percent of smokers who try to quit for the first time each year succeed. The addictive properties of nicotine and smoke make it very difficult to quit. The American Psychiatric Association and the National Institute on Drug Abuse have indicated that nicotine is perhaps the most addictive drug known to man. Smokers develop tolerance to nicotine and smoke. They become dependent on both and experience physical and psychological withdrawal symptoms when they stop smoking. While giving up smoking can be extremely difficult, cessation is by no means an impossible task.

Recent surveys have shown that between 75 and 90 percent of all smokers would like to quit. In 1986, approximately 40 million Americans had given up cigarettes. An additional 2 million quit each year. A 1984 Gallup poll indicated that only 29 percent of adult Americans smoked, down from 37 percent in 1980. More than 95 percent of the successful ex-smokers have been able to do it on their own, either by quitting cold turkey or using self-help kits available from organizations such as the American Cancer Society, the American Heart Association, and the American Lung Association. Only 3 percent of ex-smokers have done so as a result of formal cessation programs. Smoker's Information and Treatment Centers are commonly listed in the yellow pages of the telephone book. Cigarette smoking is now a declining habit in the country. During the last several years, there has been a gradual decrease among smokers of all ages with the exception of young women.

The most important factor in quitting cigarette smoking is the person's sincere desire to do so. Although some smokers can simply quit, in most instances such is not the case. Those who can easily quit are primarily light or casual smokers. They realize that the pleasure of an occasional cigarette is not worth the added risk for disease and premature death. For heavy smokers, cessation will most likely be a difficult battle. While many do not succeed the first time around, the odds of quitting are much greater for those who repeatedly try to stop. To find out a smoker's preparedness to initiate a cessation program, the test contained in Figure 8.2, also developed by the National Clearinghouse for Smoking and Health, will measure a person's attitude toward the four primary reasons why people want to quit smoking. The results will give an indication of whether the person is really ready to start the program.

Figure 8.2. *Do You Want To Quit Test.*

	Strongly Agree	Mildly Agree	Mildly Disagree	Strongly Disagree
A. Cigarette smoking might give me a serious illness.	4	3	2	1
B. My cigarette smoking sets a bad example for others.	4	3	2	1
C. I find cigarette smoking to be a messy kind of habit.	4	3	2	1
D. Controlling my cigarette smoking is a challenge to me.	4	3	2	1
E. Smoking causes shortness of breath.	4	3	2	1
F. If I quit smoking cigarettes it might influence others to stop.	4	3	2	1
G. Cigarettes cause damage to clothing and other personal property.	4	3	2	1
H. Quitting smoking would show that I have willpower.	4	3	2	1
I. My cigarette smoking will have a harmful effect on my health.	4	3	2	1
J. My cigarette smoking influences others close to me to take up or continue smoking.	4	3	2	1
K. If I quit smoking, my sense of taste or smell would improve.	4	3	2	1
L. I do not like the idea of feeling dependent on smoking.	4	3	2	1

Scoring Your Test:

Write the number you have circled after each statement on the test in the corresponding space to the right. Add the scores on each line to get your totals. For example, the sum of your scores A, E, I gives you your score for the health factor. Scores can vary from 3 to 12. Any score of 9 or over is high; and score 6 or under is low.

A _____ + E _____ + I _____ = _____ Health

B _____ + F _____ + J _____ = _____ Example

C _____ + G _____ + K _____ = _____ Aesthetics

D _____ + H _____ + L _____ = _____ Mastery

From *A Self-Test for Smokers.* U.S. Department of Health and Human Services, 1983.

INTERPRETING THE RESULTS OF THE DO YOU WANT TO QUIT TEST

On this test, the higher you score on any category, say health, the more important that reason is to you. A score of nine or above in one of these categories indicates that this is one of the most important reasons why you may want to quit.

1. Health. Knowing the harmful consequences of cigarettes, many people have stopped smoking and many others are considering it. If your score on the health factor is nine or above, the health hazards of smoking may be enough to make you want to quit now.

   If your score on this factor is low (six or less), look over the hazards of smoking. You may be lacking important information or may even have incorrect information. If so, health considerations are not playing the important role that they should in your decision to keep on smoking or to quit.

2. Example. Some people stop smoking because they want to set a good example for others. Parents quit to make it easier for their children to resist starting to smoke, doctors to influence their patients, teachers to help their students, sports stars to set an example for their young fans, husbands to influence their wives, and vice versa.

   Such examples are an important influence on our behavior. Research shows that almost twice as many high school students smoke if both parents are smokers compared to those whose parents are nonsmokers or former smokers.

   If your score is low (six or less), it may mean that you are not interested in giving up smoking in order to set an example for others. Perhaps you do not appreciate how important your example could be.

3. Aesthetics (the unpleasant aspects). People who score high, that is, nine or above, in this category, recognize and are disturbed by some of the unpleasant aspects of smoking. The smell of stale smoke on their clothing, bad breath, and stains on their fingers and teeth might be reason enough to consider breaking the habit.

4. Mastery (self-control). If you score nine or above on this factor, you are bothered by the knowledge that you cannot control your desire to smoke. You are not your own master. Awareness of this challenge to your self-control may make you want to quit.

BREAKING THE HABIT

The following seven-step plan has been developed as a guide to help you quit smoking. The total program should be completed in four weeks or less. Steps one through four should take no longer than two weeks. A maximum of two additional weeks are allowed for the rest of the program.

Step One. The first step in breaking the habit is to decide positively that you want to quit. Avoid negative thoughts of how difficult this can be. Think positive. You can do it. Now prepare a list of the reasons why you smoke and why you want to quit (use Figure 8.3). Make several copies of the list and keep them in places where you commonly smoke. The reasons for quitting should be reviewed frequently, as this will motivate and psychologically prepare you for cessation. When the reasons for quitting outweigh the reasons for smoking, it will become a lot easier to quit. At this time you should also try to read as much information as possible on the detrimental effects of tobacco and the benefits of quitting.

Step Two. Initiate a personal diet and exercise program. About one-third of the people who quit smoking gain weight. This could be caused by one or a combination of several reasons: (a) food becomes a substitute for cigarettes, (b) there may be an increased appetite, and (c) basal metabolism may slow down. If the person initiates an exercise and weight control program prior to smoking cessation, weight gain should not be a problem. If anything, exercise and decreased body weight cause a greater awareness of healthy living and increase motivation for giving up cigarettes. Even if some weight is gained, the harmful effects of cigarette smoking are much more detrimental to human health than a few extra pounds of body weight. Experts have indicated that as far as the extra load on the heart is concerned, giving up one pack of cigarettes per day is the equivalent of losing between fifty and seventy-five pounds of excess body fat!

Figure 8.3. *Smoking Versus Quitting Reasons.*

Today's Date: _____ Quit Date: _____ Decision Date: _____

Cigarettes to be Smoked Today: _____ Brand: _____

No.	Time	Activity	Rating[a]	Amount Smoked[b]	Remarks/Substitutes
1.					
2.					
3.					
4.					
5.					
6.					
7.					
8.					
9.					
10.					
11.					
12.					
13.					
14.					
15.					
16.					
17.					
18.					
19.					
20.					

Additional comments, list of friends and/or activities to avoid

_____

_____

_____

_____

_____

_____

[a]Rating: 1 = desperately needed, 2 = moderately needed, 3 = no real need
[b]Amount Smoked: entire cigarette, two-thirds, half, etc.

Step Three. Decide on the approach that you will use to stop smoking. You may quit cold turkey or gradually decrease the number of cigarettes smoked daily. Your decision should be based on the scores obtained on the "why do you smoke test." If you scored eleven points or higher in either the "Crutch: Tension Reduction" or the "Craving: Psychological Addiction" categories, your best chance for success is quitting cold turkey. For any of the other four categories, you may choose either approach.

There is still argument as to which approach may be more effective. Quitting cold turkey may cause less withdrawal symptoms than gradually tapering off. When cutting down, the fewer the cigarettes smoked, the more important each one becomes. Therefore, there is a greater chance for relapse and returning to the original amount smoked. However, when the cutting down approach is used with a definite target date for quitting, the technique has shown to be quite effective. Smokers who taper off without a target date for quitting are the most likely to relapse.

Step Four. For a few days, keep a daily log of your smoking habit. This will help you understand the situations under which you smoke. To assist you in doing so, make copies of Figure 8.4 or develop your own form. Keep this form with you,

Figure 8.4. *Daily Cigarette Smoking Log.*

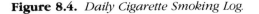

Name: _____ Date: _____

Reasons for Smoking Cigarettes

1. _____
2. _____
3. _____
4. _____
5. _____
6. _____
7. _____
8. _____

Reasons for Quitting Cigarette Smoking

1. _____
2. _____
3. _____
4. _____
5. _____
6. _____
7. _____
8. _____

and every time you smoke, record the required information. You should keep track of the number of cigarettes smoked, time of day when smoked, event associated with smoking, the amount of cigarette smoked, and a rating of how badly you needed that cigarette. Rate each cigarette from one to three. A number one means desperately needed, a two means moderately needed, and a three means no real need. This daily log will assist you in three ways. First, you will get to know your habit. Second, it will help you eliminate cigarettes that you really do not need. Third, it will aid you in finding positive substitutes for situations that trigger your desire to smoke.

Step Five. Set the target date for quitting. If you are going to taper off gradually, read the instructions under the cutting down section of this chapter before you proceed to Step Six. In setting the target date, choosing a special date may add a little extra incentive. An upcoming birthday, anniversary, vacation, graduation, family reunion, etc. are all examples of good dates to free yourself from smoking. Dates when you are going to be away from events that trigger your desire to smoke may be especially helpful. Once you have set the date, do not change it. Do not let anyone or anything interfere with this date. Let your friends and relatives know of your intentions and ask for their support. You may also consider asking someone else to quit with you. This way you can support each other in your efforts to stop. Also, avoid anyone who will not support you in your effort to quit. It is unfortunate, but in many cases other people can be a prime obstacle when attempting to quit. Since many smokers can get quite "intolerable" when they first stop smoking, some friends and relatives prefer that the individual continue to smoke rather than make the extra effort and show increased patience for a few days.

Step Six. Stock up on low-calorie foods — carrots, broccoli, cauliflower, celery, popcorn (butter and salt free), fruits, sunflower seeds (in the shell), sugarless gum, and plenty of water. Keep such food handy on the day you stop and the first few days following cessation. Replace such food for cigarettes when you want one.

Step Seven. On your quit day and the first few days thereafter, do not keep cigarettes handy. Stay away from friends and events that trigger your desire to smoke, and drink large amounts of water and fruit juices. An important factor in breaking the habit is to replace the old behavior with new behavior. You will need to replace smoking time with new positive substitutes that will make smoking difficult or impossible. When you desire a cigarette, take a few deep breaths and then occupy yourself by doing a number of things such as talking to someone else, washing your hands, brushing your teeth, eating a healthy snack, chewing on a straw, doing dishes, playing sports, going for a walk or bike ride, going swimming, and so on. Engage in activities that will necessitate the use of your hands. Try gardening, sewing, writing letters, drawing, doing household chores, washing the car. Visit nonsmoking places like libraries, museums, stores, theaters. Plan an outing or a trip away from home. Record your choice of activity or substitute under the remarks/substitute column in Figure 8.3. All these activities have shown to keep your mind away from cigarettes.

Quitting Cold Turkey

Many people have found that quitting all at once is the easiest way to do it. Most smokers have tried this approach at least once. While it may not work the first time, they do not allow themselves to get discouraged and eventually succeed. Many times after several attempts, all of a sudden they are able to overcome the habit without too much difficulty. On the average, as few as three smoke-less days are sufficient to break the physiological addiction to nicotine. The psychological addiction may linger on for years but will get weaker as time goes by.

Cutting Down Gradually

Tapering off cigarettes can be done in several ways. You may start by eliminating cigarettes that you do not necessarily need (those ranked as number three and two on your daily log); you can switch to a brand lower in nicotine and/or tar every couple of days; you can smoke less off each cigarette; or you can simply decrease the total number of cigarettes smoked each day.

Most people prefer using a combination of the four methods. When planning your strategy, it is important that you set a target date for quitting before you start cutting down. Remember — once the date is set, it is not to be changed. The total process until your quit date should not take longer than two weeks. You should reduce the total number of cigarettes smoked each day by 10 to 25 percent. As the number is decreased, be careful not to take more puffs or inhale more deeply as you smoke. This would offset the principle of cutting down.

As an aid in tapering off, make several copies of Figure 8.3 (by now you should have already completed the initial daily log of your smoking habit — see Step Four under breaking the habit). Start a new daily log, and every night review your data and set goals for the following day. You will need to decide which cigarettes will be easiest to give up, what brand you will smoke, the total number of cigarettes to be smoked, and how much of each you will smoke. You may also write down any comments or situations that you may want to avoid, as well as any substitutes that you could use to help you in the program. For example, if you always smoke with coffee, substitute juice for coffee. If you smoke while driving, arrange for a ride or take a bus to work. If you smoke with a given friend at lunch, avoid having lunch with that friend for a week or so. Continue using this log until you have completely stopped smoking.

LIFE AFTER CIGARETTES

When you first quit smoking, you can expect to experience a series of withdrawal symptoms. Among the physiological and psychological reactions that you will experience the first few days are a decrease in heart rate and blood pressure; and most likely headaches, gastrointestinal discomfort, changes in mood, irritability, aggressiveness, and difficulty in sleeping. The physiological addiction to nicotine is broken only three days following your last cigarette. As a result, you should not crave cigarettes as much on a regular basis. However, for the habitual smoker, the psychological dependency could be the most difficult to break. The first few days may not be as difficult as the first few months. Any of the activities in daily life that have been associated with smoking, either stress or relaxation, joy or unhappiness,

may cause a relapse even months or at times years after cessation.

Ex-smokers should realize that even though some harm may have already been done, it is never too late to quit. The greatest early benefit is a decrease in the risk of sudden death. Furthermore, the risk for illness starts to decrease the moment you stop smoking. You will experience a decrease in sore throats, sores in the mouth, hoarseness, cigarette cough, and peptic ulcer risk. There also will be an improvement in blood circulation to the hands and feet, improved gastrointestinal function, and improved kidney and bladder function. In addition, everything will taste and smell better, you will have more energy, and you will experience a sense of freedom, pride, and well-being. You will no longer have to worry whether you have enough cigarettes to last you through a day, a party, a meeting, a weekend, a trip, etc. When you first quit, and you think how tough it is and how miserable you feel because you cannot have a cigarette, try the opposite — think of the benefits and how great it is not to smoke! A final note of encouragement is that the ex-smoker's risk for heart disease approaches that of a lifetime nonsmoker ten years following cessation, and cancer fifteen years after cessation.

If you have been successful and stopped smoking, remember that there are a lot of events that can still trigger your urge to smoke. When confronted with such events, people rationalize and think, "One will not hurt, I have been off for months (years in some cases)" or, "I can handle it, I will just smoke today." It will not work! Before you know, you will be back to the regular nasty habit. Therefore, be prepared to take action in those situations. Find adequate substitutes. In addition to the many things that have already been discussed in this chapter, the list of tips given in Figure 8.5 should aid you in retraining yourself to live without cigarettes. You have to start thinking of yourself as a nonsmoker. There are no "buts." Remind yourself of how difficult it has been and how long it has taken you to get to this point. If you have come this far, you can certainly resist "but" small moments of temptation. Remember that it will only get easier rather than worse as times goes on.

References

1. American Cancer Society. *1986 Cancer Facts and Figures.* New York: The Society, 1986.
2. American Cancer Society. *Fifty Most Often Asked Questions About Smoking and Health . . . and the Answers.* New York: The Society, 1982.
3. American Cancer Society. *Quitter's Guide: Seven-Day Plan to Help You Stop Smoking Cigarettes.* New York: The Society, 1978.
4. American Cancer Society. *Why Quit Quiz* (VHS tape). New York: The Society, 1979.
5. American Heart Association. *Heart at Work: Smoking Reduction Program-Coordinator's Guide.* Dallas, TX: The Association, 1984.
6. American Heart Association. *How to Quit.* Dallas, TX: The Association, 1984.
7. American Heart Association. *Smoking and Heart Disease.* Dallas, TX: The Association, 1981.
8. American Heart Association. *The Good Life: A Guide to Becoming a Nonsmoker.* Dallas, TX: The Association, 1984.
9. Carroll, C. R. *Drugs in Modern Society.* Dubuque, IA: Wm. C. Brown, 1985.
10. Channing L. Bete Co., Inc. *Smoking and Your Heart.* South Deerfield, MA: The Author, 1982.
11. Girdano, D. A., D. Dusek, and G. S. Everly. *Experiencing Health.* Englewood Cliffs, NJ: Prentice-Hall, 1985.
12. Halper, M. S. *How to Stop Smoking: A Preventive Medicine Institute/ Strang Clinic Health Action Plan.* New York: Holt Rinehart and Winston, 1980.
13. Hodgson, R. J., and P. Miller. *Self-watching: Addictions, Habits, Compulsions, What to Do.* New York: Facts on File, 1982.
14. National Cancer Institute. *Clearing the Air: A Guide to Quitting Smoking.* Bethesda, MD: The Institute, 1979.
15. Public Health Service. *A Self-Test for Smokers.* Rockville, MD: U.S. Department of Health and Human Services, 1983.
16. Public Health Service. *Chronic Obstructive Lung Disease: A Report of the Surgeon General.* Rockville, MD: U.S. Department of Health and Human Services, 1984.
17. Public Health Service. *Why People Smoke Cigarettes.* Rockville, MD: U.S. Department of Health and Human Services, 1982.
18. Public Health Service. *Smoking Tobacco and Health: A Fact Book.* Rockville, MD: U.S. Department of Health and Human Services, 1981.
19. U.S. Office on Smoking and Health. *Smoking and Health: A Report of the Surgeon General.* Washington, D.C.: U.S. Department of Health, Education and Welfare, 1979.

Figure 10.6. *Tips for Smoking Cessation*

The following are different way smokers retrained themselves to live without cigarettes. Any one or several of these methods in combination might be helpful to you. Check the ones you like and from these develop your own retraining program.

1. Before you quit smoking, try wrapping your cigarettes with a sheet of paper like a Christmas present. Every time you want a cigarette, unwrap the pack and write down what you are doing, how you feel, and how important this cigarette is to you. Do this for two weeks and you'll have cut down as well as developed new insights into your smoking.

2. If cigarettes give you an energy boost, try gum, modest exercise, a brisk walk, or a new hobby. Avoid eating new foods that are high in calories.

3. If cigarettes help you relax, try eating, drinking new beverages, or social activities within reasonable bounds.

4. When you crave cigarettes, you must quit suddenly. Try smoking an excess of cigarettes for a day or two before you quit so that the taste of cigarettes is spoiled. Or, an opportune time to quit is when you are ill with a cold or influenza, and have lost your taste for cigarettes.

5. On a 3" x 5" card, make a list of what you like and dislike about smoking. Add to it and read it daily.

6. Make up a short list of luxuries you have wanted or items you would like to purchase for a loved one. Next to each item write down the cost. Now convert the cost to "packs of cigarettes." If you save the money each day from packs of cigarettes, you will be able to purchase these items. Use a special "piggy" bank for saving your money or start a "Christmas Club" account at your bank.

7. Never smoke after you get a craving for a cigarette until three minutes have passed since you got the urge. During those three minutes, change your thinking or activity. Telephone an ex-smoker or somebody you can talk to until the craving subsides.

8. Plan a memorable date for stopping. You might choose your vacation, New Year's Day, your birthday, a holiday, the birthday of your child, your anniversary. But, don't make the date so distant that you lose momentum.

9. If you smoke under stress at work, pick a date for stopping when you will be away from your work.

10. Decide whether you are going to stop suddenly or gradually. If it is to be gradual, work out a tapering system so that you have intermediate goals on your way to an "I.Q." day.

11. Don't store up cigarettes. Never buy a carton. Wait until one pack is finished before you buy another.

12. Never carry cigarettes about with you at home or at work. Keep your cigarettes as far from you as possible. Leave them with someone or lock them up.

13. Until you quit, make yourself a "smoking corner" that is far from anything interesting. If you like to smoke with others, always smoke alone. If you like to smoke alone, always smoke with others, preferably if they are nonsmokers. Never smoke while watching television.

14. Never carry matches or a lighter with you.

15. Put away your ashtrays or fill them with objects so they cannot be used for ashes. Plant flowers in them or fill them with walnuts. The latter will give you something to do with your hands.

16. Change your brand of cigarettes weekly so that you are always smoking a brand of lower tar and nicotine content than the week before.

17. Never say, "I quit smoking," because your resolution is broken if you have a cigarette. Better to say, "I don't want to smoke." This way you maintain your resolution even if you accidentally have a cigarette.

18. Try to help someone else quit smoking, particularly your spouse.

19. Always ask yourself, "Do I need this cigarette or is this just a reflex!"

Figure 10.6. *Tips for Smoking Cessation (continued).*

20. Each day try to put off lighting your first cigarette.

21. Decide arbitrarily that you will smoke only on even- or odd-numbered hours of the clock.

22. Try going to bed early and rising a half hour earlier than usual to avoid hurrying through breakfast and rushing to work.

23. Keep your hands occupied. Try playing a musical instrument, knitting, or fiddling with hand puzzles.

24. Take a shower. You cannot smoke in the shower.

25. Brush your teeth frequently to get rid of the tobacco taste and stains.

26. If you have a sudden craving for a cigarette, take ten deep breaths, holding the last breath while you strike a match. Exhale slowly, blowing out the match. Pretend the match was a cigarette by crushing it out in an ashtray. Now immediately get busy on some work or activity.

27. Only smoke half a cigarette.

28. After you quit, start using your lungs. Increase your activities and indulge in moderate exercise, such as short walks before or after a meal.

29. Bet with someone that you can quit. Put the cigarette money in a jar each morning and forfeit it if you smoke. You keep the money if you don't smoke by the end of the week. Try to extend this period to a month.

30. If you gain weight because you are not smoking, wait until you get over the craving before you diet. Dieting is easier then.

31. If you are depressed or have physical symptoms that might be related to your smoking, relieve your mind by discussing this with your physician. It is easier to quit when you know your health status.

32. Visit your dentist after you quit and have your teeth cleaned to get rid of the tobacco stains.

33. If the cost of cigarettes is your motivation for quitting, try purchasing a money order equivalent to a year's supply of cigarettes. Give it to a friend. If you smoke in the next year, he cashes the money order and keeps the money. If you don't smoke, he gives back the money order at the end of the year.

34. After you have quit, never face the confusion of "craving a cigarette" alone. Find someone who you can call or visit at this critical time.

35. When you feel irritable or tense, shut your eyes and count backward from ten to zero as you imagine yourself descending a flight of stairs, or imagine that you are looking at the horizon as the sun sets in the west.

36. Get out of your old habits. Seek new activities or perform old activities in a new way. Don't rely on the old ways of solving problems. Do things differently.

37. If you are a "kitchen smoker" in the morning, volunteer your services to schools or nonprofit organizations to get you out of the house.

38. Stock up on light reading materials, crossword puzzles, and vacation brochures that you can read during your coffee breaks.

39. Frequent places where you can't smoke, such as libraries, buses, theatres, swimming pools, department stores, or just going to bed during the first weeks you are off cigarettes.

40. Give yourself time to think and get fit by walking one-half hour each day. If you have a dog, take him for a walk with you.

A P P E N D I X   A

Coronary Heart Disease Risk and Physical Fitness Norms

Table A.1.
Cardiovascular Endurance* Risk Points and Risk Categories.

Risk Category	Risk Points	Age					
		19	20-29	30-39	40-49	50-59	60>
Men							
Very Low	0.0	55>	52>	49>	46>	43>	40>
	.3	54	51	48	45	42	39
	.6	53	50	47	44	41	38
Low	.9	52	49	46	43	40	37
	1.2	51	48	45	42	39	36
	1.5	50	47	44	41	38	35
	1.8	49	46	43	40	37	34
	2.1	48	45	42	39	36	33
Moderate	2.4	47	44	41	38	35	32
	2.7	46	43	40	37	34	31
	3.0	45	42	39	36	33	30
	3.3	44	41	38	35	32	29
	3.6	43	40	37	34	31	28
High	3.9	42	39	36	33	30	27
	4.2	41	38	35	32	29	26
	4.5	40	37	34	31	28	25
	4.8	39	36	33	30	27	24
	5.1	38	35	32	29	26	23
Very High	5.4	37	34	31	28	25	22
	5.7	36	33	30	27	24	21
	6.0	<35	<32	<29	<26	<23	<20
Women							
Very Low	0.0	46>	44>	42>	40>	38>	36>
	.3	45	43	41	39	37	35
	.6	44	42	40	38	36	34
	.9	43	41	39	37	35	33
	1.2	42	40	38	36	34	32
	1.5	41	39	37	35	33	31
	1.8	40	38	36	34	32	30
	2.1	39	37	35	33	31	29
Moderate	2.4	38	36	34	32	30	28
	2.7	37	35	33	31	29	27
	3.0	36	34	32	30	28	26
	3.3	35	33	31	29	27	25
	3.6	34	32	30	28	26	24
High	3.9	33	31	29	27	25	23
	4.2	32	30	28	26	24	22
	4.5	31	29	27	25	23	21
	4.8	30	28	26	24	22	20
	5.1	29	27	25	23	21	19
Very High	5.4	28	26	24	22	20	18
	5.7	27	25	23	21	19	17
	6.0	<26	<24	<22	<20	<18	<16

* Oxygen uptake expressed in ml/kg/min

Table A.2.
Electrocardiogram Risk Points and Risk Categories (men and women of all ages).

Risk Category	Results	EKG Risk Points	
		Resting	Stress
Very Low	Normal	0.0	0.0
Moderate	Equivocal	1.0	4.0
Very High	Abnormal	3.0	8.0

Table A.3.
Total Cholesterol-HDL Ratio Risk Points and Risk Categories (men and women of all ages).

Risk Category	Risk Points	Men	Women
Very Low	0.0	<4.5	<4.0
	0.4	4.6	4.1
	0.8	4.7	4.2
	1.2	4.8	4.3
	1.6	4.9	4.4
	2.0	5.0	4.5
Low	2.2	5.1	4.6
	2.4	5.2	4.7
	2.6	5.3	4.8
	2.8	5.4	4.9
	3.0	5.5	5.0
	3.2	5.6	5.1
	3.4	5.7	5.2
	3.6	5.8	5.3
	3.8	5.9	5.4
	4.0	6.0	5.5
Moderate	4.2	6.1	5.6
	4.4	6.2	5.7
	4.6	6.3	5.8
	4.8	6.4	5.9
	5.0	6.5	6.0
	5.2	6.6	6.1
	5.4	6.7	6.2
	5.6	6.8	6.3
	5.8	6.9	6.4
	6.0	7.0	6.5
High	6.2	7.1	6.6
	6.3	7.2	6.7
	6.5	7.3	6.8
	6.6	7.4	6.9
	6.8	7.5	7.0
	6.9	7.6	7.1
	7.0	7.7	7.2
	7.2	7.8	7.3
	7.3	7.9	7.4
	7.5	8.0	7.5
	7.6	8.1	7.6
	7.8	8.2	7.7
	7.9	8.3	7.8
	8.0	8.4	7.9
	8.1	8.5	8.0
Very High	8.3	8.6	8.1
	8.4	8.7	8.2
	8.5	8.8	8.3
	8.7	8.9	8.4
	8.8	9.0	8.5
	8.9	9.1	8.6
	9.0	9.2	8.7
	9.1	9.3	8.8
	9.3	9.4	8.9
	9.4	9.5	9.0
	9.5	9.6	9.1
	9.7	9.7	9.2
	9.8	9.8	9.3
	9.9	9.9	9.4
	10.0	10.0>	9.5>

Table A.4.
Triglycerides* Risk Points and Risk Categories (men and women of all ages).

Risk Category	Risk Points	Results
Very Low	0.0	<100
Low	0.1	101-109
	0.2	110-118
	0.3	119-127
	0.4	128-136
	0.5	137-145
Moderate	0.6	146-154
	0.7	155-163
	0.8	164-172
	0.9	173-181
	1.0	182-190
High	1.1	191-199
	1.2	200-208
	1.3	209-217
	1.4	218-226
	1.5	227-235
Very High	1.6	236-244
	1.7	245-253
	1.8	254-262
	1.9	263-271
	2.0	272>

* **Expressed in mg/dl**

Table A.5.
Blood Glucose* Risk Points and Risk Categories (men and women of all ages).

Risk Category	Risk Points	Results
Very Low	0.0	<120
Low	0.1	121
	0.2	122
	0.3	123
	0.4	124
	0.5	125
	0.6	126
	0.7	127
	0.8	128
Moderate	0.9	129
	1.0	130
	1.1	131
	1.2	132
	1.3	133
	1.4	134
	1.5	135
	1.6	136
High	1.7	137
	1.8	138
	1.9	139
	2.0	140
	2.1	141
	2.2	142
	2.3	143
	2.4	144
Very High	2.5	145
	2.6	146
	2.7	147
	2.8	148
	2.9	149
	3.0	150>
	3.0	Known Diabetic**

*Expressed in mg/dl

**Three points are added for known diabetics regardless of current
blood glucose level

Table A.6.
Blood Pressure* Risk Points and Risk Categories (men and women of all ages).

Risk Category	Risk Points	Systolic Pressure	Diastolic Pressure
Very Low	0.0	<120	<80
Low	0.1	121	81
	0.2	122	82
	0.3	123	83
	0.4	124	84
	0.5	125	85
	0.6	126	---
	0.7	127	86
	0.8	128	87
	0.9	129	88
	1.0	130	89
Moderate	1.1	131	---
	1.2	132	90
	1.3	133	91
	1.4	134	92
	1.5	135	93
	1.6	136	94
	1.7	137	95
	1.8	138	96
	1.9	139	97
	2.0	140	98
High	2.1	141	---
	2.2	142	99
	2.3	143	100
	2.4	144	101
	2.5	145	102
	2.6	146	103
	2.7	147	---
	2.8	148	104
	2.9	149	105
	3.0	150	106
Very High	3.1	151	107
	3.2	152	108
	3.3	153	109
	3.4	154	110
	3.5	155	111
	3.6	156	112
	3.7	157	113
	3.8	158	114
	3.9	159	115
	4.0	160>	116>

* Expressed in mmHg

Table A.7.
Body Composition* Risk Points and Risk Categories — Men.

Risk Category	Risk Points	Age 19	20-29	30-39	40-49	50>
Very Low	0.0	<12.0	<13.0	<14.0	<15.0	<16.0
	0.1	12.5	13.5	14.5	15.5	16.5
	0.2	13.0	14.0	15.0	16.0	17.0
	0.3	13.5	14.5	15.5	16.5	17.5
	0.4	14.0	15.0	16.0	17.0	18.0
Low	0.5	14.5	15.5	16.5	17.5	18.5
	0.6	15.0	16.0	17.0	18.0	19.0
	0.7	15.5	16.5	17.5	18.5	19.5
	0.8	16.0	17.0	18.0	19.0	20.0
	0.9	16.5	17.5	18.5	19.5	20.5
	1.0	17.0	18.0	19.0	20.0	21.0
	1.1	17.5	18.5	19.5	20.5	21.5
	1.2	18.0	19.0	20.0	21.0	22.0
	1.3	18.5	19.5	20.5	21.5	22.5
	1.4	19.0	20.0	21.0	22.0	23.0
Moderate	1.5	19.5	20.5	21.5	22.5	23.5
	1.6	20.0	21.0	22.0	23.0	24.0
	1.7	20.5	21.5	22.5	23.5	24.5
	1.8	21.0	22.0	23.0	24.0	25.0
	1.9	21.5	22.5	23.5	24.5	25.5
	2.0	22.0	23.0	24.0	25.0	26.0
	2.1	22.5	23.5	24.5	25.5	26.5
	2.2	23.0	24.0	25.0	26.0	27.0
	2.3	23.5	24.5	25.5	26.5	27.5
	2.4	24.0	25.0	26.0	27.0	28.0
High	2.5	24.5	25.5	26.5	27.5	28.5
	2.6	25.0	26.0	27.0	28.0	29.0
	2.7	25.5	26.5	27.5	28.5	29.5
	2.8	26.0	27.0	28.0	29.0	30.0
	2.9	26.5	27.5	28.5	29.5	30.5
	3.0	27.0	28.0	29.0	30.0	31.0
	3.1	27.5	28.5	29.5	30.5	31.5
	3.2	28.0	29.0	30.0	31.0	32.0
	3.3	28.5	29.5	30.5	31.5	32.5
	3.4	29.0	30.0	31.0	32.0	33.0
Very High	3.5	29.5	30.5	31.5	32.5	33.5
	3.6	30.0	31.0	32.0	33.0	34.0
	3.7	30.5	31.5	32.5	33.5	34.5
	3.8	31.0	32.0	33.0	34.0	35.0
	3.9	31.5	32.5	33.5	34.5	35.5
	4.0	<32.0	<33.0	<34.0	<35.0	<36.0

*Expressed in percent body fat

Table A.8.
Body Composition* Risk Points and Risk Categories — Women.

Risk Category	Risk Points	Age 19	20-29	30-39	40-49	50>
Very Low	0.0	<17	<18	<19	<20	<21
	0.1	17.5	18.5	19.5	20.5	21.5
	0.2	18.0	19.0	20.0	21.0	22.0
	0.3	18.5	19.5	20.5	21.5	22.5
	0.4	19.0	20.0	21.0	22.0	23.0
Low	0.5	19.5	20.5	21.5	22.5	23.5
	0.6	20.0	21.0	22.0	23.0	24.0
	0.7	20.5	21.5	22.5	23.5	24.5
	0.8	21.0	22.0	23.0	24.0	25.0
	0.9	21.5	22.5	23.5	24.5	25.5
	1.0	22.0	23.0	24.0	25.0	26.0
	1.1	22.5	23.5	24.5	25.5	26.5
	1.2	23.0	24.0	25.0	26.0	27.0
	1.3	23.5	24.5	25.5	26.5	27.5
	1.4	24.0	25.0	26.0	27.0	28.0
Moderate	1.5	24.5	25.5	26.5	27.5	28.5
	1.6	25.0	26.0	27.0	28.0	29.0
	1.7	25.5	26.5	27.5	28.5	29.5
	1.8	26.0	27.0	28.0	29.0	30.0
	1.9	26.5	27.5	28.5	29.5	30.5
	2.0	27.0	28.0	29.0	30.0	31.0
	2.1	27.5	28.5	29.5	30.5	31.5
	2.2	28.0	29.0	30.0	31.0	32.0
	2.3	28.5	29.5	30.5	31.5	32.5
	2.4	29.0	30.0	31.0	32.0	33.0
High	2.5	29.5	30.5	31.5	32.5	33.5
	2.6	30.0	31.0	32.0	33.0	34.0
	2.7	30.5	31.5	32.5	33.5	34.5
	2.8	31.0	32.0	33.0	34.0	35.0
	2.9	31.5	32.5	33.5	34.5	35.5
	3.0	32.0	33.0	34.0	35.0	36.0
	3.1	32.5	33.5	34.5	35.5	36.5
	3.2	33.0	34.0	35.0	36.0	37.0
	3.3	33.5	34.5	35.5	36.5	37.5
	3.4	34.0	35.0	36.0	37.0	38.0
Very High	3.5	34.5	35.5	36.5	37.5	38.5
	3.6	35.0	36.0	37.0	38.0	39.0
	3.7	35.5	36.5	37.5	38.5	39.5
	3.8	36.0	37.0	38.0	39.0	40.0
	3.9	36.5	37.5	38.5	39.5	40.5
	4.0	37.0>	38.0>	39.0>	40.0>	41.0>

*Expressed in percent body fat

Table A.9.
Smoking Risk Points and Risk Categories (men and women of all ages).

Risk Category	Risk Points	Questionnaire Results
Very Low	0.0	(1)* Lifetime non-smoker
	0.0	(2) Ex-smoker over one year
Low	1.0	(4) Ex-smoker less than one year
	1.0	(6) Less than one cigarette/day
	2.0	(5) Pipe, cigar smoker or chew tobacco
	2.0	(3) Non-smoker in smoking environment
Moderate	3.0	(7) 1-9 cigarettes/day
High	4.0	(8) 10-19 cigarettes/day
	5.0	(9) 20-29 cigarettes/day
Very High	6.0	(10) 30-39 cigarettes/day
	8.0	(11) 40+ cigarettes/day

*Number in parenthesis indicates response given in the wellness questionnaire

Table A.10.
Tension and Stress Risk Points and Risk Categories (men and women of all ages).

Risk Category	Risk Points	Questionnaire Results
Very Low	0.0	(1)* Hardly ever tense
Low	1.0	(2) Sometimes tense
Moderate	2.0	(3) Often tense
High	3.0	(4) Nearly always tense
Very High	4.0	(5) Always tense

*Number in parenthesis indicates response given in wellness questionnaire

Table A.11.
Personal History Risk Points and Risk Categories (men and women of all ages).

Risk Category	Risk Points	Questionnaire Results
Very Low	0.0	(1)* Never
Low	2.0	(2) Over 5 years ago
Moderate	3.0	(3) 2-5 years ago
High	5.0	(4) 1-2 years ago
Very High	8.0	(5) Within last year

*Number in parenthesis indicates response given in the wellness questionnaire

Table A.12.
Family History Risk Points and Risk Categories (men and women of all ages).

Risk Category	Risk Points	Questionnaire Results
Very Low	0.0	(1)* None
Low	1.0	(2) After age 60
Moderate	2.0	(3) Between 50 and 60
Very High	4.0	(4) Prior to age 50

*Number in parenthesis indicates response given in the wellness questionnaire

Table A.13.
Estrogen Use Risk Points and Risk Categories.

Risk Category	Risk Points	Questionnaire Results
Low	0.0	(1)* No use
Moderate	1.0	(2) 35 or younger and using for less than 5 years
Very High	2.0	(3) Used for 5+ years
	2.0	(4) 35 or older and using them

*Number in parenthesis indicates response given in the wellness questionnaire

Table A.14.
Age Risk Points and Risk Categories (men and women of all ages).

Risk Category	Risk Points	Age
Very Low	0.0	<20
	0.1	21
	0.2	22
	0.3	23
	0.4	24
Low	0.5	25
	0.6	26
	0.7	27
	0.8	28
	0.9	29
	1.0	30
	1.1	31
	1.2	32
	1.3	33
	1.4	34
Moderate	1.5	35
	1.6	36
	1.7	37
	1.8	38
	1.9	39
	2.0	40
	2.1	41
	2.2	42
	2.3	43
	2.4	44
High	2.5	45
	2.6	46
	2.7	47
	2.8	48
	2.9	49
	3.0	50
	3.1	51
	3.2	52
	3.3	53
Very High	3.4	54
	3.5	55
	3.6	56
	3.7	57
	3.8	58
	3.9	59
	4.0	60>

Table A.15.
Overall Coronary Heart Disease Risk Categories*.

Risk Category	Total Risk Points
Very Low	0 - 5
Low	6 - 15
Moderate	16 - 25
High	26 - 35
Very High	36>

*Total risk score obtained from the sum of the risk points for all the risk factors

Table A.16.
Cardiovascular Endurance* Standards for Men.

Percentile Rank	Age				
	20-29	30-39	40-49	50-59	60>
99	60.0	54.4	52.5	51.6	49.5
95	51.4	49.5	48.0	45.4	44.5
90	47.5	46.5	45.0	43.7	41.0
85	46.5	45.0	43.7	41.0	36.6
80	45.0	43.7	42.5	39.0	35.6
75	43.8	42.5	41.0	37.0	35.0
70	43.8	41.3	40.0	36.0	33.6
65	42.5	41.0	39.0	35.7	32.2
60	41.8	39.0	37.0	34.6	31.0
55	41.0	39.0	36.3	33.5	30.2
50	39.1	37.0	35.7	32.9	29.0
45	38.2	37.0	35.3	32.2	29.0
40	37.0	35.7	34.3	31.5	26.2
35	36.3	35.7	33.6	30.8	29.5
30	35.6	34.6	32.9	30.2	24.5
25	35.5	33.5	31.5	29.2	22.7
20	33.5	32.9	31.1	29.0	21.8
15	32.5	31.5	30.2	26.2	20.1
10	31.5	30.2	27.6	24.5	17.5
5	29.0	27.1	24.1	21.0	15.7
1	22.8	22.7	19.6	16.5	14.0

*Oxygen uptake expressed in ml/kg/min.
Data reproduced with permission from the Cooper Clinic Coronary Risk Factor profile, which are from data collected in patients being evaluated at the Cooper Clinic and standards being established at the Institute for Aerobics Research Dallas, Texas.

Table A.17.
Cardiovascular Endurance* Standards for Women.

Percentile Rank	Age				
	20-29	30-39	40-49	50-59	60>
99	45.0	43.7	43.7	42.5	37.0
95	41.0	40.0	37.0	35.7	31.5
90	38.0	37.0	35.0	32.9	30.2
85	37.0	35.7	32.9	31.5	30.2
80	35.7	35.0	31.5	30.2	26.9
75	34.3	33.6	30.9	30.2	25.3
70	33.6	32.9	30.2	29.0	25.3
65	32.9	31.5	30.2	27.6	24.5
60	31.5	31.5	29.0	26.2	24.5
55	30.9	30.2	29.0	25.3	23.9
50	30.2	30.2	26.7	24.5	21.8
45	30.0	29.3	26.2	24.5	21.3
40	29.6	29.0	25.3	23.6	21.0
35	29.2	27.6	24.5	22.7	20.1
30	29.0	26.2	24.5	22.7	20.1
25	27.6	25.7	22.9	21.9	19.2
20	25.3	24.5	22.7	21.0	18.3
15	24.0	23.1	21.0	20.4	17.5
10	21.8	21.7	21.0	19.2	16.1
05	20.4	21.0	19.2	17.6	15.7
01	19.2	17.0	15.7	14.4	12.3

*Oxygen uptake expressed in ml/kg/min.
Data reproduced with permission from the Cooper Clinic Coronary Risk Factor profile, which are from data collected in patients being evaluated at the Cooper Clinic and standards being established at the Institute for Aerobics Research Dallas, Texas.

Table A.18.
Muscular Strength and Endurance Standards (men and women).

	Percen-tile Rank*	Age:	Exercise								
			Leg Extension			Bench Press			Sit-Up		
			<35**	36-49	50>	<35	36-49	50>	<35	36-49	50>
Men	95		20	25	20	21	36	40	26	33	30
	90		19	23	17	19	32	35	23	26	25
	80		15	20	13	16	27	29	17	23	17
	70		14	17	10	13	23	26	14	20	15
	60		13	15	9	11	20	20	12	17	11
	50		12	14	8	10	16	15	10	13	9
	40		10	12	6	7	12	12	8	10	6
	30		9	10	4	5	10	9	5	7	4
	20		7	7	3	3	6	7	3	3	1
	10		5	2	1	1	1	1	2	1	0
	05		3	1	0	0	0	0	1	0	0
Women	95		20	20	17	21	30	29	27	30	32
	90		18	17	13	20	25	25	22	26	25
	80		13	15	11	16	22	20	14	24	21
	70		11	12	8	13	20	16	11	20	18
	60		10	11	6	11	15	13	6	14	16
	50		9	10	5	10	11	9	5	11	12
	40		8	6	4	5	8	6	4	8	7
	30		7	4	2	3	6	5	2	5	6
	20		5	2	1	1	2	2	1	1	2
	10		3	1	0	0	1	1	0	0	0
	05		1	0	0	0	0	0	0	0	0

Fitness Categories:		
	Excellent	80-99 percentile
	Good	60-79 percentile
	Average	40-59 percentile
	Fair	20-39 percentile
	Poor	01-19 percentile

*Based on total number of repetitions performed according to selected percentages of body weight
(see Appendix E, Muscular Strength and Endurance test protocol).

**Norms for the thirty-five and younger age group are reproduced with permission from Hoeger,
W.W. K. Lifetime Physical Fitness & Wellness: A Personalized Program. Morton Publishing Co.,
1986. Norms for the thirty-six to forty-nine and the fifty and over age groups were developed
at Boise State University.

Table A.19.
Modified Sit-and-Reach Flexibility Standards (men and women).

	Percentile Rank*	Age Category		
		<35	36-49	50>
Men	99	24.7	18.9	16.2
	95	19.5	18.2	15.8
	90	17.9	16.1	15.0
	80	17.0	14.6	13.3
	70	15.8	13.9	12.3
	60	15.0	13.4	11.5
	50	14.4	12.6	10.2
	40	13.5	11.6	9.7
	30	13.0	10.8	9.3
	20	11.6	9.9	8.8
	10	9.2	8.3	7.8
	05	7.9	7.0	7.2
	01	7.0	5.1	4.0
Women	99	19.8	19.8	17.2
	95	18.7	19.2	15.7
	90	17.9	17.4	15.0
	80	16.7	16.2	14.2
	70	16.2	15.2	13.6
	60	15.8	14.5	12.3
	50	14.8	13.5	11.1
	40	14.5	12.8	10.1
	30	13.7	12.2	9.2
	20	12.6	11.0	8.3
	10	10.1	9.7	7.5
	05	8.1	8.5	3.7
	01	2.6	2.0	1.5

Fitness Categories:		
	Excellent	80-99 percentile
	Good	60-79 percentile
	Average	40-59 percentile
	Fair	20-39 percentile
	Poor	01-19 percentile

*Based on the average score of three trials (see Appendix F for the Modified Sit-and-Reach Flexibility Test protocol) Reproduced with permission from Hopkins, D.R., and W.W.K. Hoeger. "The Modified Sit-and-Reach Test" contained in Lifetime Physical Fitness & Wellness: A Personalized Program by W.W.K. Hoeger. Morton Publishing Co., 1986. Norms were updated using additional data collected at Boise State University.

Table A.20.
Trunk Rotation Flexibility Standards (men and women).

Percen-tile Rank* Age:	Right Trunk Rotation			Left Trunk Rotation		
	<35	36-49	50>	<35	36-49	50>
Men 99	27.8	25.2	22.2	28.0	26.6	21.0
95	25.6	23.8	20.7	24.8	24.5	20.0
90	24.1	22.5	19.3	23.6	23.0	17.7
80	22.3	21.0	16.3	22.0	21.2	15.5
70	20.7	18.7	15.7	20.3	20.4	14.7
60	19.0	17.3	14.7	19.3	18.7	13.9
50	17.2	16.3	12.3	18.0	16.7	12.7
40	16.3	14.7	11.5	16.8	15.3	11.7
30	15.0	13.3	10.7	15.0	14.8	10.3
20	13.3	11.2	8.7	13.3	13.7	9.5
10	11.3	8.0	2.7	10.5	10.8	4.3
05	8.3	5.5	0.3	8.9	8.8	0.3
01	2.9	2.0	0.0	1.7	5.1	0.0
Women 99	29.4	27.1	21.7	28.6	27.1	23.0
95	25.3	25.9	19.7	24.8	25.3	21.4
90	23.0	21.3	19.0	23.0	23.4	20.5
80	20.8	19.6	17.9	21.5	20.2	19.1
70	19.3	17.3	16.8	20.5	18.6	17.3
60	18.0	16.5	15.6	19.3	17.7	16.0
50	17.3	14.6	14.0	18.0	16.4	14.8
40	16.0	13.1	12.8	17.2	14.8	13.7
30	15.2	11.7	8.5	15.7	13.6	10.0
20	14.0	9.8	3.9	15.2	11.6	6.3
10	11.1	6.1	2.2	13.6	8.5	3.0
05	8.8	4.0	1.1	7.3	6.8	0.7
01	3.2	2.8	0.0	5.3	4.3	0.0

Fitness Categories:		
	Excellent	80-99 percentile
	Good	60-79 percentile
	Average	40-59 percentile
	Fair	20-39 percentile
	Poor	01-19 percentile

*Based on the average score of three trials (see Appendix F for Trunk Rotation Flexibility Test protocol)

Reproduced with permission from Hoeger, W.W.K. Lifetime Physical Fitness & Welllness: A Personalized Program. Morton Publishing Co., 1986. Norms were updated using additional data collected at Boise State University

Table A.21.
Shoulder Rotation Flexibility Standards (men and women).

	Percentile Rank*	Age Category		
		<35	36-49	50>
Men	99	-1.0	18.1	21.5
	95	10.4	20.4	27.0
	90	15.5	20.8	27.9
	80	18.4	23.3	28.5
	70	20.5	24.7	29.4
	60	22.9	26.6	29.9
	50	24.4	28.0	30.5
	40	25.7	30.0	31.0
	30	27.3	31.9	31.7
	20	30.1	33.3	33.1
	10	31.8	36.1	37.2
	05	33.5	37.8	38.7
	01	42.6	43.0	44.1
Women	99	-2.4	11.5	13.1
	95	6.2	15.4	16.5
	90	9.7	16.8	20.9
	80	14.5	19.2	22.5
	70	17.2	21.5	24.3
	60	18.7	23.1	25.1
	50	20.0	23.5	26.2
	40	21.4	24.4	28.1
	30	24.0	25.9	29.9
	20	25.9	29.8	31.5
	10	29.1	31.1	33.1
	05	31.3	33.4	34.1
	01	37.1	34.9	35.4

Fitness Categories:		
	Excellent	80-99 percentile
	Good	60-79 percentile
	Average	40-59 percentile
	Fair	20-39 percentile
	Poor	01-19 percentile

*Based on the final score for the Shoulder Rotation Test (see Appendix F for Shoulder Rotation Flexibility Test protocol)

Reproduced with permission from Hoeger, W.W.K. Lifetime Physical Fitness & Wellness: A Personalized Program. Morton Publishing Co., 1986. Norms were updated using additional data collected at Boise State University.

Table A.22.
Body Composition* Standards for Men.

Percentile Rank	Age				
	20-29	30-39	40-49	50-59	60>
99	7.2	7.1	9.2	9.0	10.5
95	9.6	11.1	13.0	13.1	12.3
90	11.6	13.4	14.9	15.8	14.1
85	12.9	14.8	16.6	17.4	16.2
80	13.9	16.2	17.6	18.4	17.2
75	15.3	17.2	18.8	19.6	18.0
70	16.2	18.2	19.7	20.4	18.9
65	17.1	19.2	20.7	21.4	19.9
60	18.0	20.1	21.5	22.2	20.8
55	19.1	21.1	22.2	22.9	21.5
50	20.1	22.0	23.0	23.8	22.3
45	21.2	22.8	23.8	24.6	23.3
40	22.3	23.6	24.6	25.4	24.4
35	23.4	24.4	25.4	26.1	25.4
30	25.4	25.5	26.3	27.0	26.9
25	27.4	26.4	27.4	28.0	28.0
20	28.6	28.0	28.5	29.1	28.9
15	30.5	29.8	30.0	30.9	30.1
10	32.8	32.2	32.2	32.8	32.5
05	38.0	36.0	36.1	35.9	35.6
01	49.0	45.9	44.4	44.8	42.4

*Expressed in percent of body fat.

Data reproduced with permission from the Cooper Clinic Coronary Risk Factor Profile, which are from data collected on patients being evaluated at the Cooper Clinic and standards being established at the Institute for Aerobics Research, Dallas, Texas.

Table A.23.
Body Composition* Standards for Women.

Percentile Rank	Age				
	20-29	30-39	40-49	50-59	60>
99	7.8	5.1	7.3	10.8	6.8
95	9.6	10.1	12.0	15.9	13.1
90	11.6	13.1	15.8	18.2	17.7
85	14.5	14.8	17.9	21.0	19.3
80	15.1	16.7	19.6	22.7	22.2
75	16.1	18.3	21.0	23.9	24.0
70	18.3	19.3	21.9	25.1	25.1
65	20.2	20.5	22.7	26.1	26.6
60	23.2	21.5	23.9	27.0	27.1
55	24.1	22.5	24.9	27.7	27.9
50	24.9	23.6	25.9	28.4	29.8
45	25.6	24.6	26.7	29.6	30.4
40	26.2	25.5	27.6	30.4	30.8
35	27.3	26.3	28.2	31.4	31.2
30	28.2	27.6	29.1	32.5	31.7
25	30.3	29.0	30.2	33.4	32.5
20	33.3	31.3	31.4	34.7	34.7
15	36.4	34.6	33.7	37.1	35.2
10	38.5	38.1	37.4	39.7	36.3
05	45.5	42.9	43.1	44.4	39.9
01	51.4	50.2	49.7	52.2	51.2

*Expressed in percent of body fat.

Data reproduced with permission from the Cooper Clinic Coronary Risk Factor Profile, which are from data collected on patients being evaluated at the Cooper Clinic and standards being established at the Institute for Aerobics Research, Dallas, Texas.

Table A.24.
Posture Analysis Standards (men and women).

Classification	Total Points
Excellent	45>
Good	40-44
Average	30-39
Fair	20-29
Poor	<19

*See Appendix H for posture analysis procedures.

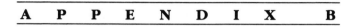

A P P E N D I X   B

Wellness Questionnaire

WELLNESS QUESTIONNAIRE (Sample)

Name _____ Birthdate _____ _____ _____

    Age _____   Sex _____   Social Security Number _____ _____ _____

    Address _____

    City _____ State _____ Zip Code _____

    Home Phone (   ) _____ Office Phone (   ) _____

    Personal Physician _____ Phone (   ) _____

Please read the following health history and lifestyle questionnaire carefully. Select the most appropriate answer to each question. All information obtained in this questionnaire will be treated strictly confidential and will not be released to any third party without your written consent. The information, however, may be used as anonymous data for publication of scientific research with your right of privacy retained.

GENERAL HEALTH HISTORY

A. Have you ever had or do you now have any of the following conditions:

1. Diabetes _____ Yes _____ No
2. Asthma _____ Yes _____ No
3. Chronic bronchitis _____ Yes _____ No
4. Pneumonia _____ Yes _____ No
5. Emphysema _____ Yes _____ No
6. Varicose veins _____ Yes _____ No
7. Phlebitis _____ Yes _____ No
8. Arthritis _____ Yes _____ No
9. Rheumatism _____ Yes _____ No
10. Gout _____ Yes _____ No
11. Gastrointestinal abnormalities _____ Yes _____ No
12. Epilepsy _____ Yes _____ No
13. Dizziness _____ Yes _____ No
14. Loss of memory _____ Yes _____ No
15. Anemia _____ Yes _____ No
16. Chronic low back pain _____ Yes _____ No
17. Kidney or bladder problems _____ Yes _____ No
18. Nervous system problems _____ Yes _____ No
19. Visual or hearing impairments _____ Yes _____ No
20. Hepatitis _____ Yes _____ No
21. Thyroid problems _____ Yes _____ No
22. Tuberculosis _____ Yes _____ No
23. Cancer _____ Yes _____ No
24. Mononucleosis _____ Yes _____ No
25. Sexually transmitted diseases _____ Yes _____ No
26. Anorexia _____ Yes _____ No
27. Bulimia _____ Yes _____ No
28. Any other major illness or surgery _____ Yes _____ No
    If yes, explain:

_____

_____

B. The following are the seven warning signals for cancer. Indicate if you have recently noticed any of these conditions:

    1. Change in bowel or bladder habits   _____ Yes _____ No

    2. A sore that does not heal   _____ Yes _____ No

    3. Unusual bleeding or discharge   _____ Yes _____ No

    4. Thickening or lump in the breast or elsewhere   _____ Yes _____ No

    5. Indigestion or difficulty in swallowing   _____ Yes _____ No

    6. Obvious change in wart or mole   _____ Yes _____ No

    7. Nagging cough or hoarseness   _____ Yes _____ No

C. Are you now taking any prescription or non-prescription drug?   _____ Yes _____ No

    If yes, indicate name of medication and reason for taking it:

    _____

D. Are you allergic to any drugs?   _____ Yes _____ No

    If yes, please list them _____

E. Are you pregnant?   _____ NA* _____ Yes _____ No

F. Have you ever or do you now smoke
(includes pipe, cigar or chewing tobacco)?   _____ Yes _____ No

    Check the appropriate category:

    ☐ 1. Lifetime non smoker

    ☐ 2. Ex-smoker over one year

    ☐ 3. Non smoker, but live or work in smoking environment

    ☐ 4. Ex-smoker less than one year

    ☐ 5. Pipe, cigar smoker or chew tobacco

    ☐ 6. Smoke less than 1 cigarette per day

    ☐ 7. Smoke 1-9 cigarettes per day

    ☐ 8. Smoke 10-19 cigarettes per day

    ☐ 9. Smoke 20-29 cigarettes per day

    ☐ 10. Smoke 30-39 cigarettes per day

    ☐ 11. Smoke 40 or more cigarettes per day

       Indicate the number of years smoked: _____ years

G. Do you consider your current body weight
as reasonable or desirable for yourself?   _____ Yes _____ No

    If no, indicate what you feel your reasonable or desirable weight should be: _____ lbs.

H. Regarding body weight:

    ☐ 1. I am frequently trying to lose weight

    ☐ 2. I have a hard time maintaining my desired weight

    ☐ 3. I am trying to lose weight (on a low-calorie diet now)

    ☐ 4. I do not worry about my weight

    ☐ 5. I don't have a problem maintaining my weight

I. When on a diet, do you try to participate
in an aerobic exercise program?   _____ NA _____ Yes _____ No

J. Do you have:

    1. A coffee addiction (or other caffeine containing beverages)   _____ Yes _____ No

    2. An alcohol problem   _____ Yes _____ No

    3. Other drug dependency   _____ Yes _____ No

K. Do you use estrogens (birth control pills and certain hormone drugs)?

    ☐ 1. Do not use estrogens (or not-applicable)

    ☐ 2. I am 35 years or younger and have used estrogens for less than five years

    ☐ 3. I have used estrogens for over five years

    ☐ 4. I am 35 years or older and currently using estrogens

*NA = Not Applicable

CARDIOVASCULAR DISEASE HISTORY

A. Have you ever suffered from cardiovascular disease
(any type of heart or blood vessel disease, including strokes)?
- ☐ 1. Never
- ☐ 2. More than 5 years ago
- ☐ 3. 2-5 years ago
- ☐ 4. 1-2 years ago
- ☐ 5. Within the last year

B. Have you ever had or do you now have any of the following*:

1. Recent acute myocardial infarction _____ Yes _____ No
2. Unstable angina _____ Yes _____ No
3. Uncontrolled ventricular dysrhythmia _____ Yes _____ No
4. Uncontrolled atrial dysrhythmia which
   compromises cardiac function _____ Yes _____ No
5. Congestive heart failure _____ Yes _____ No
6. Severe aortic stenosis _____ Yes _____ No
7. Suspected or known dissecting aneurysm _____ Yes _____ No
8. Active or suspected myocarditis _____ Yes _____ No
9. Thrombophlebitis or intracardiac thrombi _____ Yes _____ No
10. Recent systemic or pulmonary embolus _____ Yes _____ No
11. Acute infection _____ Yes _____ No
12. Third degree heart block _____ Yes _____ No
13. Significant emotional distress (psychosis) _____ Yes _____ No
14. A recent significant change in the resting ECG _____ Yes _____ No
15. Acute pericarditis _____ Yes _____ No

C. Have you ever had or now have any of these conditions**:

1. Resting diastolic blood pressure over 120 mmHg or
   resting systolic blood pressure over 200 mmHg _____ Yes _____ No
2. Moderate valvular heart disease _____ Yes _____ No
3. Digitalis or other drug effect _____ Yes _____ No
4. Electrolyte abnormalities _____ Yes _____ No
5. Fixed rate artificial pacemaker _____ Yes _____ No
6. Frequent or complex ventricular irritability _____ Yes _____ No
7. Ventricular aneurysm _____ Yes _____ No
8. Cardiomyopathy including hypertrophic cardiomyopathy _____ Yes _____ No
9. Uncontrolled metabolic disease
   (diabetes, thyrotoxicosis, myxedema, etc.) _____ Yes _____ No
10. Any serious systemic disorder (mononucleosis, hepatitis, etc.) _____ Yes _____ No
11. Neuromuscular, musculoskeletal, or rheumatoid disorders
    which would make exercise difficult _____ Yes _____ No

D. Do you have any blood relatives (brothers, sisters, parents, grandparents, uncles, aunts or cousins) that
have suffered from heart disease or strokes?
- ☐ 1. None
- ☐ 2. After age 60
- ☐ 3. Between the ages of 50 and 60
- ☐ 4. Prior to age 50

---

*Absolute contraindications for exercise testing.
**Relative contraindications for exercise testing. Reproduced with permission from Guidelines for Exercise Testing and Prescription.
American College of Sports Medicine. Philadelphia: Lea & Febiger, 1986.

E.   Have you ever had or do you now have high blood pressure?   _____ Yes _____ No

F.   Do you remember what your blood pressure was
     the last time it was taken?   _____ Yes _____ No
     If yes, do you recall what the blood pressure was? _____/_____

G.   Have you ever had:
     1. A resting electrocardiogram   _____ Yes _____ No
        If yes, was it _____ Normal _____ Equivocal _____ Abnormal?
     2. A stress electrocardiogram?   _____ Yes _____ No
        If yes, was it _____ Normal _____ Equivocal _____ Abnormal?

NUTRITION SECTION

A.   What describes your eating habits best:
     ☐ 1. I eat three regular meals a day
     ☐ 2. I skip breakfast, often miss lunch, and eat a large dinner
     ☐ 3. I only eat one meal a day
     ☐ 4. I don't have time to eat regularly and frequently snack or eat on the run

B.   How many servings of the following foods do you eat per day or week as indicated?

FOOD	SERVING SIZE	SERVINGS
Eggs	1	_____/week
Regular beef, pork or lamb	1 oz.	_____/week
Luncheon meats	1 oz.	_____/week
Poultry with skin	1 oz.	_____/week
Hard-shell fish (shrimp, lobster, oysters)	1 oz.	_____/week
Cheese (hard, such as cheddar, swiss)	1 oz.	_____/week
Salad dressings (regular, not low in calories)	1 Tbsp.	_____/week
Gravy	3 Tbsp.	_____/week
Bacon	1 slice	_____/week
Sausage	1 oz.	_____/week
Hot dogs	1 (2 oz.)	_____/week
Nuts, nut butter	1 oz. or 2 Tbsp.	_____/week
Cookies	1 small (2″)	_____/week
Ice cream	1 cup	_____/week
Pies, cakes, pastries	1 slice	_____/week
Candy bars	1	_____/week
Soft drinks (regular)	12 oz.	_____/week
Soft drinks (sugar free)	12 oz.	_____/week
Alcohol (1 beer, 4 oz. of wine, ½ jigger of whiskey or equivalent = 1)	1	_____/week
Butter, margarine or cream	1 Tbsp.	_____/day
Whole milk	8 oz. (1 cup)	_____/day
Coffee	8 oz.	_____/day

C. How many of the following do you eat per day or week as indicated?

FOOD	SERVING SIZE	SERVINGS
Fresh fruit	1 avg. piece	_____/day
Fruit juices	4 oz. or ½ cup	_____/day
Water	8 oz.	_____/day
Cooked vegetables	½ cup	_____/day
Raw vegetables	½ cup	_____/day
Low fat milk (2% or less)	8 oz.	_____/day
Low fat cheeses (such as mozzarella)	1 oz.	_____/week
Lean beef, pork or lamb	1 oz.	_____/week
Poultry without skin	3 oz.	_____/week
Fish (no hard-shell: cod, red snapper, halibut)	3 oz.	_____/week
Whole grain or unsweetened cereal	1 cup	_____/week
Whole grain bread	1 slice	_____/week
Whole grain or enriched pasta products	1 oz., dry weight	_____/week
Dried beans and peas (cooked)	½ cup	_____/week

D. How much salt do you add to your food at the table?
- ☐ 1. Do not use salt
- ☐ 2. Seldom use salt
- ☐ 3. Sometimes use a small amount
- ☐ 4. Usually add salt to food
- ☐ 5. Always add salt before tasting the food

E. How often do you eat fried foods?
- ☐ 1. Less than 3 times per week
- ☐ 2. Between 4-6 times per week
- ☐ 3. More than 7 times per week

F. How often do you eat out?
- ☐ 1. Seldom
- ☐ 2. Once a week
- ☐ 3. 2-4 times per week
- ☐ 4. 5 or more times per week

G. In terms of adequate nutrition, do you consider your present diet to be:
- ☐ 1. Poor
- ☐ 2. Fair
- ☐ 3. Good
- ☐ 4. Excellent

H. Do you take any of the following supplements?
- ☐ 1. Multiple vitamins
- ☐ 2. Multiple vitamins *and* minerals
- ☐ 3. Vitamin C
- ☐ 4. Calcium
- ☐ 5. Iron
- ☐ 6. Other, indicate _____

PHYSICAL ACTIVITY SECTION

A. Do you consider your present fitness level to be:

☐ 1. Poor
☐ 2. Fair
☐ 3. Average
☐ 4. Good
☐ 5. Excellent

B. How often do you participate in a continuous aerobic activity (or exercise) for over 20 minutes?

☐ 1. 7 or more times per week
☐ 2. 4-6 times per week
☐ 3. 3 times per week
☐ 4. 1-2 times per week
☐ 5. less than once per week

C. How would you rate the physical nature of your job?

☐ 1. Very strenuous
☐ 2. Strenuous
☐ 3. Somewhat strenuous
☐ 4. Sedentary

D. How do you feel about participating in aerobic physical activities?

☐ 1. Love it
☐ 2. Enjoy it
☐ 3. It's okay
☐ 4. Dislike it
☐ 5. Don't mention it

E. If you do or were to participate in an exercise program, name some physical activities including sports that you would choose to do:

1. _____   4. _____

2. _____   5. _____

3. _____   6. _____

F. Do you have any other physical or medical conditions that could interfere with your participation in a physical fitness program or a graded exercise stress test?   _____ Yes _____ No

If yes, indicate _____

TENSION AND STRESS SECTION

A. The Life Experiences Survey*

Listed below are a number of events which sometimes bring about change in the lives of those who experience them and which necessitate social readjustment. Please check those events which you have experienced in the past twelve months. Be sure that all check marks are directly across from the items they correspond to (only check those that apply).

Also, for each item checked below, please indicate the extent to which you viewed the event as having either a positive or negative impact on your life at the time the event occurred. That is, indicate the type and extent of impact that the event had. A rating of –3 would indicate an extremely negative impact. A rating of 0 suggests that no impact either positive or negative. A rating of +3 would indicate an extremely positive impact.

Section 1

1. Marriage	–3	–2	–1	0	+1	+2	+3
2. Detention in jail or comparable institution	–3	–2	–1	0	+1	+2	+3
3. Death of spouse	–3	–2	–1	0	+1	+2	+3
4. Major change in sleeping habits (much more or much less sleep)	–3	–2	–1	0	+1	+2	+3
5. Death of close family member:							
a. mother	–3	–2	–1	0	+1	+2	+3
b. father	–3	–2	–1	0	+1	+2	+3
c. brother	–3	–2	–1	0	+1	+2	+3
d. sister	–3	–2	–1	0	+1	+2	+3
e. grandmother	–3	–2	–1	0	+1	+2	+3
f. grandfather	–3	–2	–1	0	+1	+2	+3
g. other (specify)	–3	–2	–1	0	+1	+2	+3
6. Major change in eating habits (much more or much less food intake)	–3	–2	–1	0	+1	+2	+3
7. Foreclosure on mortgage or loan	–3	–2	–1	0	+1	+2	+3
8. Death of close friend	–3	–2	–1	0	+1	+2	+3
9. Outstanding personal achievement	–3	–2	–1	0	+1	+2	+3
10. Minor law violations (traffic tickets, disturbing the peace, etc.)	–3	–2	–1	0	+1	+2	+3
11. Male: Wife/girlfriend's pregnancy	–3	–2	–1	0	+1	+2	+3
12. Female: Pregnancy	–3	–2	–1	0	+1	+2	+3
13. Changed work situation (different work responsibility, major change in working conditions, working hours, etc.)	–3	–2	–1	0	+1	+2	+3
14. New job	–3	–2	–1	0	+1	+2	+3
15. Serious illness or injury of close family member:							
a. father	–3	–2	–1	0	+1	+2	+3
b. mother	–3	–2	–1	0	+1	+2	+3
c. sister	–3	–2	–1	0	+1	+2	+3
d. brother	–3	–2	–1	0	+1	+2	+3
e. grandfather	–3	–2	–1	0	+1	+2	+3
f. grandmother	–3	–2	–1	0	+1	+2	+3
g. spouse	–3	–2	–1	0	+1	+2	+3
h. other (specify)	–3	–2	–1	0	+1	+2	+3

*From Sarason, I.G., et al. Assessing the Impact of Life Changes: Development of the Life Experiences Survey. Journal of Consulting and Clinical Psychology 46:932-946, 1978. Copyright 1978 by the American Psychological Association. Reprinted by permission of the publisher and author.

16. Sexual difficulties	−3	−2	−1	0	+1	+2	+3
17. Trouble with employer (in danger of losing job, being suspended, demoted, etc.)	−3	−2	−1	0	+1	+2	+3
18. Trouble with in-laws	−3	−2	−1	0	+1	+2	+3
19. Major change in financial status (a lot better off or a lot worse off)	−3	−2	−1	0	+1	+2	+3
20. Major change in closeness of family members (increased or decreased closeness)	−3	−2	−1	0	+1	+2	+3
21. Gaining a new family member (through birth, adoption, family member moving in, etc.)	−3	−2	−1	0	+1	+2	+3
22. Change of residence	−3	−2	−1	0	+1	+2	+3
23. Marital separation from mate (due to conflict)	−3	−2	−1	0	+1	+2	+3
24. Major change in church activities (increased or decreased attendance)	−3	−2	−1	0	+1	+2	+3
25. Marital reconciliation with mate	−3	−2	−1	0	+1	+2	+3
26. Major change in number of arguments with spouse (a lot more or a lot less arguments)	−3	−2	−1	0	+1	+2	+3
27. Married Male: Change in wife's work outside the home (beginning work, ceasing work, changing to a new job, etc.)	−3	−2	−1	0	+1	+2	+3
28. Married Female: Change in husband's work (loss of job, beginning new job, retirement, etc.)	−3	−2	−1	0	+1	+2	+3
29. Major change in usual type and/or amount of recreation	−3	−2	−1	0	+1	+2	+3
30. Borrowing more than $10,000 (buying home, business, etc.)	−3	−2	−1	0	+1	+2	+3
31. Borrowing less than $10,000 (buying car, TV, getting school loan, etc.)	−3	−2	−1	0	+1	+2	+3
32. Being fired from job	−3	−2	−1	0	+1	+2	+3
33. Male: Wife/girlfriend having abortion	−3	−2	−1	0	+1	+2	+3
34. Female: Having abortion	−3	−2	−1	0	+1	+2	+3
35. Major personal illness or injury	−3	−2	−1	0	+1	+2	+3
36. Major change in social activities, e.g., parties, movies, visiting (increased or decreased participation)	−3	−2	−1	0	+1	+2	+3
37. Major change in living conditions of family (building new home, remodeling, deterioration of home, neighborhood, etc.)	−3	−2	−1	0	+1	+2	+3
38. Divorce	−3	−2	−1	0	+1	+2	+3
39. Serious injury or illness of close friend	−3	−2	−1	0	+1	+2	+3
40. Retirement from work	−3	−2	−1	0	+1	+2	+3
41. Son or daughter leaving home (due to marriage, college, etc.)	−3	−2	−1	0	+1	+2	+3
42. Ending of formal schooling	−3	−2	−1	0	+1	+2	+3
43. Separation from spouse (due to work, travel, etc.)	−3	−2	−1	0	+1	+2	+3
44. Engagement	−3	−2	−1	0	+1	+2	+3
45. Breaking up with boyfriend/girlfriend	−3	−2	−1	0	+1	+2	+3
46. Leaving home for the first time	−3	−2	−1	0	+1	+2	+3
47. Reconciliation with boyfriend/girlfriend	−3	−2	−1	0	+1	+2	+3
Others:							
48. _____	−3	−2	−1	0	+1	+2	+3
49. _____	−3	−2	−1	0	+1	+2	+3
50. _____	−3	−2	−1	0	+1	+2	+3

Section 2

51.	Beginning a new school experience at a higher academic level (college, graduate school, professional school, etc.)	−3	−2	−1	0	+1	+2	+3
52.	Changing to a new school at a same academic level (undergraduate, graduate, etc.)	−3	−2	−1	0	+1	+2	+3
53.	Academic probation	−3	−2	−1	0	+1	+2	+3
54.	Being dismissed from dormitory or other residence	−3	−2	−1	0	+1	+2	+3
55.	Failing an important exam	−3	−2	−1	0	+1	+2	+3
56.	Changing a major	−3	−2	−1	0	+1	+2	+3
57.	Failing a course	−3	−2	−1	0	+1	+2	+3
58.	Dropping a course	−3	−2	−1	0	+1	+2	+3
59.	Joining a fraternity/sorority	−3	−2	−1	0	+1	+2	+3
60.	Financial problems concerning school (in danger of not having sufficient money to continue)	−3	−2	−1	0	+1	+2	+3

FINAL SCORE (To interpret the final score, refer to Chapter 7, Table 7.1.)

Total number of negative points: _____

Total number of positive points: _____

Total score (add both the positive and negative scores as positive numbers): _____

B. Stress Vulnerability Scale*

The following scale has been designed to rate your vulnerability to stress. Rate each item from 1 (almost always) to 5 (never), according to how each particular statement applies to you. Make sure to mark each item. If a particular item doesn't apply to you, circle a 1 (for example, if you don't smoke, circle 1).

Item	Score					
1.	I eat at least one hot, balanced meal a day.	1	2	3	4	5
2.	I get seven to eight hours of sleep at least four nights a week.	1	2	3	4	5
3.	I give and receive affection regularly.	1	2	3	4	5
4.	I have at least one relative within 50 miles on whom I can rely.	1	2	3	4	5
5.	I exercise to the point of perspiration at least three times per week.	1	2	3	4	5
6.	I limit myself to less than half a pack of cigarettes a day.	1	2	3	4	5
7.	I take fewer than five alcoholic drinks a week.	1	2	3	4	5
8.	I am at the appropriate weight for my height.	1	2	3	4	5
9.	I have an income adequate to meet basic expenses.	1	2	3	4	5
10.	I get strength from my religious beliefs.	1	2	3	4	5
11.	I regularly attend club or social activities.	1	2	3	4	5
12.	I have a network of friends and acquaintances.	1	2	3	4	5
13.	I have one or more friends to confide in about personal matters.	1	2	3	4	5
14.	I am in good health (including eyesight, hearing, teeth).	1	2	3	4	5
15.	I am able to speak openly about my feelings when angry or worried.	1	2	3	4	5
16.	I have regular conversations with the people I live with about domestic problems — for example, chores and money.	1	2	3	4	5
17.	I do something for fun at least once a week.	1	2	3	4	5
18.	I am able to organize my time effectively.	1	2	3	4	5
19.	I drink fewer than three cups of coffee (or other caffeine-rich drinks) a day.	1	2	3	4	5
20.	I take some quiet time for myself during the day.	1	2	3	4	5

To obtain your final score, add up all of the numbers that you circled and subtract 20.

Total score: _____ − 20 = _____ Points (final score**)

---

*From "Vulnerability Scale." Stress Audit, developed by Lyle H. Miller and Alma Dell Smith. Boston University Medical Center. Copyright 1983. Biobehavioral Associates. Reprinted with permission.
**Refer to Chapter 7, Table 7.2 to obtain a stress vulnerability rating based on the final score.

C. The following is a list of typical symptoms experienced during stress. Using a scale from 1 to 3 (never, sometimes, often) rate the frequency with which you experience these symptoms:

Typical Symptoms of Stress:

_____ Headache

_____ Muscular aches

      (mainly neck, shoulders, and back)

_____ Grinding teeth

_____ Nervous tick, finger tapping,

      toe tapping

_____ Increased sweating

_____ Increase or loss of appetite

_____ Insomnia

_____ Nightmares

_____ Fatigue

_____ Dry mouth

_____ Stuttering

_____ High blood pressure

_____ Tightness or pain in the chest

_____ Impotence

_____ Hives

_____ Others that you experience (list):

_____ Dizziness

_____ Depression

_____ Irritation

_____ Anger

_____ Frustration

_____ Hostility

_____ Fear, panic, anxiety

_____ Stomach pain, flutters

_____ Nausea

_____ Cold, clammy hands

_____ Poor concentration

_____ Pacing

_____ Restlessness

_____ Rapid heart rate

_____ Low grade infection

_____ Loss of sex drive

_____ Rash or acne

_____

_____

D. How would you rate yourself as far as tension and stress is concerned?
1. Hardly ever tense.
2. Sometimes tense.
3. Often tense.
4. Nearly always tense.
5. Always tense.

WELLNESS GOALS AND OBJECTIVES

Briefly indicate what motivates you to participate in a wellness program.

_____

_____

_____

_____

_____

_____

_____

_____

APPENDIX C

Cardiovascular Endurance Test Protocols and Exercise Prescription

CARDIOVASCULAR ENDURANCE TEST PROTOCOLS

I. Procedures for The 1.5-Mile Run Test: a cardiovascular endurance test to estimate maximal oxygen uptake.

1. Make sure that the person qualifies for this test. Since the objective of this test is to cover the distance in the shortest period of time, its use must be limited to conditioned individuals who have been cleared for exercise. At least six weeks of aerobic training are recommended prior to taking the test. It is contraindicated for unconditioned beginners, individuals with symptoms of heart disease, and those with known heart disease and/or risk factors.

2. Select the testing site. Find a school track (each lap is one-fourth of a mile) or a pre-measured 1.5-mile course.

3. Have a stopwatch available to determine the time.

4. Individuals should be properly warmed up prior to the test. Some stretching exercises, walking, and slow jogging are recommended.

5. During the test the person must try to cover the distance in the fastest time possible (walking or jogging). The time required to cover the distance is recorded, and according to the performance time, the estimated maximal oxygen uptake can be found in Table C.1. If at any time during the test unusual symptoms arise, the individuals should not continue the test, but rather should slow down immediately and retake the test after another six weeks of aerobic training.

6. Make sure that at the end of the test the person cools down by walking or jogging slowly for another three to five minutes. Individuals who have taken the test should NOT sit or lie down upon completion of the test.

7. Example. A thirty-five-year-old female ran the 1.5-mile course in sixteen minutes and twenty seconds. According to

Table C.1.
Estimated Maximal Oxygen Uptake (Max. VO$_2$) in ml/kg/min for the 2.5-Mile Run Test.

Time	Max VO$_2$	Time	Max VO$_2$	Time	Max VO$_2$	Time	Max VO$_2$	Time	Max VO$_2$
6:10	80.0	8:50	59.1	11:30	44.4	14:10	35.5	16:50	29.1
6:20	79.0	9:00	58.1	11:40	43.7	14:20	35.1	17:00	28.9
6:30	77.9	9:10	56.9	11:50	43.2	14:30	34.7	17:10	28.5
6:40	76.7	9:20	55.9	12:00	42.3	14:40	34.3	17:20	28.3
6:50	75.5	9:30	54.7	12:10	41.7	14:50	34.0	17:30	28.0
7:00	74.0	9:40	53.5	12:20	41.0	15:00	33.6	17:40	27.7
7:10	72.6	9:50	52.3	12:30	40.4	15:10	33.1	17:50	27.4
7:20	71.3	10:00	51.1	12:40	39.8	15:20	32.7	18:00	27.1
7:30	69.9	10:10	50.4	12:50	39.2	15:30	32.2	18:10	26.8
7:40	68.3	10:20	49.5	13:00	38.6	15:40	31.8	18:20	26.6
7:50	66.8	10:30	48.6	13:10	38.1	15:50	31.4	18:30	26.3
8:00	65.2	10:40	48.0	13:20	37.8	16:00	30.9	18:40	26.0
8:10	63.9	10:50	47.4	13:30	37.2	16:10	30.5	18:50	25.7
8:20	62.5	11:00	46.6	13:40	36.8	16:20	30.2	19:00	25.4
8:30	61.2	11:10	45.8	13:50	36.3	16:30	29.8		
8:40	60.2	11:20	45.1	14:00	35.9	16:40	29.5		

Adapted from: Cooper, K. H. "A Means of Assessing Maximal Oxygen Intake." *JAMA* 203:201-204, 1968. Pollock, M. L., et al. *Health and Fitness Through Physical Activity.* New York: John Wiley and Sons, 1978. Wilmore, J. H. *Training for Sport and Activity.* Boston: Allyn and Bacon, Inc., 1982.

Table C.1, the estimated maximal oxygen uptake would be 30.2 ml/kg/min.

8. The respective cardiovascular endurance fitness category is determined according to Table 4.3 in Chapter 4. In this particular example, the fitness category would be fair (or "high risk" for coronary disease on this factor).

II. Procedures for the Astrand-Ryhming Test: a submaximal cardiovascular endurance test to estimate maximal oxygen uptake.

1. Adjust the bike seat so that the knees are almost completely extended as the foot goes through the bottom of the pedaling cycle.

2. During the test, the speed should be kept constant at fifty revolutions per minute. Test duration is six minutes.

3. Select the appropriate workload for the bike based on age, health, and estimated fitness level. For unconditioned individuals: women, use 300 kpm (kilopounds per meter) or 450 kpm; men, 300 kpm or 600 kpm. Conditioned adults: women, 450 kpm or 600 kpm; men, 600 kpm or 900 kpm.*

4. Have the subject ride the bike for six minutes and check the heart rate every minute, during the last ten seconds of each minute. Heart rate should be determined by recording the time it takes to count thirty pulse beats, and then converting to beats per minute using Table C.2. It is also recommended that exercise blood pressure be measured during the fourth minute of the test.

5. Average the final two heart rates (fifth and sixth minutes). If these two heart rates are not within five beats per minute of each other, continue the test for another few minutes until this is accomplished. If the heart rate continues to climb significantly after the sixth minute, stop the test and let the person rest for fifteen to twenty

minutes. You may then retest, preferably at a lower workload. The final average heart rate should also fall between the ranges given for each workload in Table C.3 (e.g., men: 300 kpm = 120 to 140 beats per minute, 600 kpm = 129 to 170 beats per minute).

6. Based on the average heart rate of the final two minutes and the workload, look up the maximal oxygen uptake in Table C.3 (e.g., men: 600 kpm and average heart rate = 145, maximal oxygen uptake = 2.4 liters/minute).

7. Correct maximal oxygen uptake using the correction factors found in Table C.4 (e.g., maximal oxygen uptake = 2.4 and age thirty-five, correction factor = .870. Multiply 2.4 x .870 and final corrected maximal oxygen uptake = 2.09 liters/minute).

8. To obtain maximal oxygen uptake in ml/kg/min, multiply the maximal oxygen uptake by 1000 (to convert liters to milliliters) and divide by body weight in kilograms (divide the weight in pounds by 2.2046 to obtain kilograms).

9. Example. Corrected maximal oxygen uptake = 2.09 liters/minute

Body weight = 132 lbs or 60 kg
$$(132/2.2046 = 60)$$

Maximal oxygen uptake in ml/kg/min:
2.09 (lts/min) x 1000 = 2090 ml/min
2090 (ml/min) divided by 60 (kg) = 34.8 ml/kg/min

The respective cardiovascular endurance fitness categories based on maximal oxygen uptake are given in Table 4.3, Chapter 4.

III. Procedures for The Step Test**: a submaximal cardiovascular endurance test to assess maximal oxygen uptake.

1. The test is conducted with a bench or gymnasium bleachers 16¼ inches high.

2. The stepping cycle is performed to a four-step cadence (up-up-down-down). Men should perform twenty-four complete

---

*On the Monarch bicycle ergometer when riding at a speed of fifty revolutions per minute, a load of 1 kp = 300 kpm, 1.5 kp = 450 kpm, 2 kp = 600 kpm, and so forth, with increases of 300 kpm to each kp.

** From McArdle, W. D. et al.: *Exercise Physiology, Energy, Nutrition, and Human Performance.* Philadelphia, Lea & Febiger, 1986.

Table C.2.
Conversion of the Time for 30 Pulse Beats to Pulse Rate per Minute (bpm).

Sec.	bpm	Sec.	bpm	Sec.	bpm
22.0	82	17.3	104	12.6	143
21.9	82	17.2	105	12.5	144
21.8	83	17.1	105	12.4	145
21.7	83	17.0	106	12.3	146
21.6	83	16.9	107	12.2	148
21.5	84	16.8	107	12.1	149
21.4	84	16.7	108	12.0	150
21.3	85	16.6	108	11.9	151
21.2	85	16.5	109	11.8	153
21.1	85	16.4	110	11.7	154
21.0	86	16.3	110	11.6	155
20.9	86	16.2	111	11.5	157
20.8	87	16.1	112	11.4	158
20.7	87	16.0	113	11.3	159
20.6	87	15.9	113	11.2	161
20.5	88	15.8	114	11.1	162
20.4	88	15.7	115	11.0	164
20.3	89	15.6	115	10.9	165
20.2	89	15.5	116	10.8	167
20.1	90	15.4	117	10.7	168
20.0	90	15.3	118	10.6	170
19.9	90	15.2	118	10.5	171
19.8	91	15.1	119	10.4	173
19.7	91	15.0	120	10.3	175
19.6	92	14.9	121	10.2	176
19.5	92	14.8	122	10.1	178
19.4	93	14.7	122	10.0	180
19.3	93	14.6	123	9.9	182
19.2	94	14.5	124	9.8	184
19.1	94	14.4	125	9.7	186
19.0	95	14.3	126	9.6	188
18.9	95	14.2	127	9.5	189
18.8	96	14.1	128	9.4	191
18.7	96	14.0	129	9.3	194
18.6	97	13.9	129	9.2	196
18.5	97	13.8	130	9.1	198
18.4	98	13.7	131	9.0	200
18.3	98	13.6	132	8.9	202
18.2	99	13.5	133	8.8	205
18.1	99	13.4	134	8.7	207
18.0	100	13.3	135	8.6	209
17.9	101	13.2	136	8.5	212
17.8	101	13.1	137	8.4	214
17.7	102	13.0	138	8.3	217
17.6	102	12.9	140	8.2	220
17.5	103	12.8	141	8.1	222
17.4	103	12.7	142	8.0	225

Table C.3.
Maximal Oxygen Uptake Estimates in Liters/Minute (Astrand-Ryhming Test).

	Work Load (kpm/min)									
	Men					Women				
Heart Rate	300	600	900	1200	1500	300	450	600	750	900
120	2.2	3.4	4.8			2.6	3.4	4.1	4.8	
121	2.2	3.4	4.7			2.5	3.3	4.0	4.8	
122	2.2	3.4	4.6			2.5	3.2	3.9	4.7	
123	2.1	3.4	4.6			2.4	3.1	3.9	4.6	
124	2.1	3.3	4.5	6.0		2.4	3.1	3.8	4.5	
125	2.0	3.2	4.4	5.9		2.3	3.0	3.7	4.4	
126	2.0	3.2	4.4	5.8		2.3	3.0	3.6	4.3	
127	2.0	3.1	4.3	5.7		2.2	2.9	3.5	4.2	
128	2.0	3.1	4.2	5.6		2.2	2.8	3.5	4.2	4.8
129	1.9	3.0	4.2	5.6		2.2	2.8	3.4	4.1	4.8
130	1.9	3.0	4.1	5.5		2.1	2.7	3.4	4.0	4.7
131	1.9	2.9	4.0	5.4		2.1	2.7	3.4	4.0	4.6
132	1.8	2.9	4.0	5.3		2.0	2.7	3.3	3.9	4.5
133	1.8	2.8	3.9	5.3		2.0	2.6	3.2	3.8	4.4
134	1.8	2.8	3.9	5.2		2.0	2.6	3.2	3.8	4.4
135	1.7	2.8	3.8	5.1		2.0	2.6	3.1	3.7	4.3
136	1.7	2.7	3.8	5.0		1.9	2.5	3.1	3.6	4.2
137	1.7	2.7	3.7	5.0		1.9	2.5	3.0	3.6	4.2
138	1.6	2.7	3.7	4.9		1.8	2.4	3.0	3.5	4.1
139	1.6	2.6	3.6	4.8		1.8	2.4	2.9	3.5	4.0
140	1.6	2.6	3.6	4.8	6.0	1.8	2.4	2.8	3.4	4.0
141		2.6	3.5	4.7	5.9	1.8	2.3	2.8	3.4	3.9
142		2.5	3.5	4.6	5.8	1.7	2.3	2.8	3.3	3.9
143		2.5	3.4	4.6	5.7	1.7	2.2	2.7	3.3	3.8
144		2.5	3.4	4.5	5.7	1.7	2.2	2.7	3.2	3.8
145		2.4	3.4	4.5	5.6	1.6	2.2	2.7	3.2	3.7
146		2.4	3.3	4.4	5.6	1.6	2.2	2.6	3.2	3.7
147		2.4	3.3	4.4	5.5	1.6	2.1	2.6	3.1	3.6
148		2.4	3.2	4.3	5.4	1.6	2.1	2.6	3.1	3.6
149		2.3	3.2	4.3	5.4		2.1	2.6	3.0	3.5
150		2.3	3.2	4.2	5.3		2.0	2.5	3.0	3.5
151		2.3	3.1	4.2	5.2		2.0	2.5	3.0	3.4
152		2.3	3.1	4.1	5.2		2.0	2.5	2.9	3.4
153		2.2	3.0	4.1	5.1		2.0	2.4	2.9	3.3
154		2.2	3.0	4.0	5.1		2.0	2.4	2.8	3.3
155		2.2	3.0	4.0	5.0		1.9	2.4	2.8	3.2
156		2.2	2.9	4.0	5.0		1.9	2.3	2.8	3.2
157		2.1	2.9	3.9	4.9		1.9	2.3	2.7	3.2
158		2.1	2.9	3.9	4.9		1.8	2.3	2.7	3.1
159		2.1	2.8	3.8	4.8		1.8	2.2	2.7	3.1
160		2.1	2.8	3.8	4.8		1.8	2.2	2.6	3.0
161		2.0	2.8	3.7	4.7		1.8	2.2	2.6	3.0
162		2.0	2.8	3.7	4.6		1.8	2.2	2.6	3.0
163		2.0	2.8	3.7	4.6		1.7	2.2	2.6	2.9
164		2.0	2.7	3.6	4.5		1.7	2.1	2.5	2.9
165		2.0	2.7	3.6	4.5		1.7	2.1	2.5	2.9
166		1.9	2.7	3.6	4.5		1.7	2.1	2.5	2.8
167		1.9	2.6	3.5	4.4		1.6	2.1	2.4	2.8
168		1.9	2.6	3.5	4.4		1.6	2.0	2.4	2.8
169		1.9	2.6	3.5	4.3		1.6	2.0	2.4	2.8
170		1.8	2.6	3.4	4.3		1.6	2.0	2.4	2.7

From Astrand, I. *Acta Physiologica Scandinavica* 49(1960). Supplementum 169:45-60.

Table C.4.
Age-Based Correction Factors for Maximal Oxygen Uptake (Astrand-Ryhming Test).

Age	Correction Factor	Age	Correction Factor
14	1.11	40	.830
15	1.10	41	.820
16	1.09	42	.810
17	1.08	43	.800
18	1.07	44	.790
19	1.06	45	.780
20	1.05	46	.774
21	1.04	47	.768
22	1.03	48	.762
23	1.02	49	.756
24	1.01	50	.750
25	1.00	51	.742
26	.987	52	.734
27	.974	53	.726
28	.961	54	.718
29	.948	55	.710
30	.935	56	.704
31	.922	57	.698
32	.909	58	.692
33	.896	59	.686
34	.883	60	.680
35	.870	61	.674
36	.862	62	.668
37	.854	63	.662
38	.846	64	.656
39	.838	65	.650

Adapted from Astrand, I. *Acta Physiologica Scandinavica* 49 (1960). Supplementum 169:45-60.

step-ups per minute, regulated with a metronome set at ninety-six beats per minute. Women perform twenty-two step-ups per minute, or eighty-eight beats per minute on the metronome.

3. Allow the participant a brief practice period of five to ten seconds to become familiar with the stepping cadence.

4. Begin the test and perform the step-ups for exactly three minutes. Upon completion of the three minutes, the subject remains standing and the heart rate (pulse) is taken for a fifteen-second interval from five to twenty seconds into recovery. This fifteen-second recovery heart rate is converted to beats per minute (multiply fifteen-second heart rate by four).

5. Maximal oxygen uptake in ml/kg/min is estimated according to the following equations:

Men: Max. VO_2 = 111.33 – (0.42 x recovery heart rate in bpm)

Women: Max. VO_2 = 65.81 – (0.1847 x recovery heart rate in bpm)

6. Example. The recovery fifteen-second heart rate for a male subject following the three-minute step test was found to be thirty-nine beats (or 39 x 4 = 156 bpm). Maximal oxygen uptake is estimated as follows:

Max. VO_2 = 111.33 – (0.42 x 156) = 45.8 ml/kg/min

7. Maximal oxygen uptake can also be obtained according to recovery heart rates in Table C.5 (the respective cardiovascular endurance fitness category for the obtained Max. VO_2 can be looked up in Table 4.3, Chapter 4).

IV. Prediction Equations to Estimate Maximal Oxygen Uptake According to Maximal Treadmill Exercise Testing.

Prediction equations have been developed to estimate maximal oxygen uptake using the Balke (modified), Bruce, and Ellestad protocols. A description of these three treadmill protocols is given in Figure C.1. As with the 1.5-mile run test, all three of these protocols are maximal exercise tests and consequently may require the presence of a physician (*see* Table 3.1, Chapter 3). The Max. VO_2 is estimated based on the duration of the test according to the following equations (also see Table C.6)*:

Balke Protocol
Max. VO_2 = (1.444 x test duration) + 14.99

Bruce Protocol
Max. VO_2 = (4.326 x test duration) – 4.66

Ellestad Protocol
Max. VO_2 = (3.933 x test duration) + 4.46

The choice of treadmill protocol selected is determined by the participant's health and level of physical condition. The Balke pro-

*From Pollock, M. L., et al. "A Comparative Analysis of Four Protocols for Maximal Treadmill Stress Testing." *American Heart Journal* 92(1):39-46, 1976.

Table C.5.
Estimated Maximal Oxygen Uptake (Max. VO$_2$) for the Three-Minute Step Test in ml/kg/min.

15-Sec HR	HR-bpm	Max VO$_2$ Men	Max VO$_2$ Women
30	120	60.9	43.6
31	124	59.3	42.9
32	128	57.6	42.2
33	132	55.9	41.4
34	136	54.2	40.7
35	140	52.5	40.0
36	144	50.9	39.2
37	148	49.2	38.5
38	152	47.5	37.7
39	156	45.8	37.0
40	160	44.1	36.3
41	164	42.5	35.5
42	168	40.8	34.8
43	172	39.1	34.0
44	176	37.4	33.3
45	180	35.7	32.6
46	184	34.1	31.8
47	188	32.4	31.1
48	192	30.7	30.3
49	196	29.0	29.6
50	200	27.3	28.9

tocol is not as strenuous, hence it is recommended for unconditioned individuals. This protocol also requires lower and more gradual increments in workloads, which may reduce the strain on the cardiovascular system, and thus may decrease the risk for abnormal heart function. The Bruce and Ellestad protocols are primarily recommended for use with conditioned or athletic individuals.

For example, the estimated maximal oxygen uptake for an individual who walked sixteen minutes and twenty-six seconds on a Balke protocol would be:

Test duration = 16:26 or 16 + (26/60)

$$= 16.43 \text{ minutes}$$

Max. VO$_2$ = (1.444 x 16.43)

$$+ 14.99 = 38.7 \text{ ml/kg/min}$$

The respective cardiovascular endurance fitness category is determined according to Table 4.3 in Chapter 4.

V. Prediction Equations to Estimate Maximal Oxygen Uptake According to Submaximal Treadmill Exercise Testing.

Maximal oxygen uptake can also be estimated using the Balke (modified), Bruce,

and Ellestad protocols, but administering the tests only to 85 percent of predicted heart rate range (maximal heart rate minus resting heart rate, times 85 percent, plus resting heart rate). Maximal oxygen uptake is then estimated according to how long (time) it takes the participant to reach the target 85 percent of predicted heart rate range. The predicting equations are the same as listed under the maximal protocols, but the final obtained values are multiplied by 1.174[*]:

Submax-Balke Protocol

Max. VO$_2$ = [(1.444 x test duration)

$$+ 14.99] \text{ x } 1.174$$

Submax-Bruce Protocol

Max. VO$_2$ = [(4.326 x test duration)

$$- 4.66] \text{ x } 1.174$$

Submax-Ellestad Protocol

Max. VO$_2$ = [(3.933 x test duration)

$$+ 4.46] \text{ x } 1.174$$

---

[*]Adapted from (a) Pollock, M. L., et al. "A Comparative Analysis of Four Protocols for Maximal Treadmill Stress Testing." *American Heart Journal* 92(1):39-46, 1976; and (b) Pollock, M. L., et al. *Health and Fitness through Physical Activity.* New York: John Wiley & Sons, 1978, pp. 300-301.

Figure C.1. *Treadmill Protocols for Exercise Testing.*

Balke (modified) Protocol

The treadmill speed is kept constant at 3.3 mph through the twenty-fifth minute. The individual walks at a 0 percent grade for the first minute, at which point the grade (treadmill inclination) is increased to 2 percent. The grade is then increased by 1 percent at the end of each subsequent minute, all the way to 25 percent at the end of the twenty-fourth minute. Thereafter, the treadmill speed is increased by 0.2 mph at the end of each additional minute until complete exhaustion is reached.

Bruce Protocol

On the Bruce protocol, both the treadmill speed and inclination are increased at the end of every third minute as follows:

1. First three minutes: speed = 1.7 mph and grade = 10%
2. Fourth through sixth minute: speed = 2.5 mph and grade = 12%
3. Seventh through ninth minute: speed = 3.4 mph and grade = 14%
4. Tenth through twelfth minute: speed = 4.2 mph and grade = 16%
5. Thirteenth through fifteenth minute: speed = 5.0 mph and grade = 18%
6. Sixteenth through eighteenth minute: speed = 5.5 mph and grade = 20%
7. Nineteenth through twenty-first minute: speed = 6.0 mph and grade = 22%

Ellestad Protocol

On the Ellestad protocol, the treadmill inclination is kept constant at 10 percent for the first ten minutes. At the end of the tenth minute the inclination is increased to 15 percent and kept at that grade for the remainder of the test. The treadmill speeds are increased as follows: first three minutes = 1.7 mph, fourth and fifth minutes = 3.0 mph, sixth and seventh minutes = 4.0 mph, eighth through twelfth minute = 5.0 mph, and starting at the end of the twelfth minute the speed is increased to 6.0 mph, at the end of the fourteenth minute to 7.0 mph, and at the end of the sixteenth to 8.0 mph.

Figure C.1a. *Balke, Bruce, and Ellestad Treadmill Protocols.*

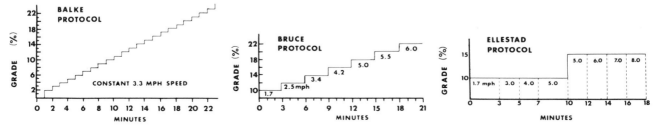

When using these equations, maximal heart rate, if unknown can be estimated by subtracting the person's age from 220 (a constant). For example, the 85 percent of predicted heart rate range for a forty-year-old male with a resting heart rate of eighty beats per minute would be:

Estimated maximal heart rate (220 – age)
    = 220 – 40 = 180 bpm
Heart rate range (maximal heart rate –
    resting heart rate) = 180 – 80 = 100 bpm
85 percent of predicted range (heart rate

range times .85, plus resting heart rate) = (100 x .85) + 80 = 165 bpm.

For instance, if in the previous example it took this person eight minutes and fifty seconds to reach the target heart rate of 165 bpm on a Bruce protocol, the maximal oxygen uptake would be estimated as follows:

Test duration = 8:50 or 8 +
    (50/60) = 8.83 minutes
Max. VO_2 = [(4.326 x 8.83) – 4.66]
    x 1.174 = 39.4 ml/kg/min

Table C.6.
Maximal Oxygen Uptake Estimates (ml/kg/min) for Selected Treadmill Protocols

Time	Maximal Protocols			Submaximal Protocols		
	Balke	**Bruce**	**Ellestad**	**Balke**	**Bruce**	**Ellestad**
3:00	19.3	8.3	16.3	22.7	9.8	19.1
3:30	20.0	10.5	18.2	23.5	12.3	21.4
4:00	20.8	12.6	20.2	24.4	14.8	23.7
4:30	21.5	14.8	22.2	25.2	17.4	26.0
5:00	22.2	17.0	24.1	26.1	19.9	28.3
5:30	22.9	19.1	26.1	26.9	22.5	30.6
6:00	23.7	21.3	28.1	27.8	25.0	32.9
6:30	24.4	23.5	30.0	28.6	27.5	35.2
7:00	25.1	25.6	32.0	29.5	30.1	37.6
7:30	25.8	27.8	34.0	30.3	32.6	39.9
8:00	26.5	29.9	35.9	31.2	35.2	42.2
8:30	27.3	32.1	37.9	32.0	37.7	44.5
9:00	28.0	34.3	39.9	32.9	40.2	46.8
9:30	28.7	36.4	41.8	33.7	42.8	49.1
10:00	29.4	38.6	43.8	34.6	45.3	51.4
10:30	30.2	40.8	45.8	35.4	47.9	53.7
11:00	30.9	42.9	47.7	36.2	50.4	56.0
11:30	31.6	45.1	49.7	37.1	52.9	58.3
12:00	32.3	47.3	51.7	37.9	55.5	60.6
12:30	33.0	49.4	53.6	38.8	58.0	63.0
13:00	33.8	51.6	55.6	39.6	60.6	65.3
13:30	34.5	53.7	57.6	40.5	63.1	67.6
14:00	35.2	55.9	59.5	41.3	65.6	69.9
14:30	35.9	58.1	61.5	42.2	68.2	72.2
15:00	36.7	60.2	63.5	43.0	70.7	74.5
15:30	37.4	62.4	65.4	43.9	73.2	76.8
16:00	38.1	64.6	67.4	44.7	75.8	79.1
16:30	38.8	66.7	69.4	45.6	78.3	81.4
17:00	39.5	68.9	71.3	46.4	80.9	83.7
17:30	40.3	71.0	73.3	47.3	83.4	86.0
18:00	41.0	73.2	75.3	48.1		
18:30	41.7	75.4	77.2	49.0		
19:00	42.4	77.5	79.2	49.8		
19:30	43.1	79.7	81.2	50.7		
20:00	43.9	81.9	83.1	51.5		
20:30	44.6	84.0	85.1	52.4		
21:00	45.3			53.2		
21:30	46.0			54.0		
22:00	46.8			54.9		
22:30	47.5			55.7		
23:00	48.2			56.6		
23:30	48.9			57.4		
24:00	49.6			58.3		
24:30	50.4			59.1		
25:00	51.1			60.0		
25:30	51.8			60.8		
26:00	52.5			61.7		
26:30	53.3			62.5		

Table C.6. *(continued)*
Maximal Oxygen Uptake Estimates (ml/kg/min) for Selected Treadmill Protocols

Time	Maximal Protocols			Submaximal Protocols		
	Balke	**Bruce**	**Ellestad**	**Balke**	**Bruce**	**Ellestad**
27:00	54.0			63.4		
27:30	54.7			64.2		
28:00	55.4			65.1		
28:30	56.1			65.9		
29:00	56.9					
29:30	57.6					
30:00	58.3					
30:30	59.0					
31:00	59.8					
31:30	60.5					
32:00	61.2					
32:30	61.9					
33:00	62.6					
33:30	63.4					
34:00	64.1					
34:30	64.8					
35:00	65.5					

The respective cardiovascular endurance fitness category is determined according to Table 4.3 in Chapter 4.

BASIC PRINCIPLES OF CARDIOVASCULAR EXERCISE PRESCRIPTION

All too often there are many individuals who exercise regularly, but when they take a cardiovascular endurance test are surprised to find that they may not be as conditioned as they thought they were. Although these individuals may be exercising regularly, they most likely are not following the basic principles for cardiovascular exercise prescription; therefore, they do not reap significant benefits.

For a person to develop the cardiovascular system, the heart muscle has to be overloaded like any other muscle in the human body. Just as the biceps muscle in the upper arm is developed by doing some weight-lifting exercises, the heart muscle also has to be exercised to increase in size, strength, and efficiency. To better understand how the cardiovascular system can be developed,

the four basic principles that govern this development will be discussed. These principles are intensity, mode, duration, and frequency of exercise.

INTENSITY OF EXERCISE

The intensity of exercise is perhaps the most commonly ignored factor when trying to develop the cardiovascular system. This principle refers to how hard a person has to exercise to improve cardiovascular endurance. Muscles have to be overloaded to a given point for them to develop. While the training stimuli to develop the biceps muscle can be accomplished with curl-up exercises, the stimuli for the cardiovascular system is provided by making the heart pump at a higher rate for a certain period of time. Research has shown that cardiovascular development occurs when working at about 60 to 80 percent of maximal aerobic capacity, which correlates with 70 and 85 percent of maximal heart rate. Maximal heart rate is either obtained through a maximal exercise test, or can be estimated using the following equations:

Men = 205 – one-half the age

Women = 220 – age

Using these percentages, training intensity is commonly prescribed using one of three methods:

1. Based on maximal heart rate. This is done by obtaining 70 and 85 percent of maximal heart rate (multiply maximal heart rate by .70 and .85). For example, the cardiovascular training intensity zone for a 50-year-old man would be determined in the following manner:

   Maximal heart rate = 205 – (50/2X = 180 bpm
   70 percent of maximal heart rate =
   180 x .70 = 126 bpm
   85 percent of maximal heart rate =
   180 x .85 = 153 bpm
   Training zone = 126 to 153 bpm.

2. Based on heart rate range. This method varies from the previous one in that the resting heart rate is taken into consideration when estimating the training zone. This method may yield significantly different training intensities and may be more accurate when comparing two individuals with the same maximal heart rate but with different resting heart rates (e.g., resting heart rates of 40 and 80 bpm).

   The training intensity using heart rate range is obtained by subtracting the resting heart rate from the maximal heart rate, then multiplying this value by .70 and .85 and adding the resting heart rate back to these two numbers. For example, the cardiovascular training zone for a thirty-year-old woman with a resting heart rate of eighty would be computed as follows:

   Maximal heart rate = 220 – 30 = 190 bpm
   Heart rate range = 190 – 80 = 110 bpm
   70 percent of heart rate range =
   110 x .70 = 77 bpm
   85 percent of heart rate range =
   110 x .85 = 94 bpm
   Training zone: 157 (77 + 80) to
   174 (94 + 80) bpm.

3. Based on rate of perceived exertion. Since many people do not check their heart rate during exercise, an alternate method of prescribing intensity of exercise has become more popular in recent years. This method uses a rate of perceived exertion (RPE) scale developed by Gunnar Borg. Using the scale shown in Figure C.2, a person subjectively rates the perceived exertion or difficulty of exercise when training in the appropriate target zone. The exercise heart rate is then associated with the corresponding RPE value. For example, if the training intensity requires a heart rate zone between 150 and 170 bpm, the person would associate this with training between "hard" and "very hard" (most people need to train between "somewhat hard" and "hard" or "very hard," which is the equivalent of intensity ratings between "13" and "15" or "17").

Figure C.2. *Rate of Perceived Exertion Scale.*

6			
7	Very, very light	14	
8		15	Hard
9	Very light	16	
10		17	Very hard
11	Fairly light	18	
12		19	Very, very hard
13	Somewhat hard	20	

From Borg, G. "Perceived Exertion: A Note on History and Methods." Medicine and Science in Sports and Exercise 5:90-93, 1973.

However, some individuals may perceive less exertion than others when training in the correct zone. Therefore, in the initial stages of training, the individual should self-monitor the RPE in the appropriate target heart rate zone. When the association between target heart rates and RPE are mastered, the person may proceed to exercise at that rate of perceived exertion. To help develop the association between target heart rates and RPE, individuals should be encouraged to keep a regular log of their physical activity by using a record form similar to Figure C.3. After several weeks of training, they should be able to predict their exercise heart rate just by their own perceived exertion of the exercise session.

The target training zone indicates that whenever people exercise to improve the cardiovascular system, they have to maintain their heart rate in the appropriate target zone in order to obtain adequate development. After a few months of training, they may experience a significant reduction in working heart rates at certain workloads, as well as a reduction in resting heart rate. Therefore, the target zone should be recomputed periodically. Once a person reaches an optimal level of cardiovascular endurance, training in that same zone will allow him/her to maintain the fitness level.

Exercise heart rate or RPE should be monitored regularly during exercise to make sure that the appropriate training intensity is achieved. An individual should wait about five minutes into the exercise session before taking the first heart rate (or cross-checking the RPE). When checking the heart rate, the pulse is counted for ten seconds and then multiplied by six to get the per minute pulse rate. (Exercise heart rate will remain at the same level for fifteen seconds following exercise. After fifteen seconds, heart rate will drop rapidly.) If the rate is too low, the person should increase the intensity of the exercise. If the rate is too high, he/she should slow down.

It is also important to note that in order to develop the cardiovascular system, a person does not have to exercise above the 85 percent rate. From a health standpoint, training above this intensity level will not add any extra benefits and may actually be unsafe for some individuals. For unconditioned adults, it is recommended that cardiovascular training be conducted around the 70 percent rate. This lower rate is recommended to reduce potential problems associated with high-intensity exercise.

MODE OF EXERCISE

The type of exercise that develops the cardiovascular system has to be aerobic in nature. Once the target training zone has been determined, any activity or combination of activities that will get the heart rate up to that training zone and keep it there for as long as the person exercises will yield adequate development. Examples of such activities are walking, jogging, aerobic dancing, swimming, cross-country skiing, rope skipping, cycling, racquetball, stair climbing, and stationary running or cycling.

The activity that the individual chooses should be based on personal preferences, enjoyment, and physical limitations. There may be a difference in the amount of strength or flexibility development between different activities, but as far as the

cardiovascular system is concerned, the heart doesn't know whether the person is walking, swimming, or cycling. All the heart knows is that it has to pump at a certain rate, and as long as that rate is in the desired range, cardiovascular development will occur.

DURATION OF EXERCISE

According to the existing evidence regarding the duration of exercise, it is recommended that a person train between fifteen and sixty minutes per session. The duration is based on how intensely a person trains. If the training is done around 85 percent of maximum, fifteen to twenty minutes are sufficient. At 70 percent intensity, the person should train for at least thirty minutes. As mentioned earlier, under intensity of training, unconditioned adults should train at the lower percentage; therefore, a minimum of thirty minutes of exercise is recommended.

As a part of the training session, always include a five-minute warm-up and a five minute cool-down period. Warm-up exercises should consist of general calisthenics, stretching exercises, or exercising at a lower intensity level than the actual target zone. To cool down, the exercise intensity should be decreased gradually. People should never stop abruptly. This will cause blood to pool in the exercised body parts, thereby diminishing the return of blood to the heart. A decreased blood return can cause dizziness, faintness, or even induce cardiac abnormalities.

FREQUENCY OF EXERCISE

Ideally, a person should engage in aerobic exercise four to five times per week. Research has indicated that to maintain cardiovascular endurance, a training session should be conducted about every forty-eight hours. As little as three training sessions per week, done on nonconsecutive days, will maintain cardiovascular endurance. For faster development in the initial stages, four to six times per week is recommended.

A final point of concern when developing exercise presriptions is that a progressive approach should be implemented to improve fitness. While unconditioned beginners could go ahead and attempt to train five or six times per week for thirty minutes at a time, they may find this discouraging and possibly drop out before getting too far. The reason for this is that as they initiate the program they will probably develop some muscle soreness and stiffness, and possibly minor injuries. According to one report, more than 65 percent of those who begin an exercise program drop out in the initial six weeks due to injuries. Muscle soreness and stiffness can be reduced or eliminated by gradually increasing the intensity,

duration, and frequency of exercise, such as illustrated in the computerized exercise prescription in Figure C.3. In this prescription, the initial training intensity is obtained between 50 and 60 percent of heart rate range, the next training intensity is given between 60 and 70, and the final intensity is prescribed between 70 and 85 percent. This computer software package can also be obtained through Morton Publishing Company.

Figure C.3. *Cardiovascular Exercise Record Form.*

Month _____

Date	Body Weight	Exercise Heart Rate	Type of Exercise	Distance in Miles	Time Hrs/Min	RPE
1						
2						
3						
4						
5						
6						
7						
8						
9						
10						
11						
12						
13						
14						
15						
16						
17						
18						
19						
20						
21						
22						
23						
24						
25						
26						
27						
28						
29						
30						
31						
Total						

Month _____

Date	Body Weight	Exercise Heart Rate	Type of Exercise	Distance in Miles	Time Hrs/Min	RPE*
1						
2						
3						
4						
5						
6						
7						
8						
9						
10						
11						
12						
13						
14						
15						
16						
17						
18						
19						
20						
21						
22						
23						
24						
25						
26						
27						
28						
29						
30						
31						
Total						

*Rate of perceived exertion.

Figure C.4. *Sample Computerized Exercise Prescription.*

PERSONALIZED CARDIOVASCULAR EXERCISE PRESCRIPTION

```
James L. Doe              Age: 46         Date: 03-12-1987
Maximal Heart Rate: 182 bpm   Resting Heart Rate: 76 bpm
Present Cardiovascular Fitness Level: Average
```

The following is your personal program for cardiovascular fitness development and/or maintenance. If you have been exercising regularly and you are in the average or good category,
you may start at week five. If you are in the excellent category, you can start at week ten.

Week	Time (min.)	Frequency (per week)	Heart Rate Range (beats per minute)	Pulse (10 sec. count)
1	15	3	129 to 140	22 to 23
2	15	4	129 to 140	22 to 23
3	20	4	129 to 140	22 to 23
4	20	5	129 to 140	22 to 23
5	20	4	140 to 150	23 to 25
6	25	4	140 to 150	23 to 25
7	20	5	140 to 150	23 to 25
8	30	4	140 to 150	23 to 25
9	30	5	140 to 150	23 to 25
10	20	4	150 to 166	25 to 28
11	20	5	150 to 166	25 to 28
12	30	4	150 to 166	25 to 28
13	30	5	150 to 166	25 to 28
14	30--40	5	150 to 166	25 to 28

You may participate in any combination of activities which are
aerobic and continuous in nature, such as walking, jogging,
swimming, cross country skiing, rope skipping, cycling, aerobic dancing, raquetball, stair climbing, stationary running or
cycling, etc.   As long as the heart rate reaches the desired
range, and it stays in that range for the period of time indicated, the cardiovascular system will improve its capacity.

Following the fourteen week program, in order to maintain your
fitness level, you should exercise between 150 and 166 bpm for
about 30 minutes, a minimum of three times per week on nonconsecutive days.

When you exercise, allow about 5 minutes for a gradual warm-up
period and another 5 for gradual cool-down. Also, when you
check your exercise heart rate, only count your pulse for 10
seconds (start counting with 0) and then refer to the above 10
sec. pulse count. You may also multiply by 6 to obtain your
rate in beats per minute.

Good cardiovascular fitness will greatly contribute toward the
enhancement and maintenance of good health.   It is especially
important in the prevention of coronary heart disease. We encourage you to be persistent in your exercise program and to
participate regularly. Best of luck James.

Computer software available through Morton Publishing Co.,
Englewood, CO.

Body Composition Assessment
and
Ideal Body Weight Determination

BODY COMPOSITION ASSESSMENT

Skinfold Thickness Technique for Body Composition Assessment.

1. Select the proper anatomical sites. For men, chest, abdomen, and thigh skinfolds are used. For women, use triceps, suprailium, and thigh skinfolds (*see* Figure D.1). All measurements should be taken on the right side of the body with the subject standing. The correct anatomical landmarks for skinfolds are:

    Chest:
      a diagonal fold halfway between the shoulder crease and the nipple.
    Abdomen:
      a vertical fold taken about one inch to the right of the umbilicus.
    Triceps:
      a vertical fold on the back of the upper arm, halfway between the shoulder and the elbow.
    Thigh:
      a vertical fold on the front of the thigh, midway between the knee and hip.

    Suprailium:
      a diagonal fold above the crest of the ilium (on the side of the hip).

2. Measure each site by grasping a double thickness of skin firmly with the thumb and forefinger, pulling the fold slightly away from the muscular tissue. The calipers are held perpendicular to the fold, and the measurement is taken one-half inch below the finger hold. Each site is measured three times and the values are read to the nearest .1 to .5 mm. The average of the two closest readings is recorded as the final value. The readings should be taken without delay to avoid excessive compression of the skinfold. Releasing and refolding the skinfold is required between readings.

3. When doing pre- and post-assessments, the measurement should be conducted at the same time of day. The best time is early in the morning to avoid water hydration changes resulting from activity or exercise.

4. Percent fat is obtained by adding together all three skinfold measurements and looking up the respective values in Tables D.1 for

Figure D.1. *Anatomical Landmarks for Skinfolds.*

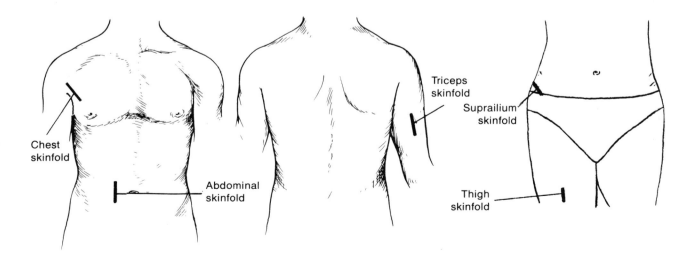

Table D.1.
Percent Fat Estimates for Women.

Sum of 3 Skinfolds	Under 22	Age to the Last Year							Over 58
		23 to 27	28 to 32	33 to 37	38 to 42	43 to 47	48 to 52	53 to 57	
23- 25	9.7	9.9	10.2	10.4	10.7	10.9	11.2	11.4	11.7
26- 28	11.0	11.2	11.5	11.7	12.0	12.3	12.5	12.7	13.0
29- 31	12.3	12.5	12.8	13.0	13.3	13.5	13.8	14.0	14.3
32- 34	13.6	13.8	14.0	14.3	14.5	14.8	15.0	15.3	15.5
35- 37	14.8	15.0	15.3	15.5	15.8	16.0	16.3	16.5	16.8
38- 40	16.0	16.3	16.5	16.7	17.0	17.2	17.5	17.7	18.0
41- 43	17.2	17.4	17.7	17.9	18.2	18.4	18.7	18.9	19.2
44- 46	18.3	18.6	18.8	19.1	19.3	19.6	19.8	20.1	20.3
47- 49	19.5	19.7	20.0	20.2	20.5	20.7	21.0	21.2	21.5
50- 52	20.6	20.8	21.1	21.3	21.6	21.8	22.1	22.3	22.6
53- 55	21.7	21.9	22.1	22.4	22.6	22.9	23.1	23.4	23.6
56- 58	22.7	23.0	23.2	23.4	23.7	23.9	24.2	24.4	24.7
59- 61	23.7	24.0	24.2	24.5	24.7	25.0	25.2	25.5	25.7
62- 64	24.7	25.0	25.2	25.5	25.7	26.0	26.2	26.4	26.7
65- 67	25.7	25.9	26.2	26.4	26.7	26.9	27.2	27.4	27.7
68- 70	26.6	26.9	27.1	27.4	27.6	27.9	28.1	28.4	28.6
71- 73	27.5	27.8	28.0	28.3	28.5	28.8	29.0	29.3	29.5
74- 76	28.4	28.7	28.9	29.2	29.4	29.7	29.9	30.2	30.4
77- 79	29.3	29.5	29.8	30.0	30.3	30.5	30.8	31.0	31.3
80- 82	30.1	30.4	30.6	30.9	31.1	31.4	31.6	31.9	32.1
83- 85	30.9	31.2	31.4	31.7	31.9	32.2	32.4	32.7	32.9
86- 88	31.7	32.0	32.2	32.5	32.7	32.9	33.2	33.4	33.7
89- 91	32.5	32.7	33.0	33.2	33.5	33.7	33.9	34.2	34.4
92- 94	33.2	33.4	33.7	33.9	34.2	34.4	34.7	34.9	35.2
95- 97	33.9	34.1	34.4	34.6	34.9	35.1	35.4	35.6	35.9
98-100	34.6	34.8	35.1	35.3	35.5	35.8	36.0	36.3	36.5
101-103	35.2	35.4	35.7	35.9	36.2	36.4	36.7	36.9	37.2
104-106	35.8	36.1	36.3	36.6	36.8	37.1	37.3	37.5	37.8
107-109	36.4	36.7	36.9	37.1	37.4	37.6	37.9	38.1	38.4
110-112	37.0	37.2	37.5	37.7	38.0	38.2	38.5	38.7	38.9
113-115	37.5	37.8	38.0	38.2	38.5	38.7	39.0	39.2	39.5
116-118	38.0	38.3	38.5	38.8	39.0	39.3	39.5	39.7	40.0
119-121	38.5	38.7	39.0	39.2	39.5	39.7	40.0	40.2	40.5
122-124	39.0	39.2	39.4	39.7	39.9	40.2	40.4	40.7	40.9
125-127	39.4	39.6	39.9	40.1	40.4	40.6	40.9	41.1	41.4
128-130	39.8	40.0	40.3	40.5	40.8	41.0	41.3	41.5	41.8

Table D.2.
Percent Fat Estimates for Men Under 40.

Sum of 3 Skinfolds	Under 19	Age to the Last Year						
		20 to 22	23 to 25	26 to 28	29 to 31	32 to 34	35 to 37	38 to 40
8- 10	.9	1.3	1.6	2.0	2.3	2.7	3.0	3.3
11- 13	1.9	2.3	2.6	3.0	3.3	3.7	4.0	4.3
14- 16	2.9	3.3	3.6	3.9	4.3	4.6	5.0	5.3
17- 19	3.9	4.2	4.6	4.9	5.3	5.6	6.0	6.3
20- 22	4.8	5.2	5.5	5.9	6.2	6.6	6.9	7.3
23- 25	5.8	6.2	6.5	6.8	7.2	7.5	7.9	8.2
26- 28	6.8	7.1	7.5	7.8	8.1	8.5	8.8	9.2
29- 31	7.7	8.0	8.4	8.7	9.1	9.4	9.8	10.1
32- 34	8.6	9.0	9.3	9.7	10.0	10.4	10.7	11.1
35- 37	9.5	9.9	10.2	10.6	10.9	11.3	11.6	12.0
38- 40	10.5	10.8	11.2	11.5	11.8	12.2	12.5	12.9
41- 43	11.4	11.7	12.1	12.4	12.7	13.1	13.4	13.8
44- 46	12.2	12.6	12.9	13.3	13.6	14.0	14.3	14.7
47- 49	13.1	13.5	13.8	14.2	14.5	14.9	15.2	15.5
50- 52	14.0	14.3	14.7	15.0	15.4	15.7	16.1	16.4
53- 55	14.8	15.2	15.5	15.9	16.2	16.6	16.9	17.3
56- 58	15.7	16.0	16.4	16.7	17.1	17.4	17.8	18.1
59- 61	16.5	16.9	17.2	17.6	17.9	18.3	18.6	19.0
62- 64	17.4	17.7	18.1	18.4	18.8	19.1	19.4	19.8
65- 67	18.2	18.5	18.9	19.2	19.6	19.9	20.3	20.6
68- 70	19.0	19.3	19.7	20.0	20.4	20.7	21.1	21.4
71- 73	19.8	20.1	20.5	20.8	21.2	21.5	21.9	22.2
74- 76	20.6	20.9	21.3	21.6	22.0	22.2	22.7	23.0
77- 79	21.4	21.7	22.1	22.4	22.8	23.1	23.4	23.8
80- 82	22.1	22.5	22.8	23.2	23.5	23.9	24.2	24.6
83- 85	22.9	23.2	23.6	23.9	24.3	24.6	25.0	25.3
86- 88	23.6	24.0	24.3	24.7	25.0	25.4	25.7	26.1
89- 91	24.4	24.7	25.1	25.4	25.8	26.1	26.5	26.8
92- 94	25.1	25.5	25.8	26.2	26.5	26.9	27.2	27.5
95- 97	25.8	26.2	26.5	26.9	27.2	27.6	27.9	28.3
98-100	26.6	26.9	27.3	27.6	27.9	28.3	28.6	29.0
101-103	27.3	27.6	28.0	28.3	28.6	29.0	29.3	29.7
104-106	27.9	28.3	28.6	29.0	29.3	29.7	30.0	30.4
107-109	28.6	29.0	29.3	29.7	30.0	30.4	30.7	31.1
110-112	29.3	29.6	30.0	30.3	30.7	31.0	31.4	31.7
113-115	30.0	30.3	30.7	31.0	31.3	31.7	32.0	32.4
116-118	30.6	31.0	31.3	31.6	32.0	32.3	32.7	33.0
119-121	31.3	31.6	32.0	32.3	32.6	33.0	33.3	33.7
122-124	31.9	32.2	32.6	32.9	33.3	33.6	34.0	34.3
125-127	32.5	32.9	33.2	33.5	33.9	34.2	34.6	34.9
128-130	33.1	33.5	33.8	34.2	34.5	34.9	35.2	35.5

Table D.3.
Percent Fat Estimates for Men Over 40.

Sum of 3 Skinfolds	Age to the Last Year							
	41 to 43	44 to 46	47 to 49	50 to 52	53 to 55	56 to 58	59 to 61	Over 62
8- 10	3.7	4.0	4.4	4.7	5.1	5.4	5.8	6.1
11- 13	4.7	5.0	5.4	5.7	6.1	6.4	6.8	7.1
14- 16	5.7	6.0	6.4	6.7	7.1	7.4	7.8	8.1
17- 19	6.7	7.0	7.4	7.7	8.1	8.4	8.7	9.1
20- 22	7.6	8.0	8.3	8.7	9.0	9.4	9.7	10.1
23- 25	8.6	8.9	9.3	9.6	10.0	10.3	10.7	11.0
26- 28	9.5	9.9	10.2	10.6	10.9	11.3	11.6	12.0
29- 31	10.5	10.8	11.2	11.5	11.9	12.2	12.6	12.9
32- 34	11.4	11.8	12.1	12.4	12.8	13.1	13.5	13.8
35- 37	12.3	12.7	13.0	13.4	13.7	14.1	14.4	14.8
38- 40	13.2	13.6	13.9	14.3	14.6	15.0	15.3	15.7
41- 43	14.1	14.5	14.8	15.2	15.5	15.9	16.2	16.6
44- 46	15.0	15.4	15.7	16.1	16.4	16.8	17.1	17.5
47- 49	15.9	16.2	16.6	16.9	17.3	17.6	18.0	18.3
50- 52	16.8	17.1	17.5	17.8	18.2	18.5	18.8	19.2
53- 55	17.6	18.0	18.3	18.7	19.0	19.4	19.7	20.1
56- 58	18.5	18.8	19.2	19.5	19.9	20.2	20.6	20.9
59- 61	19.3	19.7	20.0	20.4	20.7	21.0	21.4	21.7
62- 64	20.1	20.5	20.8	21.2	21.5	21.9	22.2	22.6
65- 67	21.0	21.3	21.7	22.0	22.4	22.7	23.0	23.4
68- 70	21.8	22.1	22.5	22.8	23.2	23.5	23.9	24.2
71- 73	22.6	22.9	23.3	23.6	24.0	24.3	24.7	25.0
74- 76	23.4	23.7	24.1	24.4	24.8	25.1	25.4	25.8
77- 79	24.1	24.5	24.8	25.2	25.5	25.9	26.2	26.6
80- 82	24.9	25.3	25.6	26.0	26.3	26.6	27.0	27.3
83- 85	25.7	26.0	26.4	26.7	27.1	27.4	27.8	28.1
86- 88	26.4	26.8	27.1	27.5	27.8	28.2	28.5	28.9
89- 91	27.2	27.5	27.9	38.2	28.6	28.9	29.2	29.6
92- 94	27.9	28.2	28.6	28.9	29.3	29.6	30.0	30.3
95- 97	28.6	29.0	29.3	29.7	30.0	30.4	30.7	31.1
98-100	29.3	29.7	30.0	30.4	30.7	31.1	31.4	31.8
101-103	30.0	30.4	30.7	31.1	31.4	31.8	32.1	32.5
104-106	30.7	31.1	31.4	31.8	32.1	32.5	32.8	33.2
107-109	31.4	31.8	32.1	32.4	32.8	33.1	33.5	33.8
110-112	32.1	32.4	32.8	33.1	33.5	33.8	34.2	34.5
113-115	32.7	33.1	33.4	33.8	34.1	34.5	34.8	35.2
116-118	33.4	33.7	34.1	34.4	34.8	35.1	35.5	35.8
119-121	34.0	34.4	34.7	35.1	35.4	35.8	36.1	36.5
122-124	34.7	35.0	35.4	35.7	36.1	36.4	36.7	37.1
125-127	35.3	35.6	36.0	36.3	36.7	37.0	37.4	37.7
128-130	35.9	36.2	36.6	36.9	37.3	37.6	38.0	38.5

women, D.2 for men under forty, and D.3 for men over forty.*

5. For example, if the skinfold measurements for an eighteen-year-old female are: (a) triceps = 16, (b) suprailium = 14, and (c) thigh = 20 (total = 50), the percent body fat would be 20.6 percent.

Hydrostatic Weighing Technique for Body Composition Assessment

1. To determine body composition by hydrostatic or underwater weighing, an autopsy scale measuring up to 10 kilograms (kg) is needed. The scale should be readable to the nearest .100 of a kg. A chair is suspended from the scale and submerged in a tank of water or a swimming pool that is at least 5 x 5 x 5 feet.

2. The subject to be weighed should fast for approximately six to eight hours and have a bladder and bowel movement prior to underwater weighing.

3. The individual's residual lung volume (RV) must be measured, preferably while the person is in the water (if measured on land, this volume should be decreased by 6 percent to account for the decrease in RV due to the hydrostatic pressure). If the residual volume cannot be measured, this volume can be estimated (which may sacrifice the accuracy of hydrostatic weighing) using the following

predicting equations** (or other predicting equations):

Men: $RV = [(0.027 \times \text{height in centimeters}) + (0.017 \times \text{age})] - 3.447$

Women: $RV = [(0.032 \times \text{height in centimeters}) + (0.009 \times \text{age})] - 3.9$

4. Weigh the subject (in kg) in a swimsuit and subtract the weight of the suit. Record the water temperature in the tank (use degrees Centigrade). The water temperature is used to determine the water density factor (*see* Table D.4) which is required in the formula to compute body density.

5. The subject, dressed in a swimsuit, should enter the tank and completely wipe off all air clinging to the skin and hair.

6. The subject sits in the chair with the water at chin level. The water and scale should remain as still as possible during the entire procedure. Decreasing scale and water movement will allow for a better underwater reading (during underwater weighing, scale movement can be decreased by holding and slowly

Table D.4.
Density of Water at Different Temperatures.

Temperature (°C)	Water Density (gr/ml)
28	0.99626
29	0.99595
30	0.99567
31	0.99537
32	0.99505
33	0.99473
34	0.99440
35	0.99406
36	0.99371
37	0.99336
38	0.99299
39	0.99262
40	0.99224

---

* Body density in tables D.1, D.2, and D.3 was calculated using the generalized equation for predicting body density of women, developed by A. S. Jackson, M. L. Pollock, and A. Ward, *Medicine and Science in Sports and Exercise* 12:175-182, 1980; and the generalized equation for predicting body density of men, developed by A. S. Jackson and M. L. Pollock, *British Journal of Nutrition* 40:497-504, 1978. These equations are:

Women: $BD = 1.0994921 - 0.0009929 (SS) + 0.0000023 (SS)^2 - 0.0001392 (A)$

Men: $BD = 1.1093800 - 0.0008267 (SS) + 0.0000016 (SS)^2 - 0.0002574 (A)$

Where: BD = body density, SS = sum of three skinfolds, and A = age

Percent body fat was determined from the calculated body density using the Siri formula (see Hydrostatic Weighing Technique for Body Composition Assessment).

**Reproduced with permission from "Respiratory Function Tests: Normal Values at Medium Altitudes and the Prediction of Normal Results" by H. L. Goldman and M. R. Becklake. *American Review of Tuberculosis* 79:457-467, 1959. (Volume is predicted in BTPS).

releasing the neck of the scale until the subject is freely floating in the water).

7. Place a clip on the subject's nose and have him/her forcefully exhale all of the air out of the lungs. The subject then totally submerges underwater, still exhaling if any air is left in the lungs while going underwater. Record the reading on the scale. This procedure is repeated eight to ten times, since practice and experience on the part of the subject will increase the accuracy of the underwater weight. The average of the three heaviest underwater weights is used as the gross underwater weight.

8. Since tare weight (chair and chain or rope used to suspend the chair) also accounts for part of the gross underwater weight, this weight has to be subtracted to obtain the subject's net underwater weight. To determine tare weight, place a clothespin on the chain or rope at the water level when the subject is completely submerged. After the subject comes out of the water, place his/her swimsuit on the chair and lower the chair into the water to the pin level. Tare weight can now be recorded. The net underwater weight can now be determined by subtracting the tare weight from the gross underwater weight.

9. Body density and percent fat is computed using the following equations:

$$\text{Body density} = \cfrac{BW}{\cfrac{BW - UW}{DW} - RV - .1}$$

$$\text{Percent fat*} = \frac{495}{BD} - 450$$

Whereby:

BW = body weight in kg

UW = net underwater weight

WD = water density (determined by water temperature)

RV = residual volume (if other lung volumes are used, such as functional residual capacity or total lung capacity, replace the RV value in the equation for the respective lung volume used — however, using other lung volumes may

also compromise the accuracy of hydrostatic weighing)

BD = body density

10. An example of percent body fat determined by hydrostatic weighing is given in Figure D.2.

LEAN BODY MASS AND IDEAL BODY WEIGHT DETERMINATION

Lean body mass and ideal body weight can be easily determined using a person's current body fat percentage and the ideal fat percentage (*see* Tables D.5 or 4.9) for that person's respective age and gender. To compute lean body mass and ideal body weight the following steps are taken:

1. Determine the pounds of body weight in fat (FW). This is done by multiplying body weight (BW) by the current percent fat (%F) expressed in decimal form (FW = BW × %F).

2. Lean body mass (LBM) is determined by subtracting the weight in fat from the total body weight (LBM = BW - FW). Remember that anything which is not fat must be part of the lean component.

3. Look up the ideal body fat percentage (IFP) in Table D.5 (or 4.9).

4. Compute ideal body weight (IBW) according to the following formula: IBW = LBM/1.0-IFP).

---

* From Siri, W. E. *Body Composition from Fluid Spaces and Density.* Berkeley, CA: Donner Laboratory of Medical Physics, University of California, March 19, 1956.

Table D.5.
Ideal Body Fat Percentages Based on Age and Gender.

Age	Percent Fat	
	Men	Women
<19	12	17
20-29	13	18
30-39	14	19
40-49	15	20
50>	16	21

Figure D.2. *Body Composition Recording Chart (sample computation).*

Name: _Jane Doe_____   Soc. Sec. _999-99-9999_____

Age: __27____   Weight: __148.5__ lbs.   ÷   2.2046 = __67.36__ kg   Date: _10-24-84_

SKINFOLD TECHNIQUE

Men

Chest:	_____ mm
Abdomen:	_____ mm
Thigh:	_____ mm
Total:	_____ mm
% Fat =	_____ %

Women

Triceps:	__25.0__ mm
Suprailium:	__14.5__ mm
Thigh:	__32.5__ mm
Total:	__72.0__ mm
% Fat =	__27.8__ %

HYDROSTATIC WEIGHING

A. Water Temperature: ____33____ °C
B. Water Density (DW): __.99473__ gr/ml
C. Residual Volume (RV): __1.36__ lit
D. Body Weight (BW): __67.36__ kg
E. Gross Underwater Weights:

1. ____6.15____ kg   6. ____6.29____ kg
2. ____6.12____ kg   7. ____6.27____ kg
3. ____6.24____ kg   8. ____6.28____ kg
4. ____6.26____ kg   9. _____ kg
5. ____6.21____ kg   10. _____ kg

F. Average Underwater Weight (Use 3 heaviest trails) (AUW) = ____6.28____ kg
G. Tare Weight (TW): __5.154__ kg
H. Net Underwater Weight (UW) = AUW - TW = __6.28__ - __5.154__ = __1.126__ kg
I. Body Density (BD):

$$BD = \frac{BW}{\frac{BW - UW}{DW} - RV - .1}$$

$$BD = \frac{67.36}{\frac{67.36 - 1.126}{.99473} - 1.36 - .1}$$

$$BD = 1.03432$$

J. Percent Fat (%F) = $\frac{495}{BD}$ - 450

$$\%F = \frac{495}{1.03432} - 450 \qquad \%F = 28.6\%$$

Figure D.3. *Body Composition Recording Chart.*

Name: _____ Soc. Sec. _____

Age: _____ Weight: _____ lbs. ÷ 2.2046 = _____ kg Date: _____

SKINFOLD TECHNIQUE

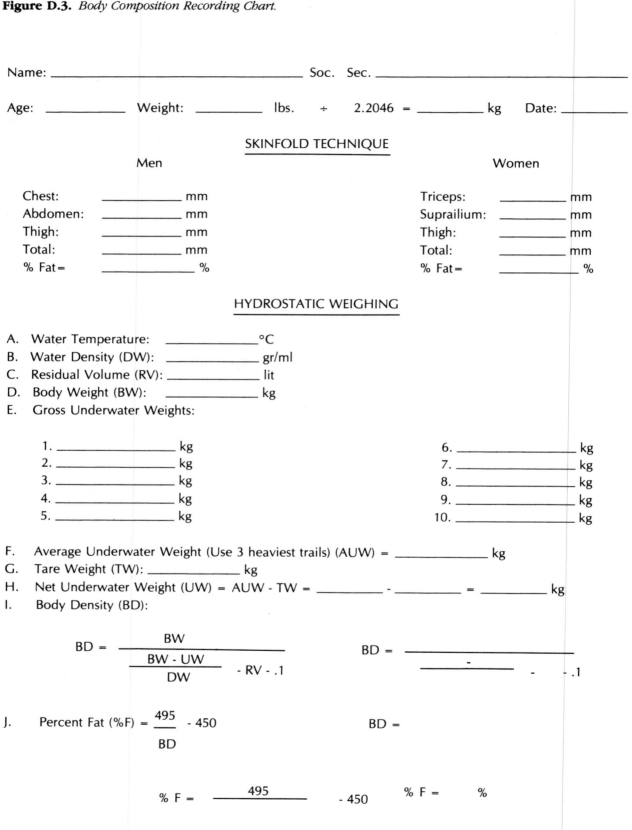

Men

Chest:	_____	mm
Abdomen:	_____	mm
Thigh:	_____	mm
Total:	_____	mm
% Fat =	_____	%

Women

Triceps:	_____	mm
Suprailium:	_____	mm
Thigh:	_____	mm
Total:	_____	mm
% Fat =	_____	%

HYDROSTATIC WEIGHING

A. Water Temperature: _____ °C

B. Water Density (DW): _____ gr/ml

C. Residual Volume (RV): _____ lit

D. Body Weight (BW): _____ kg

E. Gross Underwater Weights:

1. _____ kg   6. _____ kg
2. _____ kg   7. _____ kg
3. _____ kg   8. _____ kg
4. _____ kg   9. _____ kg
5. _____ kg   10. _____ kg

F. Average Underwater Weight (Use 3 heaviest trails) (AUW) = _____ kg

G. Tare Weight (TW): _____ kg

H. Net Underwater Weight (UW) = AUW - TW = _____ - _____ = _____ kg

I. Body Density (BD):

$$BD = \frac{BW}{\dfrac{BW - UW}{DW} - RV - .1} \qquad\qquad BD = \frac{}{\dfrac{-}{} - - .1}$$

J. Percent Fat (%F) $= \dfrac{495}{BD} - 450$ $\qquad\qquad BD =$

$$\%F = \frac{495}{} - 450 \qquad \%F = \quad\%$$

An example of these computations may be helpful. A forty-five-year-old male who weighs 186 pounds and is 25 percent fat would like to know what his ideal body weight should be.

Sex: male
Age: 19
BW = 186 lbs.
%F = 25% (.25 in decimal form)

1. FW = BW × %F
$$FW = 186 \times .25 = 46.5 \text{ lbs.}$$

2. LBM = BW - FW
$$LBM = 186 - 46.5 = 139.5 \text{ lbs.}$$

3. IFP: 15% (.15 in decimal form)

4. IBW = LBM/(1.0-IFP)
$$IBW = 139.5/(1.0-.15) = 164.1 \text{ lbs.}$$

When dieting, body composition should be reassessed periodically due to the effects of negative caloric intake on lean body mass. As explained in Chapter 6, dieting does decrease lean body mass, but this loss can be reduced or eliminated if a sensible diet is combined with physical exercise.

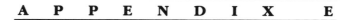

APPENDIX E

Muscular Strength Assessment and Prescription

Photography for the various strength training exercises courtesy of:

Universal Gym Equipment, Inc.
930 27th Avenue, S.W.
Cedar Rapids, Iowa

MUSCULAR STRENGTH ASSESSMENT

Muscular Strength and Endurance Test.

1. Determine the subject's weight in pounds.

2. Three exercises are performed on this test: leg extension, bench press, and sit-up (a graphic illustration of these exercises is given at the end of this Appendix). Constant resistance weight training equipment, such as Universal Gym, should be used for the leg extension and bench press exercises. For the leg extension exercise, the participant should maintain the trunk in an upright position and may use the hands to hold on to both sides of the bench. For the bench press exercise, the elbows are flexed at ninety degrees at the starting position. For the sit-up exercise, a horizontal plane is used, the feet are held in place, and the knees are flexed at a 100-degree angle. The resistance (or hands) is held behind the neck (use flat weight plates).

3. Determine the amount of resistance to be used on each lift. To obtain this number, multiply the body weight by the percent given for each exercise in Figure E.1, under the percent of body weight column.

4. The subject may then proceed to perform as many continuous repetitions as possible on each lift.

5. Based on the number of repetitions performed, the percentile rank and strength fitness category for each exercise can be found in Table A.18, Appendix A.

6. An overall strength fitness category can be obtained by determining an average percentile score for all three exercises.

MUSCULAR STRENGTH PRESCRIPTION

Physiological Factors Involved in Muscular Contraction.

There are several important physiological factors related to muscle contraction and subsequent strength gains. These factors are neural stimulation, muscle fiber type, overload principle, and specificity of training. Basic knowledge of these factors is important to understand the principles involved in strength training.

1. **Neural Stimulation.** Within the neuromuscular system, single motor neurons (nerves traveling from the central nervous system to the muscle) branch and attach to multiple muscle fibers. The combination of the motor neuron and the fibers that it innervates is called a motor neuron. The number of fibers that a motor neuron can innervate varies from just a few to as many as 200. Stimulation of a motor neuron causes the muscle fibers to contract maximally or not at all. Variations

Figure E.1. *Resistance (selected percentages of body weight) Requirements for the Muscular Strength and Endurance Test.*

Exercise	Age Group:	Percentage of body weights			
		<35	36-49	50>	
Leg Extension		.65	.55	.50	
Bench Press		.75	.60	.45	
Sit-Up		.16	.12	.10	Men
Leg Extension		.50	.42	.40	
Bench Press		.45	.35	.30	
Sit-Up		.10	.05	.00*	Women

*Since no resistance is required a maximum of one minute is allowed to perform as many repetitions as possible.

in the number of fibers innervated and the frequency of their stimulation determine the strength of the muscle contraction. As the number of fibers innervated and frequency of stimulation increase, so does the strength of the muscular contraction.

2. **Fiber Types.** There are primarily two types of muscle fibers that determine muscle response: type I or slow twitch and type II or fast twitch. Type I fibers have a greater capacity for aerobic work. Type II fibers have a greater capacity for anaerobic work and produce a greater overall force. The latter are important for quick and powerful movements, commonly used in strength training activities.

During muscular contraction, type I fibers are always recruited first. As the force and speed of muscle contraction increase, the relative importance of the type II fibers also increases. An activity must be intense and powerful for activation of the type Ii fibers to occur.

3. **Overload Principle.** Strength gains are achieved in two ways: first, through an increased ability of individual muscle fibers to elicit a stronger contraction, and second, by recruiting a greater proportion of the total available fibers for each contraction. The development of these two factors can be accomplished by the use of the overload principle. This principle states that for strength improvements to occur, the demands placed on the muscle must be systematically and progressively increased over a period of time, and the resistance must be of a magnitude significant enough to cause physiologic adaptation. In simpler terms, just like all other organs and systems of the human body, muscles have to be taxed beyond their regular accustomed loads to increase in physical capacity.

4. **Specificity of Training.** Another important aspect of training is the concept of specificity of training. This principle indicates that for a muscle to increase in strength or endurance, the training program must be specific to obtain the desired effects. In like manner, to increase static (isometric) versus dynamic (isotonic) strength, an individual must use static against dynamic training procedures to achieve the appropriate results.

Principles of Strength Training Prescription
Similar to the prescription of cardiovascular exercise, several principles need to be observed to improve muscular strength and endurance. These principles are mode, resistance and quantity, and frequency of training.

1. **Mode of Training.** There are three basic types of training methods used to improve strength: isometric, isotonic, and isokinetic. Isometric training refers to a muscle contraction producing little or no movement, such as pushing or pulling against immovable objects. Isotonic training refers to a muscle contraction with movement, such as lifting an object over the head. During isotonic training, the resistance is kept constant as the limb moves through the full range of motion at the particular joint. Isokinetic training is a form of isotonic training but uses a special apparatus that provides maximum resistance through the full range of motion.

The mode of training used by different individuals depends largely on the type of equipment available and the specific objective that the training program is attempting to accomplish.

Isometric training does not require much equipment and was commonly used several years ago, but its popularity has significantly decreased in recent years. Since strength gains with isometric training are specific to the angle at which the contraction is being performed, this type of training is beneficial in a sport like gymnastics where static contractions are regularly used during routines.

Isotonic training is the most popular mode used in weight training. The primary advantage is that strength gains occur through the full range of motion. Most daily activities are isotonic in nature. We are constantly lifting, pushing, and pulling objects, where strength is needed through a complete range of motion. Another advantage is that improvements are easily measured by the amount lifted.

The benefits of isokinetic training are similar to isotonic training. Theoretically, strength gains should be better because maximum resistance is constantly applied. However, research has not shown this type of training to be more effective than an isotonic program. Many people enjoy isokinetic training because of the impressive equipment used in the program. A real disadvantage is that the equipment is very expensive and not readily available to most people.

2. **Resistance and Quantity.** Resistance and quantity in strength training are the equivalent of intensity and duration in cardiovascular exercise prescription. The amount of resistance (or weight) used will depend on whether the individual is trying to develop muscular strength or muscular endurance.

To stimulate strength development, it is recommended that a resistance of approximately 80 percent of the maximum capacity (1 RM) be used. For example, a person who can press 150 pounds should work with at least 120 pounds (150 x .80). Using less than 80 percent will help increase muscular endurance rather than strength. Because of the time factor involved in constantly determining the 1 RM on each lift to insure that the person is indeed working above 80 percent, a rule of thumb widely accepted by many authors and coaches is that individuals should perform between six and ten repetitions maximum for adequate strength gains. In other words, if a person is training with a resistance of 100 pounds and cannot lift it more than ten times, training stimuli is adequate for strength development. Once the weight can be lifted more than ten times, the resistance should be increased by five to ten pounds and the person should again build up to ten repetitions. If training is conducted with more than ten repetitions, muscular endurance will be primarily developed.

The quantity or amount of strength training is given in number of sets rather than length of time involved. A set has been defined as a number of repetitions performed for a given exercise. For example, a person lifting 100 pounds eight times has performed one set of eight repetitions. The number of sets recommended for optimum development is anywhere from three to five sets, with about ninety seconds recovery time between each set. Due to the physiology of muscle fiber, there is a limit to the number of sets that can be done. As the number of sets increases, so does the amount of muscle fatigue and subsequent recovery time; therefore, strength gains may be lessened if too many sets are performed. A recommended program for beginners in their

first year of training is three heavy sets (up to the maximum number of repetitions) preceded by one or two light warm-up sets.

To make the exercise program more time-effective, two or three exercises that require different muscle groups may be alternated. In this manner, an individual will not have to wait the full ninety seconds before proceeding to the next set. For example, bench press, leg extensions, and sit-ups may be combined so that the person can go almost directly from one set to the next.

Additionally, to avoid muscle soreness and stiffness, new participants ought to build up gradually to the three sets of maximal repetitions. This can be accomplished by only doing one set of each exercise with a lighter resistance on the first day. On the second session, two sets of each exercise can be performed, one light, and the second with the regular resistance. On the third session three sets could be performed, one light and two heavy ones. Thereafter, a person should be able to do all three heavy sets.

3. **Frequency of Training.** Strength training should be done either with a total body workout three times per week, or more frequently if a split routine (upper body one day and lower body the next) is used. Following a maximum workout, it is necessary to rest the muscle at least forty-eight hours to allow adequate recovery. If complete recovery has not occurred in two or three days, the person is most likely overtraining and therefore not reaping the full benefits of the program. In such a case, a decrease in the total number of sets performed on the previous workout is recommended.

To achieve significant strength gains, a minimum of eight weeks of consecutive training is needed. Once an ideal level of strength is achieved, one training session per week will be sufficient to maintain the new strength level.

Strength Training Exercises

A complete strength training program will now be introduced. This program has been developed to provide a complete body workout. Most of the exercises can be performed either on gym equipment as outlined in the different pictures, or on free weights. The first eight exercises are recommended to get a complete workout, the rest are optional. However, if one of the optional exercises involves the same body parts, the person may substitute the latter for one of the basic eight (exercise 11 for 1, 9 or 10 for 2, 13 or 14 for 4, 12 for 6, and 15 for 8).

The resistance and the number of repetitions to be used are based on whether the person wishes to increase muscular strength or muscular endurance. Up to ten maximum repetitions should be used for strength gains, and more than ten for muscular endurance. Since both strength and endurance are required in daily activities, it is recommended that people conduct their training program around ten repetitions. In this manner they will obtain good strength gains and yet be close to the endurance threshold as well. Perhaps the only exercise where more than ten repetitions are recommended is the abdominal curl-up exercise. The abdominal muscles are considered primarily antigravity or postural muscles, hence, a little more endurance may be required. Usually twenty to thirty repetitions are done on this exercise. As noted earlier, three sets are recommended for each exercise.

Strength Training Exercises

Exercise 1: ARM CURL

Action: Use a supinated or palms-up grip, and start with the arms almost completely extended. Now curl up as far as possible, then return to the starting position.

Muscles Developed: Biceps, brachioradialis, and brachialis.

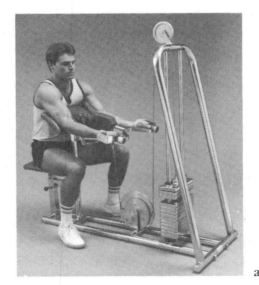

a

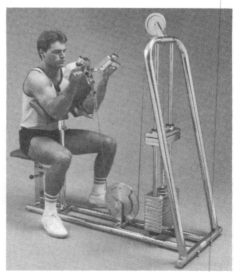

b

Exercise 2: LEG PRESS

Action: From a sitting position with the knees flexed at about ninety degrees and both feet on the footrest, fully extend the legs, then return slowly to the starting position.

Muscles Developed: Quadriceps and gluteal muscles.

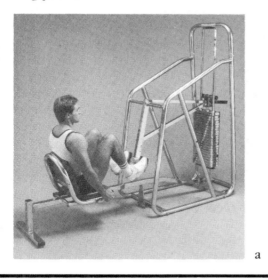

a

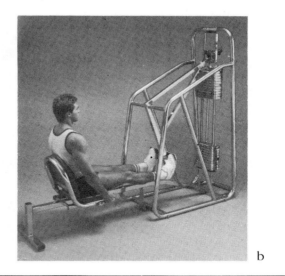

b

Exercise 3: SIT-UP

Action: Using either a horizontal or inclined board, stabilize your feet and flex the knees to about 100 to 120 degrees. Start with the head and shoulders off the board, curl all the way up, then return to the starting position without letting the head and shoulders touch the board (do not swing up, but rather curl up). You may curl straight up or use a twisting motion (twisting as you first start to come up), alternating on each sit-up.

Muscles Developed: Abdominals and hip flexors.

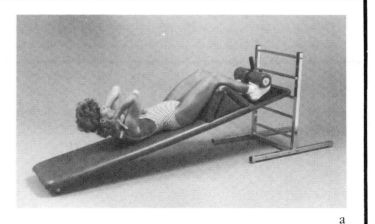

a

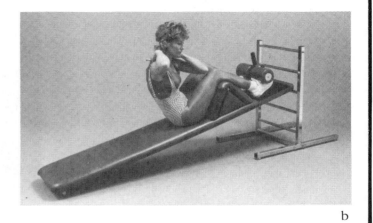

b

Exercise 4: BENCH PRESS

Action: Lie down on the bench with the head toward the weight stack, feet flat on the floor, and the bench press bar above the chest. Press upward until the arms are completely extended, then return to the starting position. Do not arch the back during the exercise.

Muscles Developed: Pectoralis major, triceps, and deltoid.

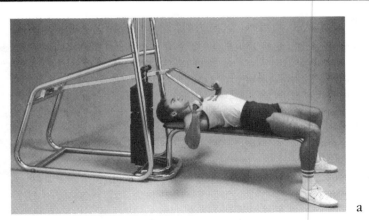

a

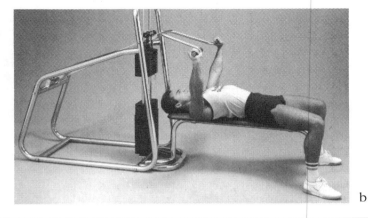

b

Exercise 5: LEG CURL

Action: Lie with the face down on the bench and legs straight with the back of the feet against the bar. Curl up to at least 90 degrees and return to the original position.

Muscles Developed: Hamstrings.

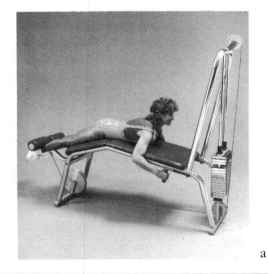

a

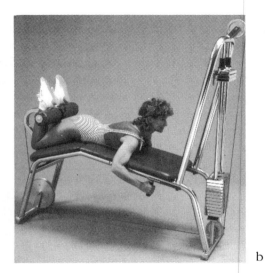

b

Exercise 6: LATERAL PULL-DOWN

Action: Start from a sitting position and hold the exercise bar with a wide grip. Pull the bar down until it touches the base of the neck, then return to the starting position (if a heavy resistance is used, stabilization of the body may be required by either using equipment as shown in the illustration or having someone else hold you down by the waist or shoulders).

Muscles Developed: Latissimus dorsi, pectoralis major, and biceps.

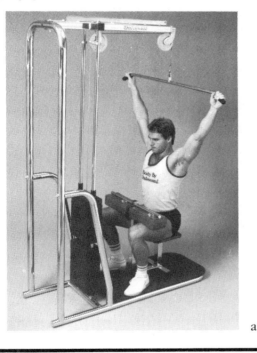

a

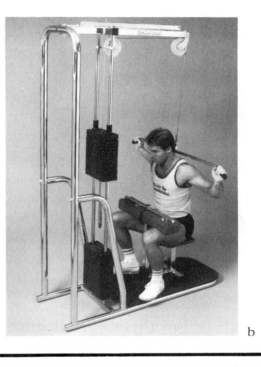

b

Exercise 7: HEEL RAISE

Action: Start with your feet either flat on the floor or the front of the feet on an elevated block, then raise and lower yourself by moving at the ankle joint only. If additional resistance is needed, you can use the squat machine, which is illustrated in Exercise 9.

Muscles Developed: Gastrocnemius and soleus.

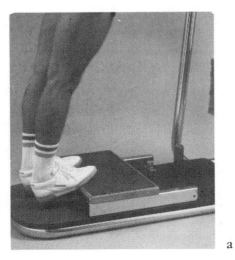

a

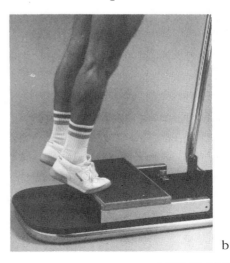

b

Exercise 8:   TRICEP EXTENSION

Action: Using a palms-down grip, grasp the bar slightly closer than shoulder width, and start with the elbows almost completely bent. Fully extend the arms, then return to starting position.

Muscle Developed: Triceps.

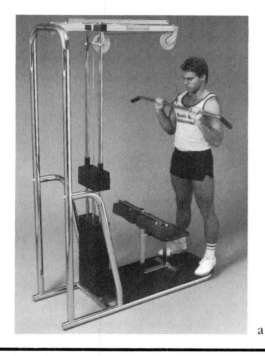

a

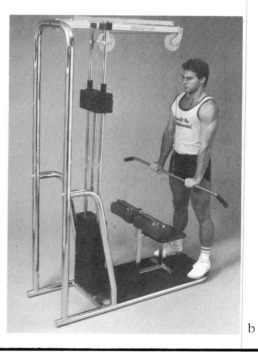

b

Exercise 9:   SQUAT

Action: Start with the knees bent at about 120 degrees and shoulders under the padded bars. Completely extend the legs, then return to the original position.

Muscles Developed: Quadriceps, gluteal muscles, hamstrings, gastrocnemius, soleus, and erector spinae.

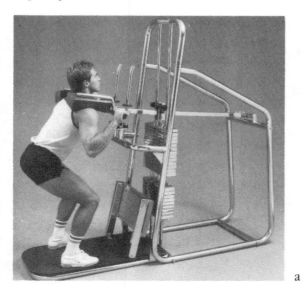

a

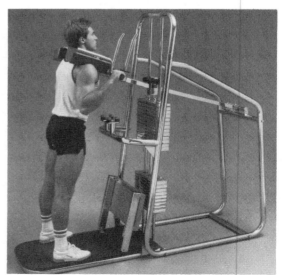

b

Exercise 10: QUADRICEPS LIFT Or LEG EXTENSION

Action: Sit in an upright position with feet under the padded bar. Extend the legs until they are completely straight, then return to the starting position.

Muscles Developed: Quadriceps.

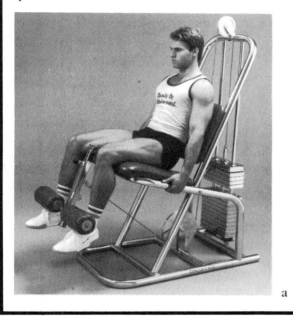

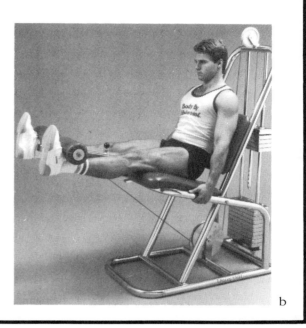

a

b

Exercise 11: UPRIGHT ROWING

Action: Start with the arms extended and grip the handles with the palms down. Pull all the way up to the chin, then return to the starting position.

Muscles Developed: Biceps, brachioradialis, brachialis, deltoid, and trapezius.

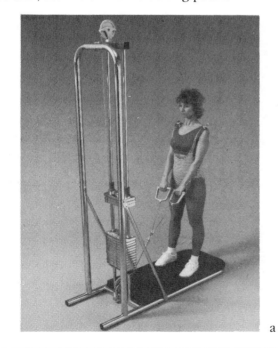

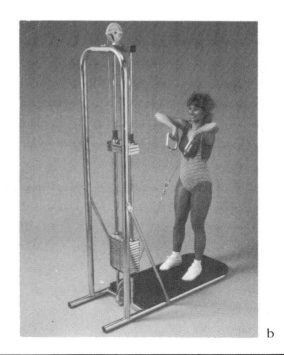

a

b

Exercise 12: BENT-ARM PULLOVER

Action: Sit back into the chair and grasp the bar behind your head. Pull the bar over your head all the way down to your abdomen and slowly return to the original position.

Muscles Developed: Latissimus dorsi, pectoral muscles, deltoid, and serratus anterior.

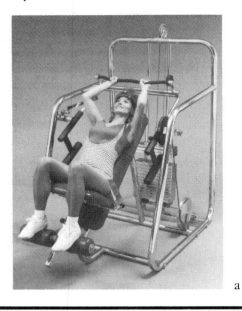

a

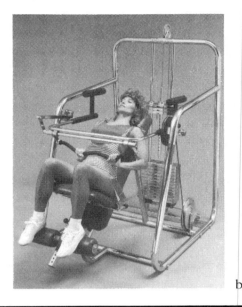

b

Exercise 13: CHEST PRESS

Action: Start with the arms to the side and elbows bent at ninety degrees. Press your arms forward until the padded bars touch in front of your chest, then return to the starting position.

Muscles Developed: Pectoralis major and deltoid.

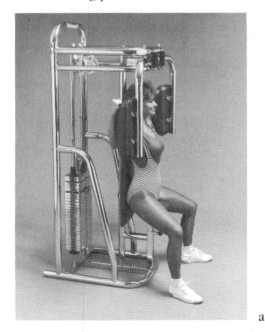

a

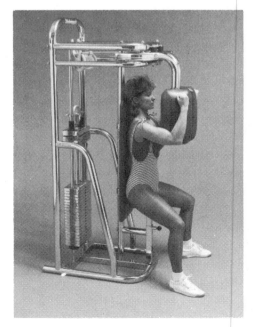

b

Exercise 14: SEATED OVERHEAD PRESS

Action: Sit in an upright position and grasp the bar wider than shoulder width. Press the bar all the way up until the arms are fully extended, then return to the initial position.

Muscles Developed: Triceps, deltoid, and pectoralis major.

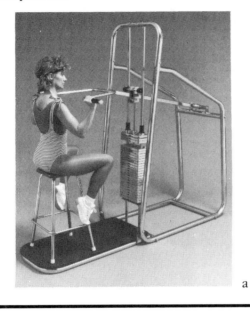

a

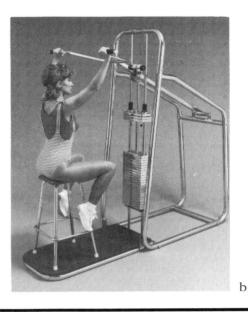

b

Exercise 15: DIP

Action: Start with your arms fully extended, knees bent, and feet crossed. Dip down at least to a ninety-degree angle at the elbow joint, then return to the initial position.

Muscles Developed: Triceps, deltoid, and pectoralis major.

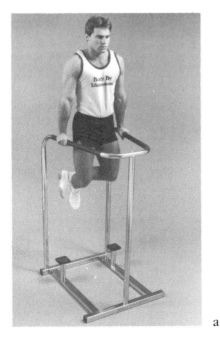

a

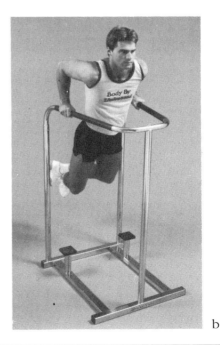

b

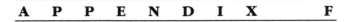

A P P E N D I X F

Muscular Flexibility Assessment and Prescription

The procedures for the Modified Sit-and-Reach Test, Trunk Rotation Test, and Shoulder Rotation Test contained in this Appendix are reproduced with permission from Hoeger, W. W. K. *Lifetime Physical Fitness & Wellness: A Personalized Program.* Englewood, CO: Morton Publishing Company, 1986. The standards for these tests (Tables A.19, A.20, and A.21 contained in Appendix A) were updated with data collected at Boise State University.

MUSCULAR FLEXIBILITY ASSESSMENT

Three flexibility tests are administered to obtain a flexibility profile.* These tests are: the Modified Sit-and-Reach Test, the Trunk Rotation Test (right and left sides), and the Shoulder Rotation Test. It is important that people warm up properly by doing some gentle stretching exercises specific to the test that will be administered.

Procedures for the Modified Sit-and-Reach Test.

1. Place a yardstick on top of a box approximately twelve inches high.

2. Have the subject sit on the floor with the back and head against a wall and the legs fully extended, and the bottom of the feet against the box (remove the shoes for this test).

3. As illustrated in Figure F.1, have the subject place the hands one on top of the other, and have him/her reach forward as far as possible without letting the head and back come off the wall (the shoulders may be rounded as much as possible, but neither head nor back should come off the wall at this time). The technician can then slide the yardstick along the top of the box until the end of the stick touches the participant's fingers. The yardstick must then be held firmly in place throughout the rest of the test.

4. The participant's head and back can now come off the wall. He/she should then bob forward three times, the third time stretching forward as far as possible on the yardstick, and holding the final position for at least two seconds (*see* Figure F.2). Record the final number of inches reached to the nearest one-half inch.

5. The subject is allowed three trials, and an average of the three scores is used as the final test score (make sure that the person is properly warmed up prior to the first trial).

---

*The equipment necessary to conduct all three of these tests can be obtained from Novel Products Figure Finder Collection, 80 Fairbanks, Unit 12, Addison, IL.

The respective percentile ranks and fitness categories for this test are given in Table A.19, Appendix A.

Figure F.1. *Starting Position for the Sit-and-Reach Test.*

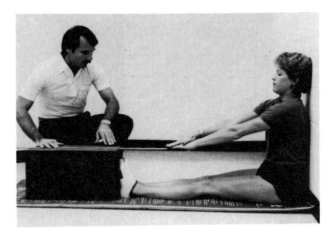

Figure F.2. *The Sit-and-Reach Test.*

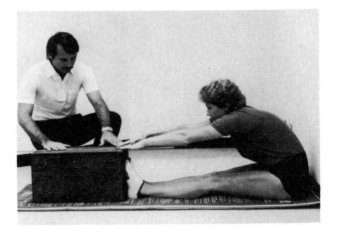

Procedures for the Trunk Rotation Test.

1. A measuring scale with a sliding panel is placed on a wall at shoulder height. The scale should be adjustable to accommodate individual differences in height. Two measuring tapes are glued in place above and below the sliding panel and centered at the fifteen-inch mark. Each tape should be at least thirty inches long. If no sliding panel is available, simply tape the measuring tapes onto the wall. A line is then drawn on the floor which must also be centered with the fifteen-inch mark (*see* Figures F.3, F.4, F.5, and F.6).

Figure F.3. *Measuring Device for the Trunk Rotation Test.*

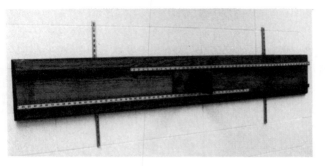

Figure F.4. *Trunk Rotation Test Using a Sliding Panel Device.*

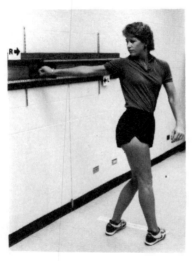

Figure F.5. *Measuring Tapes Used for the Trunk Rotation Test.*

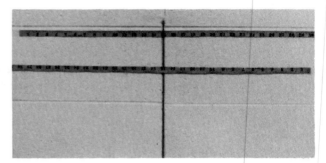

Figure F.6. *Trunk Rotation Test Using Simple Measuring Tapes.*

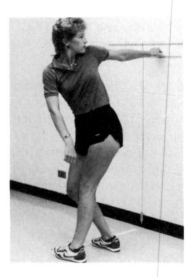

2. Have the subject stand sideways two to three feet away from the wall (depending on arm length), with the feet straight ahead and slightly separated. The arm opposite to the wall is held out horizontally from the body, making a fist with the hand. The measuring scale or tapes should be shoulder height at this time.

3. The subject can now rotate the trunk, the extended arm going backward (always maintaining a horizontal plane) and making contact with the panel, sliding it forward as far as possible. If no panel is available, slide the fist alongside the tapes (*see* Figures F.5 and F.6). The final position must be held for at least two seconds. The hand should be positioned with the little finger side forward during the entire sliding movement, as illustrated in Figure F.7

(it is crucial that the proper hand position be used, as many people will attempt to either open the hand or slide the panel with the knuckles). During the test, the knees can be slightly bent, feet should not be moved (pointing straight forward), and the body must be kept as straight (vertical) as possible.

4. The test is conducted for both the right and left sides of the body. Each participant is allowed three trials on each side. The farthest point reached, measured to the nearest one-half inch, and held for at least two seconds, is recorded (make sure that the subject is properly warmed up prior to the first trial). The average of the three trials on each side is used as the final test score. Using Table A.20 (Appendix A), determine the percentile rank

Figure F.7. *Proper Hand Position for the Trunk Rotation Test.*

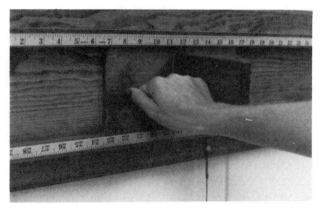

and flexibility fitness classification for both the right and left sides of the body.

Procedures for the Shoulder Rotation Test.

1. With the aid of a large caliper, measure the biacromial width to the nearest one-fourth inch (biacromial width is measured between the lateral edges of the acromion processes of the shoulders, as shown in Figure F.8). If a caliper is not available, one may be constructed by using three regular yardsticks. Nail and glue two of the yardsticks at one end at a ninety-degree angle. Use the third one as the sliding end of the caliper.

2. Place a sixty-inch measuring tape on an aluminum or wood stick, starting at about six or

Figure F.8. *Measuring Biacromial Width.*

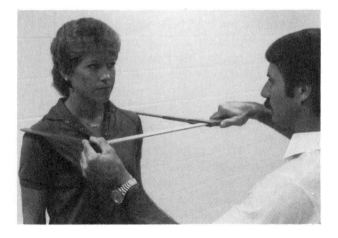

seven inches from the end to allow the subject gripping space with the hand.

3. A reverse grip is used to hold on to the stick behind the back, as shown in Figure F.9. The right hand is placed against the start of the tape and is held firmly in place throughout the test. The left hand is placed on the other end of the stick, as wide as needed.

Figure F.9. *Reverse Grip Used During the Shoulder Rotation Test.*

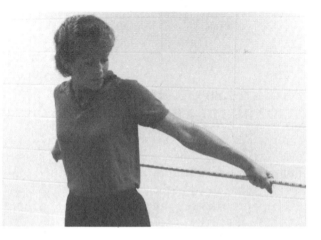

4. Standing straight up and extending both arms to full length, with elbows locked, the subject brings the stick over the head, until it can be seen in front (*see* Figure F.10). Depending on the resistance encountered when rotating the shoulders, the left grip may be moved in one-half to one inch at a time, and the task is repeated (the right-hand grip is always kept against the beginning of the tape). The trials are repeated until the subject can no longer rotate the shoulders, or starts bending the elbows to do so. Measure the last successful trial to the nearest one-half inch.

5. The final score for this test is determined by subtracting the biacromial width from the best score (shortest distance) between both hands on the rotation test. For example, if the best score is thirty-five inches and the biacromial width is fifteen inches, the final score would be twenty inches (35 – 15 = 20). Using Table A.21 (Appendix A), determine the percentile rank and flexibility fitness classification for this test.

Figure F.10. *Shoulder Rotation Test.*

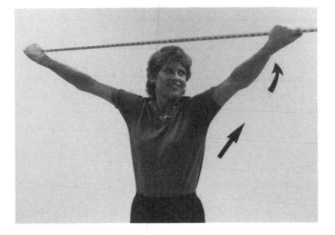

PRINCIPLES OF MUSCULAR FLEXIBILITY PRESCRIPTION

Muscular flexibility seems to be determined by heredity and exercise. Joint range of motion is limited by such factors as joint structure, ligaments, tendons, muscles, skin, tissue injury, adipose tissue, body temperature, age, sex, and index of physical activity.

The range of motion about a given joint depends largely on the structure of that particular joint. Fortunately, greater range of motion is attainable and can be accomplished through "plastic" and/or "elastic" elongation. Plastic elongation refers to a permanent elongation of soft tissue. Even though joint capsules, ligaments, and tendons are primarily nonelastic in nature, they can undergo plastic elongation. This permanent lengthening leads to increases in joint range of motion and is best attained using slow-sustained stretching exercises. Muscle tissue, on the other hand, has elastic properties and will respond to stretching exercises by undergoing elastic or temporary lengthening. This form of elongation increases the extensibility of the muscles.

The overload and specificity of training principles also apply to the development of muscular flexibility. To increase the total range of motion of a given joint, the specific muscles around the particular joint have to be progressively stretched beyond their normal accustomed length. The principles of mode, intensity, duration, and frequency of exercise are also used for the prescription of flexibility programs.

1. **Mode of Exercise.** Three modes of stretching exercises are commonly used to increase flexibility: (a) ballistic stretching, (b) slow-sustained stretching, and (c) propioceptive neuromuscular facilitation stretching. Although research has indicated that all three types of stretching are effective in developing better flexibility, there are certain advantages to each technique.

Ballistic or dynamic stretching exercises are performed using jerky, rapid, and bouncy movements that provide the necessary force to lengthen the muscles. In spite of the fact that studies have indicated that this type of stretching helps to develop flexibility, the ballistic actions may lead to increased muscle soreness and injury due to small tears to the soft tissue. In addition, proper precautions must be taken not to overstretch ligaments, since they undergo plastic or permanent elongation. If the magnitude of the stretching force cannot be adequately controlled, as in fast, jerky movements, ligaments can be easily overstretched. This, in turn, leads to excessively loose joints, increasing the risk for injuries, including joint dislocation and sublaxation (partial dislocation). Consequently, most authorities do not recommend ballistic exercises for flexibility development.

With the slow-sustained stretching technique, muscles are gradually lengthened through a joint's complete range of motion, and the final position is held for a few seconds. Using a slow-sustained stretch causes the muscles to relax; hence, greater length can be achieved. This type of stretch causes relatively little pain and has a very low risk of injury. Slow-sustained stretching exercises are the most frequently used and recommended for flexibility development programs.

Propioceptive neuromuscular facilitation (PNF) stretching has become more popular in the last few years. This technique is based on a "contract and relax" method and requires the assistance of another person. The procedure used is as follows:

A. The person assisting with the exercise provides an initial force by slowly pushing in the direction of the desired stretch. The initial stretch does not cover the entire range of motion.

B. The person being stretched then applies force in the opposite direction of the stretch, against the assistant, who will try to hold the initial degree of stretch as close as possible. In other words, an isometric contraction is being performed at that angle.

C. After four or five seconds of isometric contraction, the muscle(s) being stretched are completely relaxed. The assistant then slowly increases the degree of stretch to a greater angle.

D. The isometric contraction is then repeated for another four or five seconds, following which the muscle(s) is relaxed again. The assistant can then slowly increase the degree of stretch one more time. This procedure is repeated anywhere from two to five times until mild discomfort occurs. On the last trial, the final stretched position should be held for several seconds.

Figure F.11. *Propioceptive Neuromuscular Facilitation Stretching Technique.*

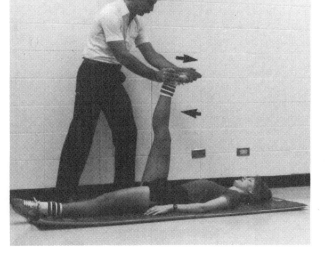

Theoretically, with the PNF technique, the isometric contraction aids in the relaxation of the muscle(s) being stretched, which results in greater muscle length. While some researchers have indicated that PNF is more effective than slow-sustained stretching, the disadvantages are that the degree of pain incurred with PNF is greater, a second person is required to perform the exercises, and a greater period of time is needed to conduct each session.

2. **Intensity of Exercise.** Before starting any flexibility exercises, always warm up the muscles adequately with some calisthenic exercises. A good time to do flexibility exercises is following aerobic workouts. Increased body temperature can significantly increase joint range of motion. Failing to conduct a proper warm up increases the risk for muscle pulls and tears.

   The intensity or degree of stretch when doing flexibiity exercises should only be to a point of mild discomfort. Pain does not have to be a part of the stretching routine. Excessive pain is an indication that the load is too high and may lead to injury. Stretching should only be done to slightly below the pain threshold. As participants reach this point, they should try to relax the muscle(s) being stretched as much as possible. After completing the stretch, the body part is brought gradually back to the original starting point.

3. **Duration of Exercise.** The duration of exercise refers to the number of repetitions for each exercise and the length of time that each repetition (final stretched position) must be held. The general recommendations are that each exercise be done four or five times, and each time the final position should be held for five to ten seconds. As the flexibility levels increase, the subject can progressively increase the time that each repetition is held, up to a maximum of one minute.

   At least one stretching exercise should be used for each major muscle group. A complete set of exercises for the development of muscular flexibility is presented at the end of this Appendix. Depending on the number and the length of the repetitions performed, a complete workout will last between fifteen and thirty minutes.

4. **Frequency of Exercise.** Flexibility exercises should be conducted five to six times per week in the initial stages of the program. After a minimum of six to eight weeks of almost daily stretching, flexibility levels can be maintained with only two or three sessions per week, using about three repetitions of ten to fifteen seconds each.

Exercise 1:
LATERAL HEAD TILT

Action: Slowly and gently tilt the head laterally. Repeat several times to each side.

Areas Stretched: Neck flexors and extensors and ligaments of the cervical spine.

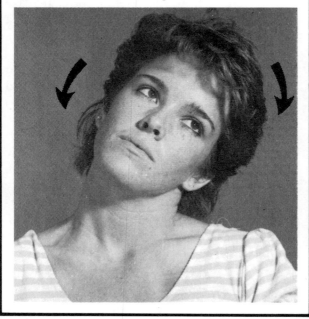

Exercise 2: ARM CIRCLES

Action: Gently circle your arms all the way around. Conduct the exercise in both directions.

Areas Stretched: Shoulder muscles and ligaments.

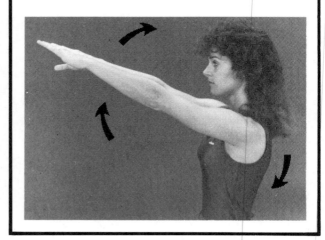

Exercise 3: SIDE STRETCH

Action: Stand straight up, feet separated to shoulder width, and place your hands on your waist. Now move the upper body to one side and hold the final stretch for a few seconds. Repeat on the other side.

Areas Stretched: Muscles and ligaments in the pelvic region.

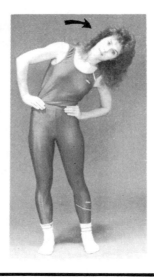

Exercise 4:
TRUNK ROTATION STRETCH

Action: Place your arms slightly away from your body and rotate the trunk as far as possible, holding the final position for several seconds. Conduct the exercise for both the right and left sides of the body. You can also perform this exercise by standing about two feet away from the wall (back toward the wall), and then rotate the trunk, placing the hands against the wall.

Areas Stretched: Hip, abdominal, chest, back, neck, and shoulder muscles. Hip and spinal ligaments.

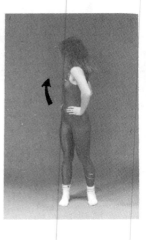

Exercise 5: CHEST STRETCH

Action: Kneel down behind a chair and place both hands on the back of the chair. Gradually push your chest downward and hold for a few seconds.

Areas Stretched: Chest (pectoral) muscles and shoulder ligaments.

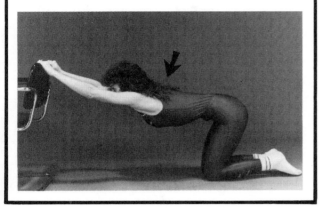

Exercise 6: SHOULDER HYPEREXTENSION STRETCH

Action: Place your hands on a table behind your back, then move your feet forward about a yard. Slowly lower your body as far as possible and hold this position for a few seconds.

Areas Stretched: Deltoid and pectoral muscles, and ligaments of the shoulder joint.

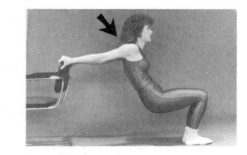

Exercise 7: SHOULDER ROTATION STRETCH

Action: With the aid of an aluminum or wood stick, place the band behind your back and grasp the two ends using a reverse (thumbs-out) grip. Slowly bring the stick over your head, keeping the elbows straight. Repeat several times (bring the hands closer together for additional stretch).

Areas Stretched: Deltoid, latissimus dorsi, and pectoral muscles. Shoulder ligaments.

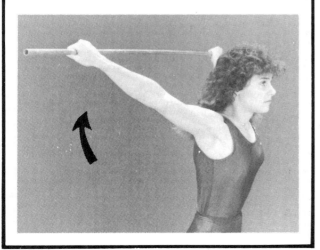

Exercise 8: QUAD STRETCH

Exercise 8: QUAD STRETCH

Action: Stand straight up and support yourself against a wall. Bring up one foot, flexing the knee. Grasp the front of the ankle and pull the ankle toward the gluteal region. Hold for several seconds. Repeat with the other leg.

Areas Stretched: Quadriceps muscle, and knee and ankle ligaments.

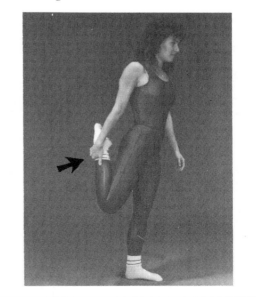

Exercise 9: HEEL CORD STRETCH

Action: Stand against the wall or at the edge of a step and stretch the heel downward, alternating legs. Hold the stretched position for a few seconds.

Areas Stretched: Heel cord (Achilles tendon), gastrocnemius, and soleus muscles.

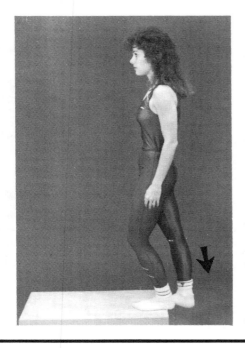

a

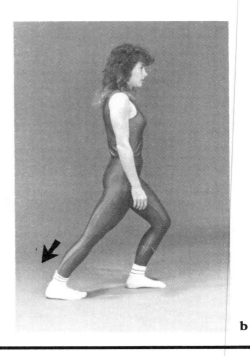

b

Exercise 10: ADDUCTOR STRETCH

Action: Stand with your feet about twice shoulder width and place your hands slightly above the knee. Flex one knee and slowly go down as far as possible, holding the final position for a few seconds. Repeat with the other leg.

Areas Stretched: Hip adductor muscles.

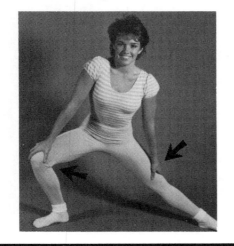

Exercise 11: SITTING ADDUCTOR STRETCH

Action: Sit on the floor and bring your feet in close to you, allowing the soles of the feet to touch each other. Now place your forearms (or elbows) on the inner part of the thigh and push the legs downward, holding the final stretch for several seconds.

Areas Stretched: Hip adductor muscles.

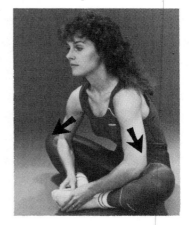

Exercise 12:
SIT AND REACH STRETCH

Action: Sit on the floor with legs together and gradually reach forward as far as possible. Hold the final position for a few seconds. This exercise may also be performed with the legs separated, reaching to each side as well as to the middle.

Areas Stretched: Hamstrings and lower back muscles, and lumbar spine ligaments.

Note: Additional stretching exercises for the lower back region are given in Appendix D.

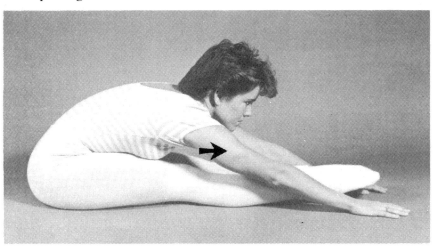

Prevention and Rehabilitation of Low Back Pain

PREVENTION AND REHABILITATION OF LOW BACK PAIN

Very few people make it through life without suffering from low back pain at some point. Current estimates indicate that 75 million Americans suffer from chronic low back pain each year. Unfortunately, approximately 80 percent of the time, backache syndrome is preventable and is caused by: (a) physical inactivity, (b) poor postural habits and body mechanics, and (c) excessive body weight.

Lack of physical activity is the most common cause contributing to chronic low back pain. The deterioration or weakening of the abdominal and gluteal muscles, along with a tightening of the lower back (erector spine) muscles, bring about an unnatural forward tilt of the pelvis. This tilt puts extra pressure on the spinal vertebrae, causing pain in the lower back. In addition, excessive accumulation of fat around the midsection of the body contributes to the forward tilt of the pelvis, which further aggravates the condition.

Low back pain is also frequently associated with faulty posture and improper body mechanics. This refers to the use of correct body positions in all of life's daily activities, including sleeping, sitting, standing, walking, driving, working, and exercising. Incorrect posture and poor mechanics, as explained in Figure G.1, lead to increased strain not only on the lower back, but on many other bones, joints, muscles, and ligaments.

The incidence and frequency of low back pain can be greatly reduced by including some specific stretching and strengthening exercises as a part of the regular fitness program. When suffering from backache, in most cases pain is only present with movement and physical activity. If the pain is severe and persists even at rest, the initial step is to consult a physician, who can rule out any disc damage and most likely prescribe correct bed rest using several pillows under the knees for adequate leg support (*see* Figure G.1). This position helps release muscle spasms by stretching the muscles involved. Additionally, a physician may prescribe a muscle relaxant, and/or anti-inflammatory medication, and/or some type of physical therapy. Once the individual is pain-free in the resting state, he/she needs to start correcting the muscular imbalance by stretching the tight muscles and strengthening weak ones (stretching exercises are always performed first).

Several exercises for the prevention and rehabilitation of the backache syndrome are introduced in this Appendix. These exercises can be conducted twice or more daily when a person suffers from backache. Under normal circumstances, three to four times per week is sufficient to prevent the syndrome.

Figure G.1.

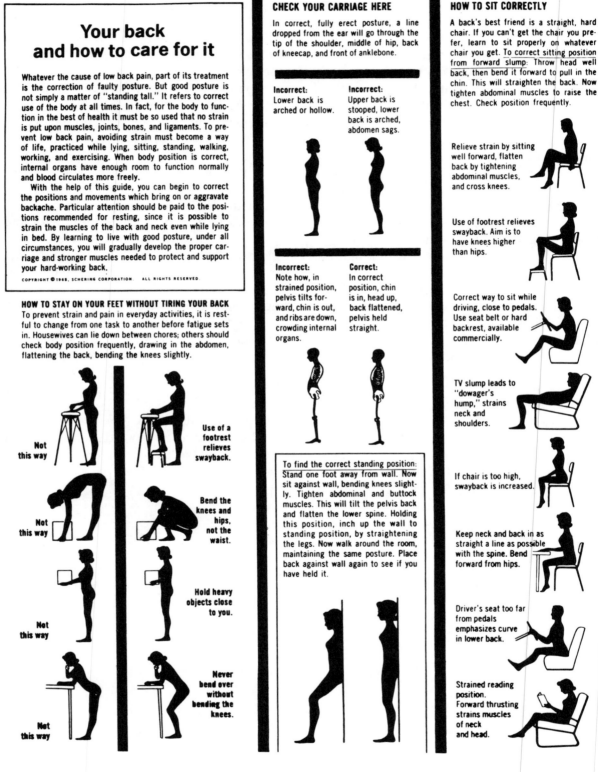

Your back
and how to care for it

Whatever the cause of low back pain, part of its treatment is the correction of faulty posture. But good posture is not simply a matter of "standing tall." It refers to correct use of the body at all times. In fact, for the body to function in the best of health it must be so used that no strain is put upon muscles, joints, bones, and ligaments. To prevent low back pain, avoiding strain must become a way of life, practiced while lying, sitting, standing, walking, working, and exercising. When body position is correct, internal organs have enough room to function normally and blood circulates more freely.

With the help of this guide, you can begin to correct the positions and movements which bring on or aggravate backache. Particular attention should be paid to the positions recommended for resting, since it is possible to strain the muscles of the back and neck even while lying in bed. By learning to live with good posture, under all circumstances, you will gradually develop the proper carriage and stronger muscles needed to protect and support your hard-working back.

COPYRIGHT © 1968, SCHERING CORPORATION.   ALL RIGHTS RESERVED.

HOW TO STAY ON YOUR FEET WITHOUT TIRING YOUR BACK
To prevent strain and pain in everyday activities, it is restful to change from one task to another before fatigue sets in. Housewives can lie down between chores; others should check body position frequently, drawing in the abdomen, flattening the back, bending the knees slightly.

Not this way

Not this way

Not this way

Not this way

Use of a footrest relieves swayback.

Bend the knees and hips, not the waist.

Hold heavy objects close to you.

Never bend over without bending the knees.

CHECK YOUR CARRIAGE HERE

In correct, fully erect posture, a line dropped from the ear will go through the tip of the shoulder, middle of hip, back of kneecap, and front of anklebone.

Incorrect:
Lower back is arched or hollow.

Incorrect:
Upper back is stooped, lower back is arched, abdomen sags.

Incorrect:
Note how, in strained position, pelvis tilts forward, chin is out, and ribs are down, crowding internal organs.

Correct:
In correct position, chin is in, head up, back flattened, pelvis held straight.

To find the correct standing position: Stand one foot away from wall. Now sit against wall, bending knees slightly. Tighten abdominal and buttock muscles. This will tilt the pelvis back and flatten the lower spine. Holding this position, inch up the wall to standing position, by straightening the legs. Now walk around the room, maintaining the same posture. Place back against wall again to see if you have held it.

HOW TO SIT CORRECTLY

A back's best friend is a straight, hard chair. If you can't get the chair you prefer, learn to sit properly on whatever chair you get. To correct sitting position from forward slump: Throw head well back, then bend it forward to pull in the chin. This will straighten the back. Now tighten abdominal muscles to raise the chest. Check position frequently.

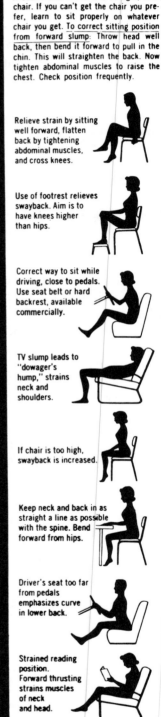

Relieve strain by sitting well forward, flatten back by tightening abdominal muscles, and cross knees.

Use of footrest relieves swayback. Aim is to have knees higher than hips.

Correct way to sit while driving, close to pedals. Use seat belt or hard backrest, available commercially.

TV slump leads to "dowager's hump," strains neck and shoulders.

If chair is too high, swayback is increased.

Keep neck and back in as straight a line as possible with the spine. Bend forward from hips.

Driver's seat too far from pedals emphasizes curve in lower back.

Strained reading position. Forward thrusting strains muscles of neck and head.

Figure G.1. *(continued).*

HOW TO PUT YOUR BACK TO BED

For proper bed posture, a firm mattress is essential. Bedboards, sold commercially, or devised at home, may be used with soft mattresses. Bedboards, preferably, should be made of ¾ inch plywood. Faulty sleeping positions intensify swayback and result not only in backache but in numbness, tingling, and pain in arms and legs.

Incorrect:
Lying flat on back makes swayback worse.

Correct:
Lying on side with knees bent effectively flattens the back. Flat pillow may be used to support neck, especially when shoulders are broad.

Use of high pillow strains neck, arms, shoulders.

Sleeping on back is restful and correct when knees are properly supported.

Sleeping face down exaggerates swayback, strains neck and shoulders.

Raise the foot of the mattress eight inches to discourage sleeping on the abdomen.

Bending one hip and knee does not relieve swayback.

Proper arrangement of pillows for resting or reading in bed.

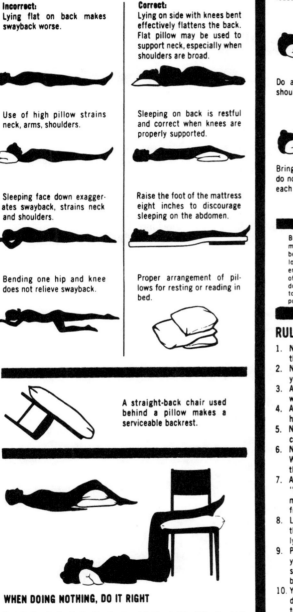

A straight-back chair used behind a pillow makes a serviceable backrest.

WHEN DOING NOTHING, DO IT RIGHT

Rest is the first rule for the tired, painful back. The following positions relieve pain by taking all pressure and weight off the back and legs.

Note pillows under knees to relieve strain on spine.

For complete relief and relaxing effect, these positions should be maintained from 5 to 25 minutes.

EXERCISE—WITHOUT GETTING OUT OF BED
Exercises to be performed while lying in bed are aimed not so much at strengthening muscles as at teaching correct positioning. But muscles used correctly become stronger and in time are able to support the body with the least amount of effort.

Do all exercises in this position. Legs should not be straightened.

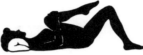

Bring knee up to chest. Lower slowly but do not straighten leg. Relax. Repeat with each leg 10 times.

Bring both knees slowly up to chest. Tighten muscles of abdomen, press back flat against bed. Hold knees to chest 20 seconds, then lower slowly. Relax. Repeat 5 times. This exercise gently stretches the shortened muscles of the lower back, while strengthening abdominal muscles. Clasp knees, bring them up to chest, at the same time coming to a sitting position. Rock back and forth.

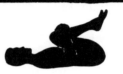

RULES TO LIVE BY—FROM NOW ON

1. Never bend from the waist only; bend the hips and knees.
2. Never lift a heavy object higher than your waist.
3. Always turn and face the object you wish to lift.
4. Avoid carrying unbalanced loads; hold heavy objects close to your body.
5. Never carry anything heavier than you can manage with ease.
6. Never lift or move heavy furniture. Wait for someone to do it who knows the principles of leverage.
7. Avoid sudden movements, sudden "overloading" of muscles. Learn to move deliberately, swinging the legs from the hips.
8. Learn to keep the head in line with the spine, when standing, sitting, lying in bed.
9. Put soft chairs and deep couches on your "don't sit" list. During prolonged sitting, cross your legs to rest your back.
10. Your doctor is the only one who can determine when low back pain is due to faulty posture. He is the best judge of when you may do general exercises for physical fitness. When you do, omit any exercise which arches or overstrains the lower back: backward bends, or forward bends, touching the toes with the knees straight.

EXERCISE—WITHOUT ATTRACTING ATTENTION
Use these inconspicuous exercises whenever you have a spare moment during the day, both to relax tension and improve the tone of important muscle groups.
1. Rotate shoulders, forward and backward.
2. Turn head slowly side to side.
3. Watch an imaginary plane take off, just below the right shoulder. Stretch neck, follow it slowly as it moves up, around and down, disappearing below the other shoulder. Repeat, starting on left side.
4. Slowly, slowly, touch left ear to left shoulder; right ear to right shoulder. Raise both shoulders to touch ears, drop them as far down as possible.
5. At any pause in the day—waiting for an elevator to arrive, for a specific traffic light to change—pull in abdominal muscles, tighten, hold it for the count of eight without breathing. Relax slowly. Increase the count gradually after the first week, practice breathing normally with the abdomen flat and contracted. Do this sitting, standing, and walking.

11. Wear shoes with moderate heels, all about the same height. Avoid changing from high to low heels.
12. Put a footrail under the desk, and a footrest under the crib.
13. Diaper the baby sitting next to him or her on the bed.
14. Don't stoop and stretch to hang the wash; raise the clothesbasket and lower the washline.
15. Beg or buy a rocking chair. Rocking rests the back by changing the muscle groups used.
16. Train yourself vigorously to use your abdominal muscles to flatten your lower abdomen. In time, this muscle contraction will become habitual, making you the envied possessor of a youthful body-profile!
17. Don't strain to open windows or doors.
18. For good posture, concentrate on strengthening "nature's corset"—the abdominal and buttock muscles. The pelvic roll exercise is especially recommended to correct the postural relation between the pelvis and the spine.

SCHERING CORPORATION • KENILWORTH, N.J.
PRINTED IN U S A   CE-504-11656900 8/76

EXERCISES FOR THE PREVENTION AND REHABILITATION OF LOW BACK PAIN

Exercise 1:   SINGLE-KNEE TO CHEST STRETCH

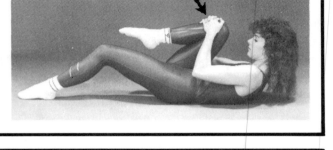

Action: Lie down flat on the floor. Bend one leg at approximately 100 degrees and gradually pull the opposite leg toward your chest. Hold the final stretch for a few seconds. Switch legs and repeat the exercise.

Areas Stretched: Lower back and hamstring muscles, and lumbar spine ligaments.

Exercise 2: DOUBLE-KNEE TO CHEST STRETCH

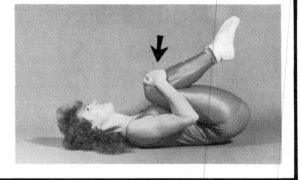

Action: Lie flat on the floor and then slowly curl up into a fetal position. Hold for a few seconds.

Areas Stretched: Upper and lower back and hamstring muscles. Spinal ligaments.

Exercise 3: UPPER AND LOWER BACK STRETCH

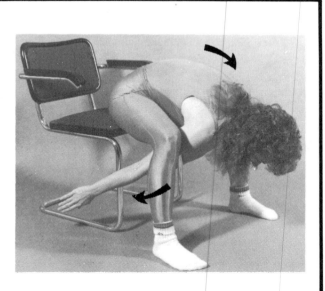

Action: Sit in a chair with feet separated greater than shoulder width. Place your arms to the inside of the thighs and bring your chest down toward the floor. At the same time, attempt to reach back as far as you can with your arms.

Areas Stretched: Upper and lower back muscles and ligaments.

Exercise 4:   SIT-AND-REACH STRETCH
(see Exercise 12 in Appendix F)

Exercise 5: PELVIC TILT

Action: Lie flat on the floor with the knees bent at about a 70-degree angle. Tilt the pelvis by tightening the abdominal muscles, flattening your back against the floor, and raising the lower gluteal area ever so slightly off the floor. Hold the final position for several seconds. The exercise can also be performed against a wall as shown in illustration c.

Areas Stretched:
Low back muscles and ligaments.

Areas Strengthened:
Abdominal and gluteal muscles.

Note: This is perhaps the most important exercise for the care of the lower back. It should be included as a part of your daily exercise routine and should be performed several times throughout the day when pain in the lower back is present as a result of muscle imbalance.

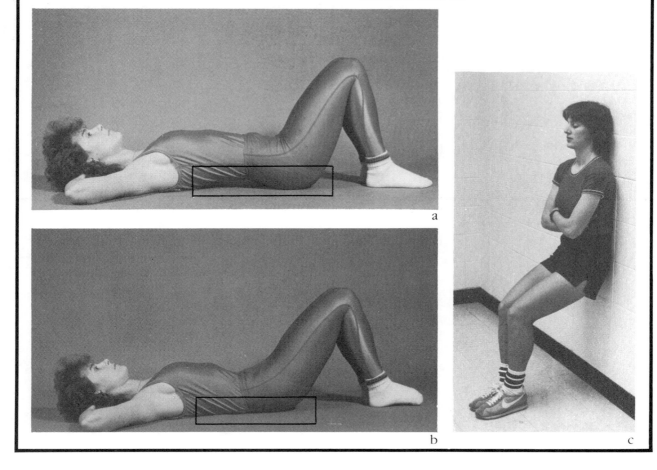

a

b

c

Exercise 6: SIT-UP

Action: Start with your head and shoulders off the floor, arms crossed on your chest, and knees slightly bent (the greater the flexion of the knee, the more difficult the sit-up). Now curl all the way up, then return to the starting position without letting the head or shoulders touch the floor, or allowing the hips to come off the floor. If you allow the hips to raise off the floor and the head and shoulders to touch the floor (*see* illustration c), you will most likely "swing up" on the next sit-up, which minimizes the work of the abdominal muscles. If you cannot curl up with the arms on the chest, place the hands by the side of the hips or even help yourself up by holding on to your thighs (illustrations d and e). Do not perform the sit-up exercise with your legs completely extended, as this will cause strain on the lower back.

Muscles Developed: Abdominal muscles and hip flexors.

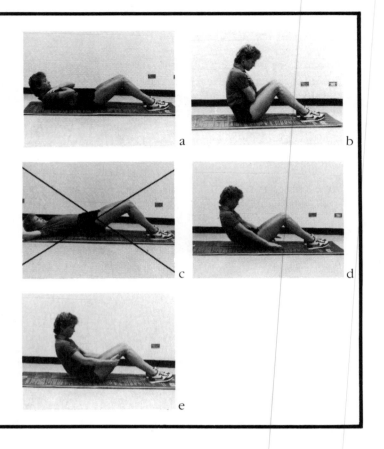

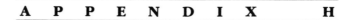

A P P E N D I X   H

Posture Analysis Form*

*Instructions on how to use the form are given in Chapter 3 (*see* Posture)

Figure H.1. *Posture Analysis Form. Adapted with permission from* **The New York Physical Fitness Test: A Manual for Teachers of Physical Education.** *New York State Education Department (Division of HPER), 1958.*

	Good — 5	Fair — 3	Poor — 1	Score
HEAD Left Right	head erect, gravity passes directly through center	head twisted or turned to one side slightly	head twisted or turned to one side markedly	
SHOULDERS Left Right	shoulders level horizontally	one shoulder slightly higher	one shoulder markedly higher	
SPINE Left Right	spine straight	spine slightly	spine markedly curved laterally	
HIPS Left Right	hips level horizontally	one hip slightly higher	one hip markedly higher	
KNEES and ANKLES	feet pointed straight ahead, legs vertical	feet pointed out, legs deviating outward at the knee	feet pointed out markedly, legs deviate markedly	
NECK and UPPER BACK	neck erect, head in line with shoulders, rounded upper back	neck slightly forward, chin out, slightly more rounded upper back	neck markedly forward, chin markedly out, markedly rounded upper back	
TRUNK	trunk erect	trunk inclined to rear slightly	trunk inclined to rear markedly	
ABDOMEN	abdomen flat	abdomen protruding	abdomen protruding and sagging	
LOWER BACK	lower back normally curved	lower back slightly hollow	lower back markedly hollow	
LEGS	legs straight	knees slightly hyper-extended	knees markedly hyper-extended	

TOTAL SCORE

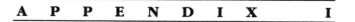

Pulmonary Function Measurement and Prediction of Normal Values

PROCEDURES FOR PULMONARY FUNCTION MEASUREMENT AND PREDICTION OF NORMAL VALUES

The following procedures are used to calculate the different lung function parameters described in Chapters 3 and 4. These parameters include forced vital capacity (FVC), forced expiratory volume at one second (FEV1), ratio of FEV1/FVC, forced mid-expiratory flow (FEF25-75%), and forced expiratory flow 75-85% (FEF75-85%).

A sample illustration of a "typical" timed FVC curve is given in Figures I.2 and I.3. The test is performed by having a subject inspire maximally, followed by a complete forced expiration into a spirometer. Care should be taken that the lungs are completely filled with air prior to forceful expiration. The expiratory phase must be as forceful and long as possible to insure rapid and complete emptying of the lungs. Cessation of change in volume (plateau) on the curve denotes that complete expiration has been reached.

Figure I.1. *Spirometry Test Using a Water Seal Bell Spirometer. (Courtesy of Fitness Monitoring Preventive Medicine Clinic. Lake Geneva, WI)*

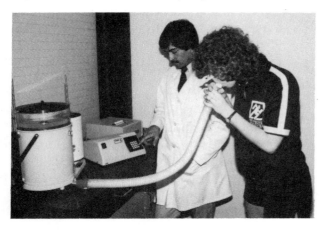

The sample curve illustrated in Figures I.2 and I.3 will be used to demonstrate the measurement techniques for the various parameters listed above. All volume measurements are made on the vertical axis of the graph (in this example, the volumes are measured in liters). Time is indicated on the horizontal axis (in

seconds). Flow rates, such as the FEF25-75%, are generated by determining the slope that represents an average flow across that portion of the curve (change in volume per second).

A point of significance when measuring pulmonary function is that the different values recorded by the spirometer are given in ATPS conditions. This indicates that the volume of gas is saturated with water vapor at ambient temperature and pressure. Since gases are affected by changes in temperature and barometric pressure, in order to make valid comparisons between measurements obtained under different environmental conditions, all pulmonary function values have to be corrected to BTPS conditions (unless a computerized spirometer is used that automatically corrects these values). BTPS implies a volume of gas saturated with water vapor at 37 °C (body temperature) and at ambient environmental pressure. ATPS to BTPS correction factors at different barometric pressures and temperatures are given in Table I.1.

Various equations to predict normal spirometric values have also been developed over the years. Most of these predicting equations are based on gender, age, and height — and were developed using healthy, lifetime non-smokers. Predicting equations are incorporated along with the description of each lung function parameter. These predicting equations are by

Figure I.2. *Forced Vital Capacity Curve (with graphic illustrations for FVC, FEV1, and FEF25-75% computations).*

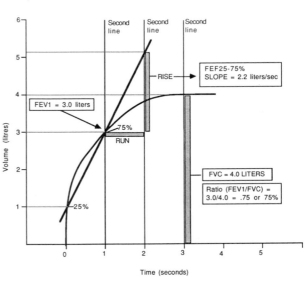

Figure I.3. *Forced Vital Capacity Curve (with graphic illustration for FEF75-85% computation).*

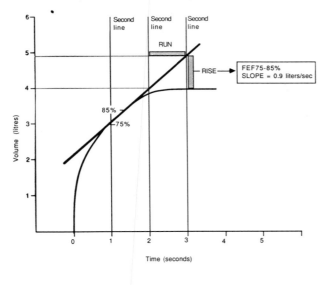

on the curve where one second of expiration has taken place. Since this is also a volume, it must be measured on the vertical axis. In the sample curve in Figure I.2 the measured FEV1 equals 3.0 liters. The corrected FEV1 would be 3.3 liters.

Prediction Equations[1] (predicted volume expressed in liters per one second - BTPS):

Men: FEV1 = [(.092 × height in inches) - (.032 × age)] - 1.26

Women: FEV1 = [(.089 × height in inches) - (.025 × age)] - 1.932

III. Ratio of FEV1/FVC

Measurement Technique: The ratio is obtained by dividing the FEV1 by FVC. In this example, the ratio would be 75 percent (3.3/4.4 = .75). In other words, the subject has exhaled 75 percent of the FVC in the first second. The prediction of the normal ratio is obtained by dividing the predicted FEV1 by the predicted FVC.

IV. Forced Expired Flow 25-75%

Measurement Technique: This parameter represents the average flow rate across the middle half of the expiratory curve (it is not a volume). This rate is determined by marking the graph at the points where 25 percent and 75 percent of FVC have been exhaled. These points are determined by multiplying FVC by .25 and .75 respectively. The 25 and 75 percent points are connected by a straight line which is extrapolated across two time lines 1 second apart, allowing calculation of the change in volume (rise) per 1 second (run). Since a straight line is generated, any portion of that line which crosses two time lines may be used. The measured FEF25-75% in Figure I.2 is approximately 2.2 liters/second. The corrected value would be 2.4 liters/second.

Prediction Equations[1] (predicted volume expressed in liters - BTPS):

Men: FEF25-75% = [(.047 × height in inches) - (.045 × age)] + 2.513

Women: FEF25-75% = [(.06 × height in inches) - (.03 × age)] + .551

no means the only ones developed, but are among the most frequently used. All estimated values generated through these equations are already given in BTPS (no ATPS to BTPS correction is necessary).

I. Forced Vital Capacity

Measurement Technique: The FVC is measured by determining the change in volume from the beginning of expiration (time 0) to the end of maximal expiration (plateau of the curve). The volume change is measured on the vertical axis. In Figure I.2, the measured FVC (ATPS) equals 4.0 liters. Assuming an environmental temperature of 22 °C and a barometric pressure of 700 mmHg, the ATPS to BTPS correction factor would be 1.095 (*see* Table I.1). Hence, the corrected FVC volume (in BTPS) would be 4.4 liters (4.0 × 1.095).

Prediction Equations[1] (predicted volume expressed in liters – BTPS):

Men: FVC = [(.148 × height in inches) - (.025 × age)] - 4.241

Women: FVC = [(.115 × height in inches) - (.024 × age)] - 2.852

II. Forced Expiratory Volume in One Second

Measurement Technique: FEV1 is measured by determining the change in volume from the beginning of expiration to the point

Table I.1.
Factors to Convert Gas Volumes from ATPS to BTPS.

Barometric Pressure	Temperature (°C)						
	20	**21**	**22**	**23**	**24**	**25**	**26**
760	1.102	1.096	1.091	1.085	1.080	1.074	1.068
750	1.102	1.097	1.092	1.086	1.080	1.075	1.069
740	1.103	1.097	1.092	1.086	1.081	1.075	1.069
730	1.104	1.098	1.093	1.087	1.081	1.076	1.070
720	1.104	1.099	1.093	1.088	1.082	1.076	1.070
710	1.105	1.099	1.094	1.088	1.082	1.077	1.071
700	1.106	1.100	1.095	1.089	1.083	1.077	1.071
690	1.107	1.101	1.095	1.089	1.084	1.078	1.072
680	1.107	1.102	1.096	1.090	1.084	1.078	1.072
670	1.108	1.102	1.097	1.091	1.085	1.079	1.073
660	1.109	1.103	1.097	1.092	1.086	1.080	1.074
650	1.110	1.104	1.098	1.092	1.086	1.080	1.074
640	1.111	1.105	1.099	1.093	1.087	1.081	1.075
630	1.112	1.106	1.100	1.094	1.088	1.082	1.076
620	1.112	1.106	1.101	1.095	1.089	1.082	1.076
610	1.113	1.107	1.102	1.095	1.089	1.083	1.077
600	1.114	1.108	1.103	1.096	1.090	1.084	1.078
590	1.116	1.109	1.103	1.097	1.091	1.085	1.078
580	1.117	1.110	1.104	1.098	1.092	1.086	1.079
570	1.118	1.111	1.105	1.099	1.093	1.086	1.080
560	1.119	1.113	1.107	1.100	1.094	1.087	1.081
550	1.120	1.114	1.108	1.101	1.095	1.088	1.082
540	1.121	1.115	1.109	1.102	1.096	1.089	1.083
530	1.123	1.116	1.110	1.103	1.097	1.090	1.084
520	1.124	1.118	1.111	1.105	1.098	1.091	1.085
510	1.125	1.119	1.113	1.106	1.099	1.092	1.086
500	1.127	1.120	1.114	1.107	1.100	1.094	1.087

V.   Forced Expired Flow 75-85%

Measurement Technique: Analogous to FEF25-75%, to determine the FEF75-85%, the 75 and 85 percent points are marked on the curve. The 85 percent point is determined by multiplying FVC by .85. The volume obtained represents the point where 85 percent of the FVC has been exhaled. A line can then be drawn between these two points (75 and 85%) and extrapolated across two time lines. Its slope (therefore flow rate) may then be determined and the volume change in 1 second is measured. The measurement of FEF75-85% is illustrated in Figure I.3 and represents approximately 0.9 liters/second. The corrected value would be 1.0 liters/second.

Prediction Equations[2] (predicted volume expressed in liters - BTPS):

Men: FEF75-85% = [(.013 × height in inches) - (.023 × age)] + 1.21

Women: FEF75-85% = [(.025 × height in inches) - (.021 × age)] + .321

PERCENTAGE OF PREDICTED VALUES

In addition to the actual (corrected) values and the predicted values, physicians frequently use percentage of predicted values to interpret diagnostic spirometry. Percentage of predicted figures are determined by dividing the actual values by the predicted values. These percentages of predicted are quite valuable because values below certain percentages may indicate pulmonary ob-struction (see pulmonary function in Chapter 4). If we assume that the previous pulmonary function values were obtained on a twenty-nine-year-old female who is sixty-eight inches tall, the pulmonary function profile would be as follows:

Parameter	Actual Value	Predicted Value	Percentage of Predicted
FVC	4.4	4.3	102
FEV1	3.3	3.4	97
RATIO	75%	79%	NA*
FEF25-75%	2.4	3.8	64
FEF75-85%	1.0	1.4	70

*Not applicable.

VARIATIONS IN SPIROMETERS

Principles of operation may vary among different types of spirometers, but all of them still generate equivalent values. Some spirometers use direct volume displacement such as a water sealed bell, a wedge bellows, or rolling seal. Others, such as a pneumotach, a heated wire, or a vortex generator may integrate flow and time to yield the respective values.

Volume displacement spirometers and their recording paper are designed in such a way that the vertical volume displacement may be read directly in liters or measured in millimeters (mm) and converted to volume (in liters) by using a bell factor. For instance, a 13-liter Collins bell utilizes a factor of 41.27 milliliters per millimeter of vertical displacement. Similarly, the horizontal axis on the graph is calibrated in seconds such that increments of time can be precisely measured. Speeds may also vary between spirometers. The fastest speed available is generally used for FVC maneuvers.

REFERENCES

1. Morris, J. F., et al. "Spirometric Standards for Health Nonsmoking Adults." *American Review of Respiratory Disease* 103:1, 1971.

2. Morris, J. F., et al. "Normal Values and Evaluation of Forced End-Expiratory Flow." *American Review of Respiratory Disease* 111:757, 1975.

(all prediction equations are reproduced with permission)

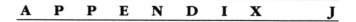

Nutritional Analysis

INSTRUCTIONS

To conduct the following nutritional analysis, the participant should be instructed to keep a three-day record* of everything that he/she eats during that period of time. The information can be recorded on a form such as that given in Figure J.1. At the end of each day, the person should look up the nutrient content for all foods that were consumed (*see* the nutritive value of selected foods list given in this Appendix). This information should be recorded in the respective spaces provided on the form. If a particular food is not found in the list, the information is often provided on the food container itself, or may be available in one of the references given at the end of the list. After recording the nutritive values for each day, the values in each column are totaled and recorded at the bottom of the form. After the third day, Figure J.2 is used to compute the average intake for the three days. The results can then be compared against the Recommended Dietary Allowances (RDA) given at the end of the Figure. The results of the analysis will give a good indication of areas of strength and deficiency in a person's current diet. Figure J.3 (Daily Diet Record Form) is to be used in conjunction with Figure 6.4 (Chapter 6): The New American Eating Guide.

---

* If the computer software available with this textbook is used, up to seven days may be analyzed (*see* Figures J.4 and J.5). In addition, the person would only have to record the code for each food and number of servings (amount) consumed (*see* the nutritive value of selected foods list).

Code	Food	Amount	Weight gm	Calories	Protein gm	Fat gm	Sat. Fat gm	Cholesterol mg	Carbohydrate gm	Calcium mg	Iron mg	Sodium mg	Vit A I.U.	Vit B1 mg	Vit B2 mg	Niacin mg	Vit C mg
001.	Almonds, shelled	1/4 c	36	213	6.6	19	1.4	0	9	83	1.7	2	0	0.09	0.33	1.3	0
002.	Apple, raw, unpared	1 med	150	80	0.3	1	0	0	20	10	0.4	1	120	0.04	0.03	0.1	6
003.	Apple juice, canned or bottled	1/2 c	124	59	0.1	0	0	0	15	8	0.7	1	0	0.01	0.03	0.1	1
004.	Apple pie	1 piece (3½")	118	302	2.6	13	3.5	120	45	9	0.4	355	40	0.02	0.02	0.5	1
005.	Applesauce, canned, sweetened	1/2 c	128	116	0.3	0	0	0	31	5	0.7	3	50	0.02	0.01	0	2
006.	Apricots, raw	3 (12 per lb)	114	55	1.1	0	0	0	14	18	0.5	1	2,890	0.06	0.04	0.6	11
007.	Apricots, canned, heavy syrup	3 halves; 1¾ tbsp liq.	85	73	0.5	0	0	0	19	9	0.3	1	1,480	0.02	0.02	0.3	3
008.	Apricots, dried, sulfured, uncooked	10 med halves	35	91	1.8	0	0	0	23	23	1.9	9	3,820	0	0.06	1.2	4
009.	Asparagus, cooked green spears	4 med	60	12	1.3	0	0	0	2	13	0.4	1	540	0.10	0.11	0.8	16
010.	Avocado, raw	1/8 med	120	185	2.4	19	3.2	0	7	11	0.6	4	310	0.12	0.22	1.7	15
011.	Bacon, cooked, drained	2 slices	15	86	3.8	8	2.7	30	1	2	0.5	153	0	0.08	0.05	0.8	0
012.	Banana, raw	1 sm (7¼")	140	81	1.0	0	0	0	21	8	0.7	1	180	0.05	0.06	0.7	10
013.	Beans, green snap, cooked	1/2 c	65	16	1.0	0	0	0	3	32	0.4	4	340	0.05	0.06	0.3	8
014.	Beans, lentils	1/4 c	50	53	3.9	0	0	0	10	12	1.0	0	10	0.03	0.04	0.4	0
015.	Beans, lima (Fordhook), froz., cooked	1/2 c	85	84	6	0	0	0	17	40	2.1	1	240	0.15	0.08	1.1	15
016.	Beans, red kidney, cooked	1 c	185	218	14.4	1	0	0	40	70	4.4	6	10	0.20	0.11	1.3	0
017.	Bean sprouts, mung, raw	1/2 c	52	18	2.0	0	0	0	4	10	0.7	3	10	0.07	0.07	0.4	10
018.	Beef-chuck, cooked, trimmed	3 oz.	85	212	25	12	7.8	80	0	11	3.1	43	20	0.05	0.19	3.8	0
019.	Beef, corned canned	3 oz.	85	163	21	10	8	70	0	22	5.0	802	0	0.02	0.27	3.9	0
020.	Beef, ground, lean	3 oz.	85	186	23.3	10	5	81	0	10	3.0	57	20	0.08	0.20	5.1	0
021.	Beef, round steak, cooked, trimmed	3 oz.	85	222	24.3	13	6	77	0	10	3.0	60	20	0.07	0.20	4.8	0
022.	Beef, rump roast	3 oz.	85	177	24.7	9	4	80	0	10	3.1	61	10	0.06	0.19	4.4	0
023.	Beef, sirloin, cooked	3 oz.	85	329	19.6	27	13	77	0	9	2.5	48	50	0.05	0.15	4.0	0
024.	Beer	12 fl. oz.	360	151	1.1	0	0	0	14	18	0	25	0	0.01	0.11	2.2	0
025.	Beets, red, canned, drained	1/2 c	80	32	0.8	0	0	0	8	15	0.6	164	15	0.01	0.02	0.1	2
026.	Beet greens, cooked	1/2 c	73	13	1.3	0	0	0	2	72	1.4	55	3,700	0.05	0.11	0.2	11
027.	Biscuits, baking powder, made from mix	1 med	35	114	2.5	6	1.1	0	18	60	0.8	272	0	0.06	0.06	0.7	0
028.	Blueberries, fresh cultivated	1/2 c	73	45	0.5	0	0	0	11	10	0.8	1	75	0.02	0.05	0.4	10
029.	Bologna	1 slice (1 oz.)	28	86	3.4	8	3	15	0	2	0.5	369	0	0.05	0.06	0.7	0
030.	Bouillon, broth	1 cube	4	5	.8	0	0	0	0	0	0	960	0	0	0	0	0
031.	Bran Cereal	1/2 c	30	72	3.8	1	0	0	22	25	3	247	2,000	1.0	0.80	3.0	20
032.	Bread, Corn	1 slice	78	161	5.8	6	0.1	0	23	94	0.9	490	120	0.10	0.15	0.5	1
033.	Bread, French enriched	1 slice	35	102	3.2	1	0.2	0	19	15	0.8	203	0	0.10	0.08	0.9	0
034.	Bread, rye (American)	1 slice	25	61	2.3	0	0	0	13	19	0.4	139	0	0.05	0.02	0.4	0
035.	Bread, white enriched	1 slice	25	68	2.2	1	0.2	0	13	21	0.6	127	0	0.06	0.05	0.6	0

(Continued)

Code	Food	Amount	Weight gm	Calories	Protein gm	Fat gm	Sat. Fat gm	Cholesterol mg	Carbohydrate gm	Calcium mg	Iron mg	Sodium mg	Vit A I.U.	Vit B₁ mg	Vit B₂ mg	Niacin mg	Vit C mg
036.	Bread, whole wheat	1 slice	25	61	2.6	1	0.6	0	12	25	0.8	132	0	0.06	0.03	0.7	0
037.	Broccoli, raw	1 sm stalk	114	38	4.1	0	0	0	7	117	1.3	17	2,835	0.10	0.23	0.9	125
038.	Broccoli, cooked drained	1 sm stalk	140	36	4.3	0	0	0	6	123	1.1	14	3,500	0.13	0.28	1.1	126
039.	Brussels sprouts, froz., cooked drained	1/2 c	78	28	3.2	0	0	0	5	25	0.8	8	405	0.06	0.11	0.5	63
040.	Bulgur, wheat	1 c	135	227	8.4	1	0	0	47	27	1.8	809	0	0.07	0.04	3.2	0
041.	Burrito, combination, Taco Bell	1	175	404	21	16	0	0	43	91	3.7	300	1,666	0.34	0.31	4.6	15
042.	Butter	1 tsp	5	36	0	4	0.4	12	0	1	0	46	160	0	0	0	0
043.	Buttermilk, cultured	1 c	245	88	8.8	0	1.3	5	12	296	0.1	319	10	0.10	0.44	0.2	2
044.	Cabbage, raw chopped	1/2 c	45	11	0.6	0	0	0	3	22	0.2	9	60	0.03	0.03	0.2	21
045.	Cabbage, boiled, drained wedge	1/2 c	85	16	0.9	0	0	0	3	36	0.3	10	100	0.02	0.02	0.1	21
046.	Cake, angel food, plain	1 piece	60	161	4.3	0	0	0	36	5	0.1	170	0	0.01	0.08	0.1	0
047.	Cake, devil's food, iced	1 piece	99	365	4.5	16	5	68	55	69	1.0	233	160	0.02	0.10	0.2	0
048.	Candy, hard	1 oz.	28	109	0	0	0	0	28	9	0.5	9	0	0	0	0	0
049.	Cantaloupe	1/4 melon 5" diam.	239	35	2.0	0	0	0	10	20	0.8	17	4,620	0.06	0.04	0.6	45
050.	Caramel (candy, plain or choc.)	1 oz.	28	113	1.1	3	1.6	0	22	42	0.4	64	0	0.01	0.05	0.1	0
051.	Carrots, raw	1 carrot 7½" long	81	30	0.8	0	0	0	7	27	0.5	34	7,930	0.04	0.04	0.4	6
052.	Carrots, cooked, drained	1/2 c	73	23	0.7	0	0	0	5	24	0.5	10	7,615	0.04	0.04	0.4	5
053.	Cauliflower, cooked, drained	1/2 c	63	14	1.5	0	0	0	3	13	0.5	6	40	0.06	0.05	0.4	35
054.	Celery, green, raw, long	1 outer stalk 8"	40	7	0.4	0	0	0	2	16	0.1	50	110	0.01	0.01	0.1	4
055.	Cheese, American	1 oz. slice	28	100	6	8	5.6	27	0	188	0.1	307	343	0.01	0.10	0	0
056.	Cheese, blue	1 oz.	28	100	6	8	5.3	25	1	89	0.1	510	204	0.01	0.11	0.3	0
057.	Cheese, cheddar	1 oz.	28	114	7	9	6	30	0	204	0.2	171	300	0.01	0.11	0	0
058.	Cheese, cottage, creamed	1/2 cup	105	112	14	5	6.4	15	3	99	0.3	241	180	0.03	0.26	0.1	0
059.	Cheese, creamed	1 oz.	28	99	6	8	3	31	1	71	0.3	71	320	0.02	0.14	0	0
060.	Cheese, souffle	1 portion	110	240	10.9	19	9.5	189	7	221	1.1	400	880	0.06	0.26	0.2	0
061.	Cheesecake	1 piece (3½")	85	257	4.6	16	9.0	150	24	48	0.4	189	216	0.03	0.11	0.4	4
062.	Cherries	10	75	47	0.9	0	0	0	12	15	0.3	8	450	0.20	0.24	1.6	41
063.	Cherry Pie	1 piece (3½")	118	308	3.1	13	5.0	137	45	17	0.4	355	40	0.02	0.02	0.5	1
064.	Chicken, drumstick Kentucky Fried	1	54	136	14	8	2.2	73	2	20	0.9	320	30	0.04	0.12	2.7	0
065.	Chicken, wing, Kentucky Fried	1	45	151	11	10	2.9	70	4	0	0.6	300	0	0.03	0.07	0	0
066.	Chicken, roast, light meat without skin	3 oz.	85	141	27	3	0.4	45	0	10	1.2	54	51	0.03	0.09	9.9	0
067.	Chicken, roast, dark meat without skin	3 oz.	85	149	24	5	0.8	50	0	11	1.5	54	127	0.06	0.19	4.7	0
068.	Chocolate, milk	1 oz.	28	147	2	9	3.6	5	16	65	0.3	27	80	0.02	0.10	0.1	0
069.	Clam, canned drained	3 oz.	85	83	13	2	0.2	50	2	46	3.5	750	93	0.01	0.09	0.9	9
070.	Cocoa, plain, dry	1 tbsp	5	14	0.9	1	0	0	3	7	0.6	0	0	0.01	0.02	0.1	0
071.	Coconut, shredded, packed	1/2 c	65	225	2.3	23	20	0	6	8	1.1	165	0	0.03	0.01	0.3	2

No.	Food	Serving															
072.	Cod, cooked	3 oz.	85	144	24.3	4	1.5	60	0	27	0.9	63	150	0.06	0.09	2.7	0
073.	Cola	12 oz.	369	144	0	0	0	0	37	27	0	30	0	0	0	0	0
074.	Coffee	3/4 cup	180	1	0	0	0	0	0	1	0.2	2	0	0	0	0.1	0
075.	Coleslaw	1 c	120	173	1.6	17	1	5	6	53	0.5	144	190	0.06	0.06	0.4	35
076.	Collards, leaves without stems, cooked, drained	1/2 c	95	32	3.4	1	2	0	5	178	0.8	28	7,410	0.01	0.19	1.2	72
077.	Cookies, chocolate chip homemade	2 2¼" diam.	20	103	1	6	1.7	14	12	7	0.4	70	20	0.02	0.02	0.2	0
078.	Cookies, vanilla	5 1¾" diam.	20	93	1	3	0.8	10	15	8	0.1	50	25	0	0.01	0	0
079.	Corn, boiled on cob	1 ear 5" long	140	70	2.5	1	0	0	16	2	0.5	1	310	0.09	0.08	1.1	7
080.	Corn, canned, drained	1/2 c	83	70	2.2	1	0	0	16	4	0.4	195	290	0.03	0.04	0.8	4
081.	Cornflakes	1 c	25	97	2.0	0	0	0	21	3	0.6	251	180	0.29	0.55	2.9	9
082.	Cornmeal, degermed, yellow, enriched cooked	1/2 c	120	60	1.3	0	0	0	13	1	0.5	264	70	0.07	0.05	0.6	0
083.	Crackers, graham	2 squares	14	55	1.1	1	0.3	0	10	6	0.2	95	0	0.01	0.03	0.2	0
084.	Crackers, saltines	4 squares	11	48	1.0	1	0.3	0	8	2	0.1	123	0	0	0	0.1	0
085.	Cream, light coffee or table	1 tbsp	15	20	0.5	2	0.5	5	1	16	0	7	70	0	0.02	0	0
086.	Cream, heavy whipping	1 tbsp	15	53	0.3	6	1.3	12	1	11	0	5	230	0	0.02	0	0
087.	Croissants (Sara Lee)	1 roll	18	59	1.6	2	0.3	0	8	22	0.6	105	0	0.14	0.09	0.8	3
088.	Cucumbers, raw pared	9 sm slices	28	4	0.3	0	0	0	1	7	0.3	2	70	0.01	0.01	0.1	0
089.	Dates hydrated	5	46	110	0.9	0	0	0	29	24	1.2	1	20	0.04	0.04	0.9	0
090.	Doughnuts, plain	1	42	164	1.9	8	2	19	22	17	0.6	210	30	0.07	0.07	0.5	0
091.	Eggs, hard cooked	1 large	50	72	6	5	1.8	250	1	24	1.0	54	520	0.05	0.13	0	0
092.	Eggs, White	1 large	33	17	3.6	0	0	0	0	3	0	48	0	0	0.09	0	0
093.	Farina, enriched, quick cooking, cooked	1/2 c	123	51	1.6	0	0	0	11	5	6	176	0	0.06	0.03	0.5	0
094.	Figs, dried	1 large	21	60	1.0	0	0	0	15	26	0.6	1	20	0.16	0.17	3.9	0
095.	Filet of Fish, McDonald's	1	131	402	15	23	7.9	43	34	105	1.8	709	152	0.28	0.28	3.9	4
096.	Flounder	3 oz.	85	171	25.5	7	1	60	0	21	1.2	201	0	0.06	0.06	2.1	3
097.	Flour, all purpose enriched	1 c	125	455	13	1	0	0	95	20	3.6	3	0	0.55	0.33	4.4	0
098.	Flour, whole wheat	1 c	120	400	16	2	0	0	85	49	4.0	4	0	0.66	0.14	5.2	0
099.	Frankfurters, cooked	1	57	176	7	16	5.6	45	1	4	1.1	627	0	0.09	0.11	1.5	0
100.	Fruit cocktail	1 c	245	91	1	0	0	0	24	22	1.0	12	370	0.05	0.02	1.2	5
101.	Ginger ale	12 oz.	366	113	0	0	0	0	29	0	0	45	0	0	0	0	5
102.	Grapefruit, raw white	1/2 med	301	56	1	0	0	0	15	22	0.5	1	10	0.05	0.03	0.3	52
103.	Grapefruit, juice unsweetened canned	1/2 c	124	50	0.6	0	0	0	12	11	0.2	2	10	0.05	0.03	0.3	46
104.	Grapes, raw seedless European	10 grapes	50	34	0.3	0	0	0	9	6	0.2	2	50	0.03	0.03	0.2	2
105.	Grape juice, unsweetened bottled	1/2 c	127	84	0.3	0	0	0	21	14	0.4	3	0	0.05	0.03	0.3	0
106.	Haddock, fried (dipped in egg, milk, bread crumbs)	3 oz.	85	141	17	5	1	54	5	33	0.9	150	0	0.03	0.06	2.7	3
107.	Halibut, broiled with butter or margarine	3 oz.	85	144	21	6	2.1	55	0	15	0.6	114	570	0.03	0.06	7.2	1
108.	Hamburger, McDonald's	1	99	257	13	9	3.7	26	30	63	3.0	526	231	0.23	0.23	5.1	2

(Continued)

Code	Food	Amount	Weight gm	Calories	Protein gm	Fat gm	Sat. Fat gm	Cholesterol mg	Carbohydrate gm	Calcium mg	Iron mg	Sodium mg	Vit A I.U.	Vit B₁ mg	Vit B₂ mg	Niacin mg	Vit C mg
109.	Ham (cured pork) baked, trimmed	3 oz.	85	318	20	26	9.4	77	0	9	2.6	48	0	0.43	0.20	3.8	0
110.	Honey	1 tbsp	21	64	0	0	0	0	17	1	0.1	1	0	0	0.01	0.1	0
111.	Ice cream, vanilla	1/2 c	67	135	3	7	4.4	27	14	97	0.1	42	295	0.03	0.14	0.1	1
112.	Ice cream cone, Dairy Queen	medium	142	230	6	7	4.6	15	35	200	0	150	300	0.09	0.26	0	0
113.	Ice milk, vanilla	1/2 c	61	100	3	3	1.8	13	15	102	0.1	45	140	0.04	0.15	0.1	1
114.	Jelly	1 tbsp	18	49	0	0	0	0	13	4	0.3	3	0	0	0.01	0	1
115.	Kale, fresh cooked, drained	1/2 c	55	22	2.5	0	0	0	3	103	0.9	24	4,565	0.06	0.10	0.9	51
116.	Lamb leg, roast, trimmed	3 oz.	85	237	22	16	7.3	60	0	9	1.4	53	0	0.13	0.23	4.7	0
117.	Lemon juice, fresh	1 tbsp	15	4	0.1	0	0	0	1	1	0	0	0	0	0	0	7
118.	Lentils, cooked	1/2 c	100	106	8	0	0	0	19	25	2.1	0	20	0.07	0.06	0.6	0
119.	Lettuce, crisp head	1 c sm chunks	75	10	0.7	0	0	0	2	15	0.4	7	250	0.05	0.05	0.2	5
120.	Lettuce, cos or romaine	1 c chopped	55	10	0.7	0	0	0	2	37	0.8	5	1,050	0.08	0.04	0.2	10
121.	Liver, beef, fried	1 slice 3 oz.	85	195	22	9	2.5	345	5	9	7.5	156	45,390	0.22	3.56	14.0	23
122.	Liverwurst, fresh	1 slice 1 oz.	28	87	5	7	3.5	50	1	3	1.5		1,800	0.06	0.37	1.6	0
123.	Lobster	1 c	145	138	27	2	1	293	0	94	1.2	305	0	0.15	0.10	0	0
124.	Macaroni, enriched cooked	1/2 c	70	78	2.4	0	0	0	16	6	0.7	1	0	0.10	0.06	0.8	0
125.	Macaroni and cheese	1/2 c	100	215	8.2	11	4	21	20	181	0.9	543	430	0.10	0.20	0.9	0
126.	Margarine	1 tsp	5	34	0	4	0.7	2	0	1	0	46	160	0	0	0	0
127.	Matzo	1 piece	30	117	3.0	0	0	0	25	*	*	0	*	*	*	*	*
128.	Mayonnaise	1 tsp	5	36	0	4	0.7	3	0	1	0	28	13	0	0	0	0
129.	Milk, evaporated whole	1/2 c	126	172	9	10	5.8	40	13	329	0.2	149	405	0.05	0.43	0.2	2
130.	Milk, lowfat (2% fat)	1 c	246	145	10	5	3.1	5	15	352	0.1	150	200	0.10	0.52	0.2	2
131.	Milk shake, vanilla (McDonald's)	1	289	323	10	8	5.1	29	52	346	0.2	250	346	0.12	0.66	0.6	3
132.	Milk skim	1 c	245	88	9	0	0.3	5	12	296	0.1	126	10	0.09	0.44	0.2	2
133.	Milk, whole (3.5% fat)	1 c	244	159	9	9	5.1	34	12	288	0.1	120	350	0.07	0.40	0.2	2
134.	Molasses, medium	1 tbsp	20	50	0	0	0	0	13	33	0.9	3	0	0.01	0.01	0	0
135.	Mushrooms, fresh cultivated	1/2 c sliced	35	12	1.0	0	0	0	2	4	0.5	4	0	0.04	0.12	2.4	1
136.	Mustard greens, cooked drained	1/2 c	70	16	1.7	0	0	0	3	96	1.2	13	4,060	0.05	0.10	0.4	33
137.	Noodles, egg, enriched cooked	1/2 c	80	100	3.3	1	0	0	19	8	0.7	2	55	0.11	0.07	1.0	0
138.	Nuts, Brazil	1 oz. (6-8 nuts)	28	185	4.1	19	4.8	0	3	53	1.0	0	0	0.27	0.03	0.5	0
139.	Nuts, pecans	1 oz.	28	195	2.6	20	1.4	0	4	21	0.7	0	40	0.24	0.04	0.3	1
140.	Nuts, walnuts	1 oz. (14 halves)	28	185	4.2	18	1	0	5	28	0.9	1	10	0.09	0.4	0.3	1
141.	Oatmeal, quick, cooked	1/2 c	120	66	2.4	1	0.2	0	12	11	0.7	262	0	0.10	0.03	0.1	0
142.	Oil, soybean	1 tsp.	5	44	0	5	2	0	0	0	0	0	0	0	0	0	0
143.	Okra, cooked drained	1/2 c	80	23	1.6	0	0	0	5	74	0.4	2	390	0.11	0.15	0.7	16
144.	Olives, black ripe	10 extra large	55	61	0.5	7	1	0	1	40	0.8	385	30	0	0	0	0
145.	Onions, mature cooked, drained	1/2 c sliced	105	31	1.3	0	0	0	7	25	0.4	8	40	0.03	0.03	0.2	8
146.	Onion rings (Brazier) Dairy Queen	1 serving	85	360	6	17	6	15	33	20	0.4	125	0	0.09	0	0.4	2

#	Food	Portion															
147.	Orange, raw (medium skin)	1 med	180	64	1.3	0	0	0	16	54	0.5	1	260	0.13	0.05	0.5	66
148.	Orange juice, froz. reconstituted	1/2 c	125	61	0.9	0	0	0	15	13	0.1	1	270	0.12	0.02	0.5	60
149.	Oysters, raw Eastern	1/2 c (6-9 med)	120	79	10	2	1.3	60	4	113	6.6	145	370	0.17	0.22	3.0	0
150.	Pancakes	6" diam x 1/2" thick	73	169	5.2	5	1	36	25	74	0.9	310	90	0.12	0.16	0.9	0
151.	Papaya, raw	1/2 med	227	60	0.9	0	0	0	15	31	0.5	5	2,660	0.06	0.06	0.5	85
152.	Parsnips, cooked	1 large 9" long	160	106	2.4	1	0	0	24	72	1.0	13	50	0.11	0.13	0.2	16
153.	Peaches, raw, peeled	1 2¾" diam.	175	58	0.9	0	0	0	15	14	0.8	2	2,030	0.03	0.08	1.5	11
154.	Peaches, canned, heavy syrup	1 half 2⅛ tbsp liq.	96	75	0.4	0	0	0	19	4	0.3	2	410	0.01	0.02	0.6	3
155.	Peanut butter	2 tbsp	32	188	8	16	1	0	6	18	0.6	194	0	0.04	0.04	4.8	0
156.	Peanuts, roasted	1 oz.	28	166	7	14	1	0	5	21	0.6	119	0	0.09	0.04	4.9	0
157.	Pears, Bartlett, raw	1 pear	180	100	1.1	1	0	0	25	13	0.5	2	30	0.03	0.07	0.2	7
158.	Pears, canned, heavy syrup	1 half 2¼ tbsp liq.	103	78	0.2	0	0	0	20	5	0.2	1	0	0.01	0.02	0.1	1
159.	Pears, frozen, cooked drained	1/2 c	80	55	4.1	0	0	0	10	15	1.5	92	480	0.22	0.07	1.4	11
160.	Peas, early, canned, drained	1/2 c	85	75	4.0	0	0	0	14	22	1.6	200	585	0.08	0.05	0.7	7
161.	Peppers, sweet, raw	1 pepper 3¼"x3" diam.	200	36	2.0	0	0	0	8	15	1.1	21	690	0.13	0.13	0.8	210
162.	Pickles, dill	1 large 4" long	135	15	0.9	0	0	0	3	35	1.4	1,928	140	0	0.03	0	8
163.	Pickles, sweet	1 large 3" long	35	51	0.2	0	0	0	13	4	0.4	0	30	0	0.01	0	2
164.	Pineapple, raw	1/2 c diced	78	41	0.3	0	0	0	11	13	0.4	1	55	0.07	0.03	0.2	13
165.	Pineapple, canned, heavy syrup	1/2 c	128	95	0.4	0	0	0	25	14	0.4	2	65	0.10	0.03	0.3	9
166.	Pizza, Cheese, Thin 'n Crispy, Pizza Hut	1/2 10" pie	*	450	25	15	7	125	54	450	4.5	1,200	750	0.30	0.51	5.0	1
167.	Pizza, Cheese, Thick 'n Chewy, Pizza Hut	1/2 10" pie	*	560	34	14	6	110	71	500	5.4	1,100	1,000	0.68	0.68	7.0	1
168.	Plums, Japanese and hybrid, raw	1 plum 2⅛" diam.	70	32	0.3	0	0	0	8	8	0.3	1	160	0.02	0.02	0.3	4
169.	Popcorn, popped, plain, large kernel	1 c	6	12	0.8	0	0	0	5	1	0.2	0	0	0	0.01	0.1	0
170.	Pork, roast, trimmed	2 slices 3 oz.	85	179	24	8	2.2	65	0	11	3.1	863	0	0.55	0.22	4.3	0
171.	Pork, sausage, cooked	1 sm link	17	72	2.8	6	2.1	13	1	0	0.3	221	0	0	0	0	0
172.	Potato, baked in skin	1 potato 2 1/3x4¼"	202	145	4.0	8	0	0	33	14	1.1	6	0	0.15	0.07	2.7	31
173.	Potato chips	10 chips	20	114	1.1	8	2.1	0	10	8	0.4	150	0	0.04	0.01	1.0	3
174.	Potato, French fried long	10 strips 3½-4"	78	214	3.4	10	1.7	0	28	12	1.0	5	0	0.10	0.06	2.4	16
175.	Potato, mashed, milk added	1/2 c	105	69	2.2	1	0.4	8	14	25	0.4	316	20	0.09	0.06	1.1	11
176.	Prunes, dried "softenized" without pits	5 prunes	61	137	1.1	0	0	0	36	26	0.1	4	860	0.05	0.09	0.9	2
177.	Prune juice, canned or bottled	1/2 c	128	99	0.5	0	0	0	24	18	5.3	3	0	0.02	0.02	0.5	3
178.	Pumpkin Pie	1 (3½")	114	241	4.6	13	3	70	28	58	0.6	244	2,810	0.03	0.11	0.6	0
179.	Raisins, unbleached, seedless	1 oz.	28	82	0.7	0	0	0	22	18	1.0	8	10	0.03	0.02	0.1	0
180.	Rice, brown, cooked	1/2 c	96	116	2.5	1	0	0	25	12	0.5	275	0	0.09	0.02	1.3	0
181.	Rice, white enriched, cooked	1/2 c	103	113	2.1	0	0	0	25	11	0.9	384	0	0.12	0.01	1.1	0
182.	Salami, dry	1 oz.	28	128	7	11	1.6	24	0	4	1.0	349	20	0.10	0.07	1.5	0
183.	Salmon, broiled with butter or margarine	3 oz.	85	156	23	6	2.2	53	0	0	0.9	99	150	0.15	0.06	8.4	0

(Continued)

Code	Food	Amount	Weight gm	Calories	Protein gm	Fat gm	Sat. Fat gm	Cholesterol mg	Carbohydrate gm	Calcium mg	Iron mg	Sodium mg	Vit A I.U.	Vit B1 mg	Vit B2 mg	Niacin mg	Vit C mg
184.	Salmon, canned Chinook	3 oz.	85	179	16.6	12	0.8	30	0	131	0.7	105	197	0.03	0.01	6.2	0
185.	Sardines, canned drained	1 oz.	28	58	7	3	1	20	0	124	0.8	233	60	0.01	0.06	1.5	0
186.	Sauerkraut, canned	1/2 c	118	21	1.2	0	0	0	5	43	0.6	878	60	0.04	0.05	0.3	17
187.	Shrimp, boiled	3 oz.	85	99	18	1	0.1	128	1	99	2.7	0	60	0	0.03	1.5	0
188.	Soup, cream of mushroom condensed, prepared with equal volume of milk	1 c	245	216	7	14	5.4	15	16	191	0.5	955	250	0.05	0.34	0.7	1
189.	Soup, split pea, condensed, prepared with equal volume of water	1 c	245	145	9	3	1.1	0	21	29	1.5	941	440	0.25	0.15	1.5	1
190.	Soup, tomato, condensed, prepared with equal volume of water	1 c	245	88	2.0	3	0.5	0	16	15	0.7	970	1,000	0.05	0.05	1.2	12
191.	Soup, vegetable beef, condensed, prepared with equal volume of water	1 c	245	78	5	2	0	0	10	12	0.7	1,046	2,700	0.05	0.05	1.0	0
192.	Spaghetti, in tomato sauce with cheese	1 c	250	260	8.8	9	2	10	37	80	2.3	955	1,080	0.25	0.18	2.3	13
193.	Spaghetti, with meatballs and tomato sauce	1 c	248	332	18.6	11.7	3	75	39	124	3.7	1,009	1,590	0.25	0.30	4.0	22
194.	Spareribs, cooked	3 oz.	85	377	17.8	33	12	73	0	8	2.2	31	0	0.37	0.18	2.9	0
195.	Spinach, raw, chopped	1 c	55	14	1.8	0	0	0	2	51	1.7	39	4,460	0.06	0.11	0.3	28
196.	Spinach, canned, drained	1/2 c	103	25	2.3	1	0	0	4	121	2.6	242	8,200	0.02	0.12	0.3	15
197.	Spinach, froz., cooked, drained	1/2 c	103	24	3.1	0	0	0	4	116	2.2	54	8,100	0.07	0.16	0.4	20
198.	Squash, summer, cooked	1/2 c	90	13	0.8	0	0	0	3	23	0.4	1	350	0.05	0.07	0.7	9
199.	Squash, winter, baked mashed	1/2 c	103	70	1.9	1	0	0	18	41	1.0	1	6,560	0.05	0.14	0.7	8
200.	Strawberries, raw	1 c	149	55	1.0	1	0	0	13	31	1.5	1	90	0.04	0.10	0.9	88
201.	Sundae, choc. Dairy Queen	medium	184	300	6	7	4.9	79	53	200	1.1	175	300	0.06	0.26	0	0
202.	Sugar, white granulated	1 tsp	4	15	0	0	0	0	4	0	0	0	0	0	0	0	0
203.	Sweet potato, baked	1 potato 5" long	146	161	2.4	1	0	0	37	46	1.0	14	9,230	0.10	0.08	0.8	25
204.	Syrup (maple)	1 tbsp	20	50	0	0	0	0	13	33	0.2	3	0	0	0	0	0
205.	Taco, Taco Bell	1	83	186	15	8	0	0	14	120	2.4	79	120	0.09	0.16	2.9	0
206.	Tangerine	1 med 2⅜" diam.	116	39	0.7	0	0	0	10	34	0.3	2	360	0.05	0.02	0.1	27
207.	Tea, brewed	1/4 c	180	0	0	0	0	0	0	0	0	0	0	0	0	0	0
208.	Tomato sauce (catsup)	1 tbsp	15	16	0.3	0	0	0	4	3	0.1	156	105	0.01	0.01	0.2	2
209.	Tomatoes, raw	1 tomato 3½ oz.	100	20	1.0	0	0	0	4	12	0.5	3	820	0.05	0.04	0.6	21
210.	Tomatoes, canned	1/2 c	121	26	1.2	0	0	0	5	7	0.6	157	1,085	0.06	0.04	0.9	21
211.	Tortillas, corn, lime	6" diam.	30	63	1.5	1	0	0	14	60	0.9	0	6	0.04	0.02	0.3	0
212.	Tuna, canned, oil pack, drained	3 oz.	85	167	25	7	1.7	60	0	7	1.6	0	70	0.04	0.10	10.1	0
213.	Tuna, canned, water pack, solids and liquid	3½ oz.	99	126	27.7	1	0	55	0	16	1.6	161	0	0	0.10	13.2	0
214.	Turkey, roast (light and dark mixed)	3 oz.	85	162	27	5	1.5	73	0	7	1.5	111	0	0.04	0.15	6.5	0

#	Food	Portion															
215.	Turnip, cooked, drained	1/2 c cubed	78	18	0.6	0	0	0	4	27	0.3	27	0	0.03	0.04	0.3	17
216.	Turnip greens, cooked drained	1/2 c	73	19	2.1	0	0	0	3	98	1.3	14	5,695	0.04	0.08	0.4	16
217.	Veal, cooked loin	3 oz.	85	199	22	11	4	90	0	9	2.7	55	0	0.06	0.21	4.6	0
218.	Vegetables, mixed, cooked	1 c	182	116	5.8	0	0	0	24	46	2.4	348	4,505	0.22	0.13	2.0	15
219.	Watermelon	1 c diced	160	42	0.8	0	0	0	10	11	0.8	2	940	0.05	0.05	0.3	11
220.	Wheat germ, plain toasted	1 tbsp	6	23	1.8	1	0	0	3	3	0.5	0	10	0.11	0.05	0.3	1
221.	Whiskey, gin, rum, vodka 90 proof	1/2 11 oz (jigger)	42	110	0	0	0	0	0	0	0	0	0	0	0	0	0
222.	Whole wheat cereal, cooked	1/2 c	123	55	2.2	0	0	0	12	9	0.06	9	0	0.08	0.03	0.8	0
223.	Whole wheat flakes, ready-to-eat	1 c	30	106	3.1	1	0	0	24	12	2	310	1,410	0.35	0.42	3.5	11
224.	Whopper, Burger King	1	*	606	29	32	10.5	100	51	37	6.0	909	641	0.02	0.03	5.2	13
225.	Wine, dry table 12% alc.	3½ fl. oz.	102	87	0.1	0	0	0	4	9	0.4	5	0	0	0.01	0.1	0
226.	Wine, red dry 18.8% alc.	2 fl. oz.	59	81	0.1	0	0	0	5	5	0	4	0	0.01	0.02	0.2	0
227.	Yeast, brewers	1 tbsp	8	23	3.1	0	0	0	3	17	1.4	10	0	1.25	0.34	3.0	0
228.	Yogurt, plain low fat	1 8-oz. container	226	113	7.7	4	2.3	15	12	271	0.1	115	150	0.09	0.41	0.2	2

Adapted from:

Nutritive Value of American Foods in Common Units. Agriculture Handbook No. 456. U.S. Dept. of Agriculture. Washington, D.C. November 1975.

Young, E. A., E. H. Brennan, and G. L. Irving, Guest Eds. Perspectives on Fast Foods. Public Health Currents, 19(1), 1979, Published by Ross Laboratories, Columbus, OH.

Dennison, D. The Dine System: the Nutrition Plan For Better Health. C. V. Mosby Comp. St. Louis, Mo., 1982.

Pennington, S. A. T. and H. N. Church. Food Values of Portions Commonly Used. Harper and Row Publishers, New York, 1985.

Kullman, D. A. ABC Milligram Cholesterol Diet Guide. Merit Publications, Inc. North Miami Beach, Florida 1978.

Figure J.1. *Dietary Analysis.*

Date: _____

Foods	Amount	Calories	Protein (gm)	Fat (total) (gm)	Sat. Fat (gm)	Chol-esterol (mg)	Carbo-hydrates (gm)	Cal-cium (mg)	Iron (mg)	Sodium (mg)	Vit. A (I.U.)	Vit. B₁ (mg)	Vit B₂ (mg)	Nia-cin (mg)	Vit. C (mg)
Totals															

Figure J.2. *Three-Day Nutritional Analysis.*

Name: _____

Day	Calories	Protein (gm)	Fat (gm)	Sat. Fat (gm)	Chol-esterol (mg)	Carbo-hydrates (gm)	Calcium (mg)	Iron (mg)	Sodium (mg)	Vit. A (I.U.)	Vit. B1 (mg)	Vit. B2 (mg)	Niacin (mg)	Vit. C (mg)
One														
Two														
Three														
Totals														
Averagea														
Percentagesb														

Recommended Daily Dietary Allowances

	Calories	Protein	Fat	Sat. Fat	Chol-esterol	Carbo-hydrates	Calcium	Iron	Sodium	Vit. A	Vit. B1	Vit. B2	Niacin	Vit. C
Men 15-18 yrs.	See belowc,*	< 20%*	< 30%*	See belowd,* →	< 300*	50%*>	1,200	18	3,000*	5,000	1.4	1.7	18	60
Men 19-22 yrs.		< 20%	< 30%		< 300	50% >	800	10	3,000	5,000	1.5	1.7	19	60
Men 23-50 yrs.		< 20%	< 30%		< 300	50% >	800	10	3,000	5,000	1.4	1.6	18	60
Women 15-18 yrs.		< 20%	< 30%		< 300	50% >	1,200	18	3,000	4,000	1.1	1.3	14	60
Women 19-22 yrs.		< 20%	< 30%		< 300	50% >	800	18	3,000	4,000	1.1	1.3	14	60
Women 23-50 yrs.		< 20%	< 30%		< 300	50% >	800	See belowe →	3,000	4,000	1.0	1.2	13	60
Pregnant		25%	< 30%		< 300	50% >	+ 400		3,000	5,000	+ 0.4	+ 0.3	+ 2	+ 20
Lactating		22%	< 30%		< 300	50% >	+ 400		3,000	6,000	+ 0.5	+ 0.5	+ 5	+ 40

aDivide totals by 3 or number of days assessed.

bPercentages: Protein and Carbohydrates = multiply avg. by 4 and divide by avg. calories, Fat = multiply avg. by 9 and divide by avg. calories, Saturated Fat = divided avg. grams of saturated fat by avg. grams of fat.

*Amounts based on recommendations by nutrition experts.

cUse Figure 6.5 for all categories.

dLess than 10% of total calories. Multiply avg. by 9 and divide by avg. calories.

eAdd 30 to 60 mg of supplemental iron during and 3 months after pregnancy.

Figure J.3. *Daily Diet Record Form. (Use in conjunction with Figure 6.4, Chapter 6, The New American Eating Guide).*

Name: _____ Dates: _____ to _____

Daily Caloric Intake: _____ calories[1]

Day of Month

Food Group	Code[2]	Scr.[3]	Cal.[4]	Code	Scr.	Cal.	Code	Scr.	Cal.	Code	Scr.	Cal.	Code	Scr.	Cal.	Code	Scr.	Cal.	Code	Scr.	Cal.
Group 1 **Beans, Grains** **& Nuts** **4 Servings**																					
Meet Req. Serv.																					
Group 2 **Fruits &** **Vegetables** **4 Servings**																					
Meet Req. Serv.																					
Group 3 **Milk Products** **2 Servings** (children 3-4 Serv.)																					
Meet Req. Serv.																					
Group 4 **Poultry, Meat** **Fish & Eggs** **2 Servings**																					
Meet Req. Serv.																					
Totals																					

[1]**Refer to Figure 6.5.** [2]**Code, see food list.** [3]**Scr. = Score ("+", "NP", "–"), use Figure 6.4.** [4]**Cal. + Calories, refer to food list.**

Figure J.4. *Computerized Nutritional Analysis. Sample Food List.* *

```
                    John Doe                      Date: 02-18-1987
                    Age: 44
                    Body Weight: 180 lbs ( 81.6 Kg)
                    Activity Rating: Sedentary
```

Food Intake Day One

Food	Amount	Calo-ries	Pro-tein gm	Fat gm	Sat Fat gm	Cho-les-terol mg	Car-bohy-drate gm	Cal-cium mg	Iron mg	Sodium mg	Vit A I.U.	Thi-amin mg	Ribo-fla-vin mg	Nia-cin mg	Vit C mg
Coffee	.75 c	1	0.0	0	0.0	0	0	1	0.2	2	0	0.00	0.00	0.1	0
Eggs/hard/cooked	2 large	144	12.0	10	3.6	500	2	48	2.0	108	1,040	0.10	0.26	0.0	0
Bacon/cooked	3 slices	129	5.7	12	4.1	45	2	3	0.8	230	0	0.12	0.08	1.2	0
Croissants	1 roll	59	1.6	2	0.3	0	8	22	0.6	105	0	0.14	0.09	0.8	0
Butter	2 tsp	72	0.0	8	0.8	24	0	2	0.0	92	320	0.00	0.00	0.0	0
Bread/white	2 slice(s)	136	4.4	2	0.4	0	26	42	1.2	254	0	0.12	0.10	1.2	0
Mayonnaise	1 tsp.	36	0.0	4	0.7	3	0	1	0.0	28	13	0.00	0.00	0.0	0
Cheese/american	1 oz./slice	100	6.0	8	5.6	27	0	188	0.1	307	343	0.01	0.10	0.0	0
Bologna	1 slice (oz.)	86	3.4	8	3.0	15	0	2	0.5	369	0	0.05	0.06	0.7	0
Cola	12 oz.	144	0.0	0	0.0	0	37	27	0.0	30	0	0.00	0.00	0.0	0
Cookies/choc. chip	5 cookies	258	2.5	15	4.3	35	30	18	1.0	175	50	0.05	0.05	0.5	0
Beef/sirloin/cooked	3 oz.	329	19.6	27	13.0	77	0	9	2.5	48	50	0.05	0.15	4.0	0
Potato/baked in skin	1 med	145	4.0	0	0.0	0	33	14	1.1	6	0	0.15	0.07	2.7	31
Butter	3 tsp	108	0.0	12	1.2	36	0	3	0.0	138	480	0.00	0.00	0.0	0
Bread/french	3 slice(s)	306	9.6	3	0.6	0	57	45	2.4	609	0	0.30	0.24	2.7	0
Tomato sauce(catsup)	2.5 tbsp.	40	0.8	0	0.0	0	10	8	0.3	390	263	0.02	0.02	0.5	5
Mayonnaise	1 tsp.	36	0.0	4	0.7	3	0	1	0.0	28	13	0.00	0.00	0.0	0
Tomatoes/raw	.5 med	10	0.5	0	0.0	0	2	6	0.3	2	410	0.03	0.02	0.3	11
Lettuce/head	1 c sm. chunks	10	0.7	0	0.0	0	2	15	0.4	7	250	0.05	0.05	0.2	5
Milk whole	2 c	318	18.0	18	10.2	68	24	576	0.2	240	700	0.14	0.80	0.4	4
Apple pie	1 pc. (3.5 in.)	302	2.6	13	3.5	120	45	9	0.4	355	40	0.02	0.02	0.5	1
Totals Day One		2,769	91.4	146	51.9	953	278	1,039	13.9	3,522	3,972	1.4	2.1	15.8	57

*Nutrition Analysis software available through Morton Publishing Company. Englewood, Colorado.

Figure J.5. *Computerized Nutritional Analysis. Sample Daily Analysis, Average, and Recommended Dietary Allowance Comparison.* *

NUTRITIONAL ANALYSIS: DAILY ANALYSIS, AVERAGE, AND
RECOMMENDED DIETARY ALLOWANCE (RDA) COMPARISON

	Calo-ries	Pro-tein gm	Fat %	Sat Fat %	Cho-les-terol mg	Car-bohy-drate %	Cal-cium mg	Iron mg	Sodium mg	Vit A I.U.	Thi-amin mg	Ribo-fla-vin mg	Nia-cin mg	Vit C mg
Day One	2,769	91.4	47	17	953	40	1,039	13.9	3,522	3,972	1.4	2.1	15.8	57
Day Two	1,917	101.0	27	11	240	52	1,103	16.4	5,942	7,412	1.4	2.7	26.2	81
Day Three	2,236	77.1	29	10	432	56	1,073	10.7	2,629	4,337	1.2	2.1	18.1	163
Three Day Average	2,307	89.8	36	13	542	48	1,071	13.6	4,031	5,240	1.3	2.3	20.0	100
RDA	2,340*	65.3	<30	<10	<300	50>	800	10.0	2,340	5,000	1.4	1.6	18.0	60

*Estimated caloric value based on gender, current body weight, and activity rating (does not include additional calories burned through a physical exercise program).

OBSERVATIONS

Daily caloric intake should be distributed in such a way that 50 to 60 percent of the total calories come from carbohydrates and less than 30 percent of the total calories from fat. Protein intake should be about .8 grams per kilogram of body weight or about 15 to 20 percent of the total calories. Pregnant women need to consume an additional 30 grams of daily protein, while lactating women should have an extra 20 grams of daily protein, or about 25 and 22 percent of total calories respectively (these additional grams of protein are already included in the RDA values for pregnant and lactating women). Saturated fats should constitute less than 10 percent of the total daily caloric intake. Please note that the daily listings of food intake express the amount of carbohydrates, fat, saturated fat, and protein in grams. However, on the daily analysis and the RDA, only the amount of protein is given in grams. The amount of carbohydrates, fat, and saturated fat are expressed in percent of total calories.

If your average intake for protein, fat, saturated fat, cholesterol, or sodium is high, refer to the daily listings and decrease the intake of foods that are high in those nutrients. If your diet is deficient in carbohydrates, calcium, iron, vitamin A, thiamin, riboflavin, niacin, or vitamin C, refer to the statements below and increase your intake of the indicated foods, or consult Appendix E in the textbook Lifetime Physical Fitness & Wellness: A Personalized Program.

Total fat intake is too high.

Saturated fat intake is too high, which increases your risk for coronary heart disease.

Dietary cholesterol intake is too high. An average consumption of dietary cholesterol above 300 mg/day increases the risk for coronary heart disease. Do you know your blood cholesterol level?

Carbohydrate intake is low. Good sources of carbohydrates are whole grain breads and cereals, pasta, rice, fruits, and vegetables such as potatoes and peas.

Sodium intake is high.

Thiamin (Vit. B1) intake is low. Good sources of thiamin are whole grain enriched breads, lean meats, fish, poultry, liver, legumes, nuts, and dried yeast.

---

*Nutrition Analysis software available through Morton Publishing Company. Englewood, Colorado.

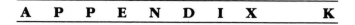

A P P E N D I X   K

Case Study

CASE STUDY

Using the data provided in Figure K.1, this case study on "Jane Doe" is provided to help you go through the different computations required to obtain a complete coronary heart disease (CHD) risk profile and physical fitness profile (*see* Figure 3.12, which contains a computer printout of the actual test results).

Coronary Heart Disease Risk Profile

1. Cardiovascular Endurance. According to the data sheet, Jane was tested using a Balke treadmill protocol — maximal test — (*see* Appendix C for predicting equation) and she walked on the treadmill for eleven minutes and thirty seconds. Her cardiovascular endurance level is determined as follows:

   Treadmill time = 11:30 = 11 + (30/60) = 11.5 minutes

   Max. VO2 = (4.326 × 11.5) + 14.99 = 31.6 ml/kg/min

   According to Table A.1 in Appendix A, a maximal oxygen uptake of 31.6 ml/kg/min (round off to 32 ml/kg/ min) for a forty-two-year-old woman yields 2.4 risk points and a moderate CHD risk category for this factor.

2/3. Resting and Stress Electrocardiogram. According to Table A.2 in Appendix A, a normal resting ECG is assigned 0.0 risk points and a very low CHD risk category. An equivocal stress ECG is given 4.0 risk points and a moderate CHD risk category.

4. Total Cholesterol/HDL-Cholesterol Ratio. A total cholesterol of 224 mg/dl and a HDL-cholesterol of 24 mg/dl yield a ratio of 9.3 (224/24). Based on Table A.3 (Appendix A), a ratio of 9.3 for women is given 9.8 risk points and a very high CHD risk category.

5. Triglycerides. Using Table A.4 in Appendix A, a triglyceride level of 134 mg/dl is assigned 0.4 risk points and a low CHD risk category.

6. Glucose. Jane is not a diabetic according to her data provided in the wellness questionnaire in the general health history section, question A.1 (*see* diabetes question in the data sheet under wellness questionnaire data). The blood test results were also normal, revealing a blood glucose level of 97 mg/dl. Based on Table A.5 in Appendix A, no risk points are assigned for this glucose level, yielding a very low CHD risk category for this factor.

7/8. Blood Pressure. Jane's blood pressure was 144/86. According to Table A.6 in Appendix A, a systolic pressure of 144 mmHg is assigned 2.4 risk points and a high CHD risk category, and a diastolic pressure of 86 mmHg is given 0.7 risk points and a low CHD risk category.

9. Body Fat Percentage. The sum of Jane's skinfolds (SS) equals 71 mm (26.0 + 10.5 + 34.5). Using the predicting equations for body density (BD) of women and percent body fat (*see* Appendix D, Skinfold Thickness Technique for Body Composition Assessment), Jane's percent fat would be:

   BD = 1.0994921 - 0.0009929(SS) + 0.0000023(SS)^2 - 0.0001392(Age)

   BD = 1.0994921 - 0.0009929(71) + 0.0000023(71)^2 - 0.0001392(42)

   BD = 1.037528

   Percent Fat = (495/BD) - 450

   Percent Fat = (495/1.037528) - 450 = 27.1%

   Using Table A.8 in Appendix A, Jane is given 1.4 risk points (rounded off to 27.0 percent) and a moderate CHD risk category for percent body fat.

10. Smoking. Jane indicated that she is currently smoking between twenty and twenty-nine cigarettes per day (*see* wellness questionnaire data, smoking question). Based on Table A.9 in Appendix A, 5.0 risk points and a high CHD risk category are awarded for Jane's current smoking habit.

11. Tension and Stress. According to Jane's responses to the tension and stress questions in the wellness questionnaire, a final rating of 3 (question D of tension and stress section in the wellness questionnaire) was recorded for tension and stress in the wellness questionnaire data section of the data sheet. A rating of 3, using Table A.10 (Appendix A), is given 2.0 risk points and a moderate CHD risk category.

Figure K.1. *Data for Sample Case Study.*

WELLNESS TESTING DATA SHEET

Date: _0 3_-_1 2_-_1 9 8 7_   Test Type: ① II III IV V
 Month   Day   Year

General Information:

Last Name: _Doe_   First: _Jane_   Middle Initial: _____

Soc. Sec.: _9 9 9_-_9 9_-_9 9 9 9_   Birthdate: _0 1_-_2 4_-_1 9 4 5_
                                              Month Day   Year

Age: _42_   Sex: _____ Male _✓_ Female

Address: _1111 Golden Street_

City: _Boise_   State: _ID_ Zip Code: _83725_   Phone: _(999) 999-9999_

I. Wellness Questionnaire Data
   Personal History (Question A, CV Hist. Sect.) _1_
   Family History (Question D, CV Hist. Sect.) _4_
   Estrogen Use (Question K, Gen. Hist. Sect.) _4_
   Diabetes (Question A.1, Gen. Hist. Sect.) Y/N _N_
   Smoking (Question F, Gen. Hist. Sect.) _0 9_
   Tension & Stress (Question D, Stress Sect.) _3_

II. Body Composition Data
   Height _7 0.0_ in.
   Weight _1 4 4.5_ lb.
   Men Skinfolds
     Chest _ _ _._ mm
     Abdomen _ _ _._ mm
     Thigh _ _ _._ mm
   Women Skinfolds
     Triceps _2 6.0_ mm
     Suprailium _1 0.5_ mm
     Thigh _3 4.5_ mm
   Hydrostatic Weighing
     Water Temperature _ _ °C
     Residual Volume
       (if unknown enter 0) _ _._ lt
     Average Underwater Weight _ _._ _ _ kg
     Tare Weight _ _._ _ _ kg

III. Blood Chemistry
   Total Cholesterol _2 2 4_ mg/dl
   HDL-Cholesterol _ _2 4_ mg/dl
   Triglycerides _ _1 3 4_ mg/dl
   Glucose _ _9 7_ mg/dl

IV. Resting Heart Rate & Blood Pressure
   Heart Rate _ _7 8_ bpm
   Systolic Blood Pressure _1 4 4_ mmHg
   Diastolic Blood Pressure _ _8 6_ mmHg

V. Electrocardiogram
   (normal=1, equivocal=2, abnormal=3)
   Resting ECG _1_
   Stress ECG _2_

VI. Cardiovascular Endurance
   1. 1.5-Mile Run   Time=_ _:_ _
   2. Astrand-Ryhming   Work Load=_ _ _ kpm
                        Avg. Heart Rate=_ _ _ bpm
   3. Step Test   Rec. Heart Rate=_ _ _ bpm
   ④.Balke (max.)   Time=_1 1:3 0_
   5. Bruce (max.)   Time=_ _:_ _
   6. Ellestad (max.)   Time=_ _:_ _
   7. Balke (submax.)   Time=_ _:_ _
   8. Bruce (submax.)   Time=_ _:_ _
   9. Ellestad (submax.) Time=_ _:_ _

VII. Muscular Strength
   Upper Body (Bench Press) _1 0_ reps.
   Abdominal (Sit-Up) _ _6_ reps.
   Lower Body (Leg Extension) _ _7_ reps.

VIII. Muscular Flexibility
   Sit-and-Reach _1 4.0_-_1 4.0_-_1 4.0_ in.
   Right Trunk Rot. _1 1.0_-_1 3.0_-_1 2.0_ in.
   Left Trunk Rot. _1 3.0_-_1 5.0_-_1 4.0_ in.
   Shoulder Width _1 4.0_ in.
   Shoulder Rotation _3 9.0_ in.

IX. Posture Analysis
   Score _3 5_ Points

X. Pulmonary Function
   Forced Vital Capacity _4.1_ lt
   Forced Exp. Vol. 1 Sec. _2.6_ lt
   Forced Exp. Flow 25-75% _2.1_ lt
   Forced Exp. Flow 75-85% _0.8_ lt

12. Personal History of Heart Disease. Jane does not have a personal history of heart disease (a response of 1 for question A in the cardiovascular disease history section of the wellness questionnaire), consequently, no risk points and a very low CHD risk category are assigned for this factor (see Table A.11, Appendix A).

13. Family History of Heart Disease. Jane has a family history of heart disease prior to age fifty (a response of 4 for question D in the cardiovascular disease history section of the wellness questionnaire). Table A.12 in Appendix A indicates that 4.0 risk points and a very high CHD risk category are assigned for the family history.

14. Age. One-tenth of a point is assigned for each year after twenty (see Table A.14, Appendix A). If Jane is forty-two years old, 2.2 risk points and a high CHD risk category are assigned for the age factor.

15. Estrogen Use. Jane is forty-two years old and is currently using estrogens (see wellness questionnaire data, estrogen use question). According to Table A.13, Jane is awarded 2.0 risk points and is placed in the very high risk category for this factor.

Total Risk. Total CHD risk is obtained by totaling all of the risk points obtained for each individual factor. In Jane's case, the total risk score is 36.3 risk points, which, according to Table A.15, places her in the very high CHD risk category.

Physical Fitness Profile

1. Cardiovascular Endurance. The previously obtained maximal oxygen uptake of 31.6 ml/kg/min (see Cardiovascular Endurance under Coronary Heart Disease Risk Profile) places Jane at about the 80 percentile rank for her age group according to Table A.17 in Appendix A (using normative data) and in the average cardiovascular fitness category according to Table 4.3 in Chapter 4 (based on criterion standards).

2. Muscular Strength. Jane performed ten, six, and seven repetitions, respectively, for the upper body, abdominal, and lower body strength tests. Using Table A.18 (Appendix A), the percentile ranks and fitness ratings for those tests are:

Upper body (bench press): 40 percentile, average fitness
Abdoinal sit-up): 30 percentile, fair fitness
Lower body (leg extension): 40 percentile, average fitness

The overall muscular strength fitness category is obtained by taking an average of the three percentile ranks (37 percentile), which would indicate a fair fitness category.

3. Muscular Flexibility. Jane's average scores for the Sit-and-Reach, Right and Left Trunk Rotation, and Shoulder Rotation Flexibility Tests were: 14.0, 12.0, 14.0, and 25.0. According to Tables A.19, A.20, and A.21 (Appendix A) the percentile ranks and fitness ratings for these tests are:

Sit-and-Reach: 50 percentile, average fitness
Right Trunk Rotation: 30 percentile, fair fitness
Left Trunk Rotation: 30 percentile, fair fitness
Shoulder Rotation (rotation score minus shoulder width): 30 percentile, fair fitness.

As with muscular strength, the overall fitness category is obtained by taking an average of the four percentile ranks (35 percentile), which would indicate a fair fitness category for muscular flexibility.

4. Body Composition. A percent body fat of 27.1 yields an approximate 40 percentile rank according to normative data (see Table A.23, Appendix A, 40-49 age group). The fitness classification is obtained according to the criterion standards given in Table 4.9 (Chapter 4), placing Jane in an average fitness category.

5. Posture. Jane received a posture score of 35 points, which according to Table A.25 (Appendix A) places her in the average posture category.

6. Pulmonary Function. According to the data sheet, the following spirometry results were obtained from Jane's forced expiration:

Forced vital capacity (FVC) = 4.1 lt
Forced Expiratory Volume in One Second (FEV1) = 2.6 lt
Ratio FEV1/FVC = 2.6/4.1 = 63 percent
Forced Expired Flow 25-75% = 2.1 lt
Forced Expired Flow 75-85% = 0.8 lt

Using the predicting equations from Appendix I, Jane's predicted values would be the following (for a forty-two-year-old woman, seventy inches tall):

FVC = [(.115 × 70) - (.024 × 42)] - 2.852 = 4.2 lt

FEV1 = [(.089 × 70) - (.025 × 42)] - 1.932 = 3.3 lt

Ratio FEV1/FVC = 3.3/4.2 = 79 percent

FEF25-75% = [(.06 × 70) - (.03 × 42)] + .551 = 3.5 lt

FEF75-85% = [(.025 × 70) - (.021 × 42)] + .321 = 1.2 lt

Jane's percentage of predicted values would be:

FVC = 4.1/4.2 = 98 percent of predicted

FEV1 = 2.6/3.3 = 79 percent of predicted

FEF25-75% = 2.1/3.5 = 60 percent of predicted

FEF75-85% = 0.8/1.2 = 67 percent of predicted

Figure K.2. *Sample Wellness Testing Data Sheet.*

WELLNESS TESTING DATA SHEET

Date: __ __-__ __-__ __ __ __   Test Type: I II III IV V
     Month Day   Year

General Information:

Last Name: _____ First: _____ Middle Initial: _____

Soc. Sec.: __ __ __-__ __-__ __ __ __   Birthdate: __ __-__ __-__ __ __ __
                                                 Month Day   Year

Age: _____   Sex: _____ Male _____ Female

Address: _____

City: _____ State: _____ Zip Code: _____ Phone: _____

I. Wellness Questionnaire Data
  Personal History (Question A, CV Hist. Sect.)   —
  Family History (Question D, CV Hist. Sect.)   —
  Estrogen Use (Question K, Gen. Hist. Sect.)   —
  Diabetes (Question A.1, Gen. Hist. Sect.) Y/N   —
  Smoking (Question F, Gen. Hist. Sect.)   — —
  Tension & Stress (Question D, Stress Sect.)   —

II. Body Composition Data
  Height   — —.— in.
  Weight   — — —.— lb.
  Men Skinfolds
    Chest   — —.— mm
    Abdomen   — —.— mm
    Thigh   — —.— mm
  Women Skinfolds
    Triceps   — —.— mm
    Suprailium   — —.— mm
    Thigh   — —.— mm
  Hydrostatic Weighing
    Water Temperature   — °C
    Residual Volume
    (if unknown enter 0)   —.— lt
    Average Underwater Weight   —.— — — kg
    Tare Weight   —.— — — kg

III. Blood Chemistry
  Total Cholesterol   — — — mg/dl
  HDL-Cholesterol   — — — mg/dl
  Triglycerides   — — — — mg/dl
  Glucose   — — — mg/dl

IV. Resting Heart Rate & Blood Pressure
  Heart Rate   — — — bpm
  Systolic Blood Pressure   — — — mmHg
  Diastolic Blood Pressure   — — — mmHg

V. Electrocardiogram
  (normal=1, equivocal=2, abnormal=3)
  Resting ECG   —
  Stress ECG   —

VI. Cardiovascular Endurance
  1. 1.5-Mile Run   Time=__ __:__ __
  2. Astrand-Ryhming   Work Load=__ __ __ kpm
                Avg. Heart Rate=__ __ __ bpm
  3. Step Test   Rec. Heart Rate=__ __ __ bpm
  4. Balke (max.)   Time=__ __:__ __
  5. Bruce (max.)   Time=__ __:__ __
  6. Ellestad (max.)   Time=__ __:__ __
  7. Balke (submax.)   Time=__ __:__ __
  8. Bruce (submax.)   Time=__ __:__ __
  9. Ellestad (submax.)   Time=__ __:__ __

VII. Muscular Strength
  Upper Body (Bench Press)   — — reps.
  Abdominal (Sit-Up)   — — reps.
  Lower Body (Leg Extension)   — — reps.

VIII. Muscular Flexibility
  Sit-and-Reach   — —.—-— —.—-— —.— in.
  Right Trunk Rot.   — —.—-— —.—-— —.— in.
  Left Trunk Rot.   — —.—-— —.—-— —.— in.
  Shoulder Width   — —.— in.
  Shoulder Rotation   — —.— in.

IX. Posture Analysis
  Score   — — Points

X. Pulmonary Function
  Forced Vital Capacity   —.— lt
  Forced Exp. Vol. 1 Sec.   —.— lt
  Forced Exp. Flow 25-75%   —.— lt
  Forced Exp. Flow 75-85%   —.— lt

Alcohol Abuse
Are You Drinking Too Much?
How To Cut Down Your Drinking

Reproduced with permission from *Family Medical Guide* by The American Medical Association. New York: Random House, 1982.

ALCOHOL ABUSE

ALCOHOL QUESTIONNAIRE: ARE YOU DRINKING TOO MUCH?

1. When you are holding an empty glass at a party, do you always actively look for a refill instead of waiting to be offered one?

2. If given the chance, do you frequently pour out a more generous drink for yourself than seems to be the "going" amount for others?

3. Do you often have a drink or two when you are alone, either at home or in a bar?

4. Is your drinking ever the direct cause of a family quarrel, or do quarrels often seem to occur, if only by coincidence, when you have had a drink or two?

5. Do you feel that you must have a drink at a specific time every day — right after work, for instance?

6. When worried or under unusual stress, do you almost automatically take a stiff drink to "settle your nerves?"

7. Are you untruthful about how much you have had to drink when questioned on the subject?

8. Does drinking ever cause you to take time off work, or to miss scheduled meetings or appointments?

9. Do you feel physically deprived if you cannot have at least one drink every day?

10. Do you sometimes crave a drink in the morning?

11. Do you sometimes have "mornings after" when you cannot remember what happened the night before?

EVALUATION

You should regard a YES answer to any one of the above questions as a warning sign. Do not increase your consumption of alcohol. Two YES answers suggest that you may already be becoming dependent on alcohol. Three or more YES answers indicate that you may have a serious drinking problem, and you should get professional help.

HOW TO CUT DOWN YOUR DRINKING

If you gave two or more YES answers on the alcohol questionnaire, you may be jeopardizing your health through excessive consumption of alcohol. Now is the time to start limiting your intake of alcohol. For many people who are determined to control the problem, it is not that hard to do. The first and most important step is to want to cut down. If you want to cut down but find you cannot, you had better accept the probability that drink is becoming a serious problem for you, and you should seek guidance from your physician or from an organization such as Alcoholics Anonymous. The next few suggestions may also help you cut down alcohol intake.

Set Reasonable Limits For Yourself

Decide not to exceed a certain number of drinks on a given occasion, and stick to your decision. No more than two beers or two cocktails a day is a reasonable limit. You have proved to yourself that you can control your drinking if you set such a target and regularly do not exceed it.

Learn To Say No

Many people have "just one more" drink because others in the group are having one or because someone puts pressure on them, not because they really want a drink. When you reach the sensible limit you have set for yourself, politely but firmly refuse to exceed it. If you are being the generous host, pour yourself a glass of water or juice "on the rocks." Nobody will notice the difference.

Drink Slowly

Never gulp down a drink. Choose your drinks for their flavor, not their "kick," and savor the taste of each sip.

Dilute Your Drinks

If you prefer cocktails to beer, try having long drinks. Instead of downing your gin or whiskey neat or nearly so, drink it diluted with a mixer such as tonic, water or soda water, in a tall glass. That way, you can enjoy the flavor as well as the act of drinking, but it will take longer to finish each drink. Also, you can make your two-drink limit last all evening or switch to the mixer by itself.

Do Not Drink On Your Own

Make a point of confining your drinking to social gatherings. It is sometimes hard to resist the urge to pour yourself a relaxing drink at the end of a hard day, but many formerly heavy drinkers have found that a cup of coffee or a soft drink satisfies the need as well as alcohol did, and that it was just a habit. What may help you really to unwind, even with no drink at all, is a comfortable chair, loosened clothing, and perhaps a soothing record, a television program or a good book to read.

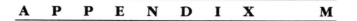

A P P E N D I X M

Safety and Environmental Health Questionnaire

Reproduced with permission from *Family Medical Guide* by The American Medical Association. New York: Random House, 1982.

SAFETY AND ENVIRONMENTAL HEALTH QUESTIONNAIRE

SECTION 1: ACCIDENT PREVENTION

1. Do you make it a point never to smoke in bed?

2. Do all your fireplaces have screens around them?

3. When cooking, do you guard against accidental tipping by positioning pan handles so that they do not extend outwards?

4. Do you keep electric cords out of the reach of children and avoid overloading the outlets?

5. Are you careful never to leave small children unsupervised in the kitchen or bathroom?

6. Are your children's nightclothes and soft toys labeled to show they are made of nonflammable materials?

7. Are medicines in your house kept in a secure place out of children's reach, and away from beds?

8. Are you careful never to store drugs or dangerous chemicals (bleach, paint-stripper, etc.) within children's reach or in incorrectly labeled containers?

9. Do you make a point of preventing your children from playing with objects small enough to be swallowed or inhaled?

10. Do you keep plastic bags away from your children?

11. When working around the house, do you wear safety glasses, ear plugs, and protective clothing such as sturdy shoes?

12. Are your carpets firmly fixed, with no ragged spots or edges, and are loose rugs placed to minimize the risk of sliding or tripping?

13. Are your stairs, halls, and other passages well lit (brightly enough to read a newspaper)?

14. Is it a rule in your house that nothing is left on the stairs?

15. If you spill or drop something that might be slippery on the floor, do you always clean it up right away?

16. Do you keep nonslip mats both in and alongside the bath or shower?

SECTION 2: SAFETY ON THE ROAD

17. Have you taught your children exactly how, when, and where to cross streets safely?

18. Have your children been taught the basic rules of the road to use when bicycling?

19. When walking in streets or open roads at twilight or in the dark, do all members of your family carry a light, or wear a markedly visible outer garment such as white or luminous jacket?

20. Do you always drive within the speed limit and drive defensively?

21. Are you always careful to drink very little alcohol or none at all if you are going to drive a car soon afterwards?

22. Do you avoid driving when you feel unusually tired or ill, or if you are taking drugs (such as antihistamines) that are known to impair alertness?

23. Do you have your car fully serviced, including lights, tires, windshield washer and wipers, brakes and steering, either every 10,000 km (6,000 miles) or at least every six months?

24. Do you check at least once a week to make sure that your car windows, lights, mirrors, and reflectors are clean?

25. When driving, do you always try to keep a gap of at least a meter (yard) for each mile-per-hour of speed between your car and the one in front?

26. Do you always make sure that you and all passengers in your car use available seat belts?

27. Are any infants or toddlers riding in your car securely strapped into infant car seats?

SECTION 3: SAFETY ON VACATIONS

28. Are all members of your family able to swim, or in the process of learning how to swim?

29. Do you test the depth of the water and go in feet first?

30. In a boat, does everyone always wear a life-jacket?

31. If you do any skiing, hiking or climbing, do you always go properly prepared with the right clothing and equipment?

32. When going on an excursion for a day or longer, do you tell someone what your route is and when you expect to be back?

33. Do you and your family take full safety precautions and have the proper equipment when you engage in contact and other possibly dangerous sports?

34. Before taking up a new and potentially dangerous activity such as hang-gliding, do you make sure you get proper instruction?

35. During a vacation, do you make sure you get adequate rest and relaxation?

EVALUATION

A NO answer to any of the above questions indicates that you are not doing all you can to minimize the risk of accidents. You can and should take all the protective steps suggested in the questions.

Index